Novel Therapeutic Strategies in the Treatment of Sepsis

INFECTIOUS DISEASE AND THERAPY

Series Editors

Brian E. Scully, M.B., B.Ch.
Harold C. Neu, M.D.

College of Physicians & Surgeons
Columbia University
New York, New York

1. Parasitic Infections in the Compromised Host, *edited by Peter D. Walzer and Robert M. Genta*
2. Nucleic Acid and Monoclonal Antibody Probes: Applications in Diagnostic Methodology, *edited by Bala Swaminathan and Gyan Prakash*
3. Opportunistic Infections in Patients with the Acquired Immunodeficiency Syndrome, *edited by Gifford Leoung and John Mills*
4. Acyclovir Therapy for Herpesvirus Infections, *edited by David A. Baker*
5. The New Generation of Quinolones, *edited by Clifford Siporin, Carl L. Heifetz, and John M. Domagala*
6. Methicillin-Resistant *Staphylococcus aureus*: Clinical Management and Laboratory Aspects, *edited by Mary T. Cafferkey*
7. Hepatitis B Vaccines in Clinical Practice, *edited by Ronald W. Ellis*
8. The New Macrolides, Azalides, and Streptogramins: Pharmacology and Clinical Applications, *edited by Harold C. Neu, Lowell S. Young, and Stephen H. Zinner*
9. Antimicrobial Therapy in the Elderly Patient, *edited by Thomas T. Yoshikawa and Dean C. Norman*
10. Viral Infections of the Gastrointestinal Tract: Second Edition, Revised and Expanded, *edited by Albert Z. Kapikian*
11. Development and Clinical Uses of Haemophilus b Conjugate Vaccines, *edited by Ronald W. Ellis and Dan M. Granoff*
12. *Pseudomonas aeruginosa* Infections and Treatment, *edited by Aldona L. Baltch and Raymond P. Smith*
13. Herpesvirus Infections, *edited by Ronald Glaser and James F. Jones*

Additional Volumes in Production

Novel Therapeutic Strategies in the Treatment of Sepsis

edited by
David C. Morrison
**University of Kansas Medical Center
Kansas City, Kansas**

John L. Ryan
**Genetics Institute, Inc.
Cambridge, Massachusetts**

Marcel Dekker, Inc.   **New York•Basel•Hong Kong**

ISBN: 0-8247-9661-6

The publisher offers discounts on this book when ordered in bulk quantities. For more information, write to Special Sales/Professional Marketing at the address below.

This book is printed on acid-free paper.

MARCEL DEKKER, INC.
270 Madison Avenue, New York, New York 10016

Current printing (last digit):
10 9 8 7 6 5 4 3 2 1

Printed in the United States of America

Series Introduction

Marcel Dekker, Inc., has for many years specialized in the publication of high-quality monographs in tightly focused areas in a variety of medical disciplines. These have been of great value to both the practicing physician and the research scientist as sources of detailed and up-to-date information presented in an attractive format. During the last decade, there has been a veritable explosion in knowledge in the various fields related to infectious diseases and clinical microbiology. Antimicrobial resistance, antibacterial and antiviral agents, AIDS, Lyme disease, infections in immunocompromised patients, and parasitic diseases are but a few of the areas in which an enormous amount of significant work has been published. The Infectious Disease and Therapy series covers carefully chosen topics that should be of interest and value to the practicing physician, the clinical microbiologist, and the research scientist.

BRIAN E. SCULLY
HAROLD C. NEU

Preface

Sepsis and septic shock remain important clinical problems for which optimal therapeutic intervention strategies have yet to be adequately established. This disease, which affects hundreds of thousands of Americans annually, is frequently initiated by microbial infection, even with appropriate and effective antimicrobial agents. Characteristic clinical manifestations of sepsis and septic shock include fever and/or hypothermia, tachypnea, tachycardia, reduced or elevated circulating white cell levels, hypotension, and evidence of inadequate organ perfusion. These conditions often lead to the more problematic multisystem organ failure, and mortality in such cases is estimated at greater than 50%. Although not reportable to the Centers for Disease Control and Prevention as a specific disease, several recent studies have estimated that, in the United States alone, between 50,000 and 100,000 patients die annually as a result of sepsis. By way of comparison, the number of deaths in the United States in 1994 due to AIDS was approximately 77,000.

The past 20 years have witnessed an explosion of knowledge in defining the underlying mechanisms that contribute to the sepsis syndrome, more recently redefined as the systemic inflammatory response syndrome (SIRS). In this respect, it is now recognized that the infectious microbe or its products can serve as a focal point for the initiation of a series of host inflammatory responses, ostensibly designed to protect the host from the invading microbe. This response may involve the normal host mediation systems, such as the complement and coagulation pathways, as well as cellular mediation systems, both of which result in the generation of a variety of inflammatory mediators. Of potential importance is the fact that the mediators so generated can themselves act as stimuli for production of additional inflammatory mediators, triggering a cascade amplification response and resulting systemic inflammation and tissue destruction.

It has long been axiomatic in the treatment of infection that elimination of the infectious microbe with appropriate antibiotic chemotherapy is an essential first step in treatment of septic patients. That effective chemotherapy alone may be insufficient to ensure patient survival is strongly suggested by the simple fact that mortality in treated patients remains at unacceptably high levels of 20 to 70%, depending on the severity of the disease. Most current efforts to reduce mortality have focused on antibiotic chemotherapy coupled with efforts to reverse the pathophysiological consequences of the systemic inflammatory responses.

A conceptually different approach to treatment of sepsis, in which efforts were focused on immune elimination of the initiating agents responsible for the systemic inflammation, was initiated approximately 30 years ago. Paradigm shifters in this approach were Drs. Abraham Braude and William McCabe. These investigators independently conceptualized that many of the deleterious sequelae of postantibiotic therapy in sepsis were the result of microbial constituents released from dying microbes. Since more than half of all infections at that time were caused by gram-negative microbes, and since gram-negative microbes contained endotoxin, a bacterial macromolecule with well-described potent inflammatory properties, it was hypothesized that endotoxin might be responsible for the multiple pathophysiological symptoms seen in septic patients. Of interest, it was at exactly this time that investigators interested in the chemistry of endotoxin, particularly Drs. Westphal, Luderitz, Rietschel, and Galanos, showed that the structure of the active principle of endotoxin, lipid A, was a highly conserved structure linked to an almost equally conserved core oligosaccharide. Braude and McCabe reasoned, therefore, that immunological targeting of the endotoxin molecule might well reduce, or even eliminate, postantibiotic mortality in patients with gram-negative sepsis.

Exhaustive studies in experimental animals by Drs. Braude, McCabe, their collaborators, and others provided compelling evidence in support of the potential efficacy of this approach using both endotoxin challenge and live infection models, although not all investigators were successful in demonstrating efficacy. Nevertheless, the data were sufficiently compelling that controlled clinical trials were initiated in the late 1970s to test human antiendotoxin antibodies in treating gram-negative sepsis. In 1982, Elizabeth Ziegler and coworkers reported a well-controlled major study using polyclonal immune serum from immunized volunteers, and provided the first strong data to suggest that this approach would work in humans. Interestingly, the publication of this study coincided with the advent and maturation of monoclonal antibody technology and set the stage for intensive efforts to develop antiendotoxin, monoclonal antibody-based drugs that would be successful in treating patients with gram-negative sepsis. While two early well-controlled studies in patients with sepsis using both a human and a mouse monoclonal IgM antiendotoxin antibody yielded data suggesting that both antibodies were effective in certain subpopulations, additional studies with these reagents have not provided the necessary data to confirm these earlier reports.

Nevertheless, the increased knowledge concerning the mechanisms of disease in sepsis, coupled with the continually growing appreciation that additional modalities are essential if reduction in mortality is to be realized, has prompted an ever-increasing number of investigations into the arena of antisepsis drugs. One of the first new and exciting areas of study was the targeting of the inflammatory mediators generated by the host in response to the endotoxin stimulus. The pioneering study of Beutler, Milsark, and Cerami, published in 1985, demonstrated in experimental animals a significant protective efficacy of neutralizing antibody to tumor necrosis factor (TNF) against endotoxin lethality. This set the stage for a series of extensive studies in both experimental animals and septic patients to reduce mortality using agents that affected the biological activity of a variety of cytokines and/or other inflammatory mediators. As with antiendotoxin strategies, the various anticytokine approaches have proved promising in experimental animal models, but more problematic when extrapolated to the septic patient.

In spite of the relatively disappointing clinical trials to date using both antiendotoxin strategies and antiinflammatory (anticytokine) strategies, there is a conviction among investigators and clinicians that the increasing knowledge concerning mechanisms of sepsis must contain the necessary clues from which effective therapeutic strategies can be developed. Our current understanding of molecular pathways involved in the development of the systemic inflammatory response syndrome is, in fact, impressive, and should serve as a cause for optimism. It is probably fair to conclude that one or more successful treatment strategies is tantalizingly close, and will be realized in the forthcoming decade by a dramatic reduction in deaths due to microbial sepsis.

Given this premise, it is of relevance to consider the state of the art of the approaches being developed in laboratories around the world to translate this existing biochemical knowledge base into an effective therapeutic treatment strategy for sepsis. The collection of chapters in this volume provides a status report on many of the most promising of these strategies by leading investigators in the field. All these strategies are based on sound scientific knowledge gained over the past decade or more about pathogenic mechanisms involved in sepsis. The approaches selected for inclusion in this volume describe technologies that have not yet been evaluated, or are just now being evaluated in the septic patient.

As the reader will quickly perceive from a review of the chapter titles, attention continues to be focused on the endotoxin molecule and the inflammatory mediators generated by the host in response to endotoxin stimulation. Although it may come as a surprise to some readers, given the history summarized above, antibody-to-endotoxin remains a promising tool in treatment of sepsis, and several extremely interesting antibodies are described in the first two chapters of this volume. In addition to antibody-to-endotoxin, however, two relatively new approaches to target the endotoxin molecule and/or reduce its ability to induce the production of inflammatory mediators are being developed. The first involves proteins/peptides that can bind to endotoxin and modulate its biological activity. Four such molecules are described in individual chapters from different laboratories, and each of these molecules has been documented to serve as a potent neutralizing agent for endotoxin activity. A second approach has derived from the growing appreciation that endotoxin interacts with specific receptors at the surface of host inflammatory cells, and that interference with such interactions can, in an indirect manner, neutralize the effects of endotoxin. Several interesting analogs representing structures related to lipid A, derived from both natural and synthetic sources, are now being intensively investigated in a number of laboratories, and are described in four chapters. In recognition of the potentially important role of CD14 in focusing endotoxin on the cell surface of inflammatory cells preparatory to cell activation, an additional effective neutralization strategy involves targeting the receptor itself in a soluble form, and this approach is described in one chapter.

Although the precise signaling pathway utilized by endotoxin in causing the production of cytokines and other inflammatory mediators from host cells has yet to be fully elucidated, there is growing recognition that interference with these pathways by selective inhibitors can serve as an effective tool to reduce inflammation caused by endotoxin, and several novel inhibitors are described in this volume. Further, efforts to target specific inflammatory mediators and use recombinant antiinflammatory cytokine mediators as therapeutic agents continue to offer new and potentially promising approaches, and these are also described, by several contributors. Finally, one novel approach, predicated upon the early concepts of Braude and McCabe, combines rational chemotherapy treatment with considerations of limiting the production of the initial inciting inflammatory agent endotoxin.

Collectively, these chapters provide a broad overview of novel, exciting, and potentially promising therapeutic approaches for the treatment of sepsis. Whether these approaches, which show considerable promise in both in vitro studies and animal models, will fulfill that promise in the more complex human gram-negative sepsis, remains to be established; nevertheless, they are strong justification for optimism that the era of high mortality in the septic patient is indeed limited, and that effective therapeutic strategies to treat such patients will be available in the foreseeable future.

DAVID C. MORRISON
JOHN L. RYAN

Contents

Contents **xiii**

Contributors

Daniel H. Albert, Ph.D.   Research Investigator, Abbott Laboratories, Abbott Park, Illinois

W. Steve Ammons, Ph.D.   Director, Department of Pharmacology, XOMA Corporation, Berkeley, California

Osamu Asano, Ph.D.   Research Chemist, Department of Research, Eisai Research Institute, Andover, Massachusetts

Robert F. Balint, Ph.D.   Senior Scientist, Palo Alto Institute of Molecular Medicine, Mountain View, California

G. Robin Barclay, B.Sc., M.Sc., Ph.D.   Principal Clinical Scientist, R&D Laboratories, Edinburgh Regional Centre, Scottish National Blood Transfusion Service, Edinburgh, Scotland, United Kingdom

Paul J. Bertics, Ph.D.   Associate Professor, Department of Biomolecular Chemistry, University of Wisconsin Medical School, Madison, Wisconsin

Apurba K. Bhattacharjee, Ph.D.   Senior Investigator, Department of Bacterial Diseases, Walter Reed Army Institute of Research, Washington, D.C.

Helmut Brade, M.D.   Professor, Department of Biochemical Microbiology, Forschungsinstitut Borstel, Borstel, Germany

John R. Bristol   Section of Chemistry, Eisai Research Institute, Andover, Massachusetts

Stuart L. Bursten, M.D.   Co-Director, Department of Second Messenger and Lipid Biochemistry, Cell Therapeutics, Inc., Seattle, Washington

Chinpan Chen   Research Associate, Division of Structural Biology, Institute of Biomedical Sciences, Academia Sinica, Nankang, Taipei, Taiwan, Republic of China

William J. Christ, Ph.D.   Principal Scientist, Department of Research, Eisai Research Institute, Andover, Massachusetts

Alan S. Cross, M.D.   Division of Infectious Diseases, Department of Medicine, University of Maryland School of Medicine, Baltimore, Maryland

Steven K. Daugherty, M.D.   Fellow, Departments of Medicine and Medical Microbiology/Immunology, University of Wisconsin Medical School, Madison, Wisconsin

Loren C. Denlinger   Research Assistant, Department of Medical Microbiology/Immunology, University of Wisconsin Medical School, Madison, Wisconsin

Franco Di Padova, M.D.   Department of Preclinical Research/Immunology, Sandoz Pharma, Basel, Switzerland

Gloria R. Dubuc   Research Chemist, Department of Research, Eisai Research Institute, Andover, Massachusetts

Philip L. Fisette   Research Assistant, Department of Biomolecular Chemistry, University of Wisconsin Medical School, Madison, Wisconsin

Hans-Dieter Flad   Director, Department of Immunology and Cell Biology, Forschungsinstitut Borstel, Borstel, Germany

Gary R. Fleisher, M.D. Associate Professor of Pediatrics, Harvard Medical School, and Chief, Division of Emergency Medicine, Children's Hospital, Boston, Massachusetts

Kristen A. Garis Research Assistant, Department of Biomolecular Chemistry, University of Wisconsin Medical School, Madison, Wisconsin

Wendy E. Gavin Research Chemist, Department of Research, Eisai Research Institute, Andover, Massachusetts

Michel Goldman, M.D. Head, Department of Immunology, Hôpital Erasme, Brussels, Belgium

Sanna M. Goyert, Ph.D. Associate Professor and Director, Laboratory of Molecular Hematology, Division of Molecular Medicine, Department of Medicine, North Shore University Hospital, Cornell University Medical College, Manhasset, New York

Hermann Gram Department of Preclinical Research/Biotechnology, Sandoz Pharma, Basel, Switzerland

Ward E. Harris, Ph.D. Co-Director, Second Messenger Laboratory, Department of Biochemistry, Cell Therapeutics, Inc., Seattle, Washington

Elda H. S. Hausmann, Ph.D. Research Assistant Professor, Department of Pathology and Laboratory Medicine, University of Kansas Medical Center, Kansas City, Kansas

Lynn D. Hawkins, Ph.D. Senior Scientist, Department of Research, Eisai Research Institute, Andover, Massachusetts

Alain Haziot, M.D., Ph.D. Assistant Professor, Division of Molecular Medicine, Department of Medicine, North Shore University Hospital, Cornell University Medical College, Manhasset, New York

Holger Heine Department of Immunology and Cell Biology, Forschungsinstitut Borstel, Borstel, Germany

Michimasa Hirata, Ph.D. Department of Bacteriology, School of Medicine, Iwate Medical University, Morioka, Iwate, Japan

Ieharu Hishinuma   Department of Exploratory Drug Research, Eisai Co. Ltd. Tsukuba Research Laboratories, Tsukuba, Japan

Jaroslav Hofman, Ph.D.   Research Associate, Department of Bacteriology, University of Wisconsin, Madison, Wisconsin

Tai-huang Huang, Ph.D.   Special Medical Research Fellow, Division of Structural Biology, Institute of Biomedical Sciences, Academia Sinica, Nankang, Taipei, Taiwan, Republic of China

J. J. Jackson   Merck Research Laboratories, Rahway, New Jersey

Kouichi Katayama   Department of Exploratory Drug Research, Eisai Co. Ltd. Tsukuba Research Laboratories, Tsukuba, Japan

Tsutomu Kawata   Section of Chemistry, Eisai Research Institute, Andover, Massachusetts

Akifumi Kimura   Department of Exploratory Drug Research, Eisai Co. Ltd. Tsukuba Research Laboratories, Tsukuba, Japan

Yoshito Kishi, Ph.D.   Professor and Chairman, Advisory Board, Eisai Research Institute, Andover, Massachusetts

Hollis D. Kleinert, Ph.D.   Division Director, Pharmaceutical Products Research & Development, Abbott Laboratories, Abbott Park, Illinois

Seiichi Kobayashi   Department of Exploratory Drug Research, Eisai Co. Ltd. Tsukuba Research Laboratories, Tsukuba, Japan

Fred R. Kohn   Senior Scientist, Department of Immunology, XOMA Corporation, Berkeley, California

H. Kropp   Merck Research Laboratories, Rahway, New Jersey

Ada H. C. Kung, Ph.D.   Skyline Technology Consulting Group, San Francisco, California

Shoichi Kusumoto, Ph.D.   Professor, Department of Chemistry, Faculty of Science, Osaka University, Osaka, Japan

James W. Larrick, M.D., Ph.D.   Scientific Director, Palo Alto Institute of Molecular Medicine, Mountain View, California

Michael D. Lewis, Ph.D.   Senior Scientist, Department of Research, Eisai Research Institute, Andover, Massachusetts

Ekke Liehl, Ph.D.   Head, Department of Immunopharmacology, Sandoz Research Institute, Vienna, Austria

Yue Lin, M.D., Ph.D.   Scientist, Departments of Pharmacology and Toxicology, XOMA Corporation, Berkeley, California

Arnaud Marchant, M.D.   Research Fellow, Department of Immunology, Hôpital Erasme, Brussels, Belgium

Marian N. Marra   Director, Department of Preclinical Research, Incyte Pharmaceuticals, Palo Alto, California

Taila Mattern, Ph.D.   Department of Immunology and Cell Biology, Forschungsinstitut Borstel, Borstel, Germany

Pamela D. McGuinness   Research Chemist, Department of Research, Eisai Research Institute, Andover, Massachusetts

David C. Morrison, Ph.D.   Professor of Cancer Research, Department of Microbiology, Molecular Genetics, and Immunology, University of Kansas Medical Center, Kansas City, Kansas

Maureen A. Mullarkey   Research Biologist, Department of Research, Eisai Research Institute, Andover, Massachusetts

Thomas J. Novitsky, Ph.D.   President and Chief Executive Officer, Associates of Cape Cod, Inc., Woods Hole, Massachusetts

Steven M. Opal, M.D.   Associate Professor, Department of Infectious Disease Division, Brown University School of Medicine, Providence, Rhode Island

Michael J. Parmely, Ph.D.   Professor, Department of Microbiology, Molecular Genetics, and Immunology, University of Kansas Medical Center, Kansas City, Kansas

Michel Perez, Ph.D.   Research Chemist, Department of Research, Eisai Research Institute, Andover, Massachusetts

Ian R. Poxton, B.Sc., Ph.D., D.Sc.   Reader in Medical Microbiology, Department of Medical Microbiology, University of Edinburgh Medical School, Edinburgh, Scotland, United Kingdom

Richard A. Proctor, M.D.   Professor, Departments of Medicine and Medical Microbiology/Immunology, University of Wisconsin Medical School, Madison, Wisconsin

Nilofer Qureshi, Ph.D.   Associate Professor, Department of Bacteriology, University of Wisconsin, Madison, Wisconsin

Glenn C. Rice, Ph.D.   Director, Department of Cell Biology, Cell Therapeutics, Inc., Seattle, Washington

Ernst Th. Rietschel   Department of Immunochemistry and Biochemical Microbiology, Forschungsinstitut Borstel, Borstel, Germany

Andrea L. C. Robidoux   Research Chemist, Department of Research, Eisai Research Institute, Andover, Massachusetts

Jeffrey R. Rose   Section of Chemistry, Eisai Research Institute, Andover, Massachusetts

Daniel P. Rossignol   Section of Chemistry, Eisai Research Institute, Andover, Massachusetts

John L. Ryan, Ph.D., M.D.   Vice President of Clinical Development, Genetics Institute, Inc., Cambridge, Massachusetts

Jerald C. Sadoff, M.D.   Director, Division of Communicable Diseases and Immunology, Walter Reed Army Institute of Research, Washington, D.C.

Richard A. Saladino, M.D.   Assistant Professor of Pediatrics, Harvard Medical School, and Assistant in Medicine, Children's Hospital, Boston, Massachusetts

Randal W. Scott, Ph.D.   Vice President, Department of Research and Development, Incyte Pharmaceuticals, Palo Alto, California

Jeffrey J. Seilhamer, Ph.D.   Vice President, Molecular Biology Research, Incyte Pharmaceuticals, Palo Alto, California

Michael P. Sherman, M.D.   Professor, Department of Pediatrics, University of Kansas Medical Center, Kansas City, Kansas

George R. Siber, M.D.   Associate Professor of Medicine, Division of Infectious Diseases, Dana-Farber Cancer Institute, Harvard Medical School, and Director, Massachusetts Public Health Biologic Laboratories, Boston, Massachusetts

Jack Silver, Ph.D.   Professor and Chief, Division of Molecular Medicine, Department of Medicine, North Shore University Hospital, Cornell University Medical College, Manhasset, New York

Richard Silverstein, Ph.D.   Professor, Department of Biochemistry and Molecular Biology, University of Kansas Medical Center, Kansas City, Kansas

James B. Summers, Ph.D.   Senior Project Leader, Abbott Laboratories, Abbott Park, Illinois

Kuni Takayama, Ph.D.   Supervisory Research Chemist, Mycobacteriology Research Laboratory, William S. Middleton Memorial Veterans Hospital, Madison, Wisconsin

Claudette Thompson   Coordinating Laboratory Supervisor, Division of Infectious Diseases, Dana-Farber Cancer Institute, Harvard Medical School, Boston, Massachusetts

William E. Truog, M.D.   Professor, Department of Pediatrics, University of Missouri–Kansas City School of Medicine, and Attending Neonatologist, Children's Mercy Hospital, Kansas City, Missouri

Artur J. Ulmer, Ph.D.   Department of Immunology and Cell Biology, Forschungsinstitut Borstel, Borstel, Germany

Jean-Louis Vincent, M.D.   Clinical Director, Department of Intensive Care, Hôpital Erasme, Brussels, Belgium

Stefanie N. Vogel, Ph.D.   Professor, Department of Microbiology and Immunology, Uniformed Services University of the Health Sciences, Bethesda, Maryland

Kenneth B. Von Eschen, Ph.D.   Vice President, Department of Clinical/Regulatory Affairs, Ribi ImmunoChem Research, Inc., Hamilton, Montana

Yuan Wang, Ph.D.   Senior Research Chemist, Department of Research, Eisai Research Institute, Andover, Massachusetts

H. Shaw Warren, M.D.   Associate Professor of Pediatrics, Departments of Medicine, Pediatrics, and Infectious Diseases, Massachusetts General Hospital, Boston, Massachusetts

Birgit Weidemann   Department of Immunology and Cell Biology, Forschungsinstitut Borstel, Borstel, Germany

Susan C. Wright, Ph.D.   Senior Scientist, Palo Alto Institute of Molecular Medicine, Mountain View, California

Isao Yamatsu   Department of Exploratory Drug Research, Eisai Co. Ltd. Tsukuba Research Laboratories, Tsukuba, Japan

Jian Zhong, M.D.   Scientist, Palo Alto Institute of Molecular Medicine, Mountain View, California

Novel Therapeutic Strategies in the Treatment of Sepsis

1

New Trends in *Escherichia coli* O111:B4 J5 Mutant (R_c Chemotype) Vaccine Development for Use in Gram-Negative Bacillary Sepsis

Apurba K. Bhattacharjee
Walter Reed Army Institute of Research
Washington, D.C.

Alan S. Cross
University of Maryland School of Medicine
Baltimore, Maryland

Steven M. Opal
Brown University School of Medicine
Providence, Rhode Island

H. Shaw Warren
Massachusetts General Hospital
Boston Massachusetts

Jerald C. Sadoff
Walter Reed Army Institute of Research
Washington, D.C.

I. INTRODUCTION

With the recognition that there was still an unacceptably high mortality rate from bacterial sepsis despite the introduction of new, potent antimicrobial agents, many investigators examined the potential of immunotherapeutic strategies to supplement the conventional treatment of this condition. This effort was facilitated by the elucidation of the structure of lipopolysaccharide (LPS) by both biochemists and bacterial geneticists. Lipid A and inner core sugar regions of the molecule were found to be widely shared by a diverse array of gram-negative bacilli, and that an outer polysaccharide region of the molecule, the 0 repeat region, provided serological specificity to the individual strains of bacteria.

Chedid et al. (1–3) and colleagues provided important data in animal models which suggested that immunization with vaccines in which the core LPS regions (i.e., "rough" LPS) were exposed could provide protection against challenge with heterologous organisms.

Further work with one of these rough LPS vaccines, the *Escherichia coli* O111:B4, J5 (R_c chemotype) mutant, led Ziegler, McCutchan, and colleagues to test the efficacy of anti-J5 antisera in patients suspected of having gram-negative bacterial sepsis (4). In this study, administration of J5 antisera led to a significant decrease in mortality, particularly in the subgroup of patients who required pressor agents for at least 6 h; however, protection did not correlate with hemagglutinating antibody titers. Moreover, since J5 antisera was prepared in normal volunteers immunized with a boiled whole-cell vaccine, the nature of the protective antigen was not clear.

The inability to determine either the protective antigen or the role of antibody in the protection observed may have contributed to the failure of investigators to confirm these results in subsequent clinical studies (5,6). Consequently, the validity of the hypothesis that antibody to the inner core region of LPS might protect against a wide array of gram-negative bacterial pathogens has been questioned (7,8). In addition, the lack of an adequate animal model made it difficult to evaluate potential therapeutic candidates before undertaking clinical trials.

In the course of our studies on the immunotherapy of gram-negative bacterial sepsis, we devised an animal model of sepsis which closely mimicked the clinical presentation of sepsis in humans both in the kinetics and level of bacteremia observed as well as in the cytokine profile generated (9). Additionally, we observed in preliminary experiments that a J5 antisera prepared from a whole-cell vaccine administered to rabbits was protective in this neutropenic rat model of sepsis (10). Using this animal model of sepsis, we assessed the ability of antibody fractions directed against the J5 *E. coli* to protect against lethal *Pseudomonas aeruginosa* sepsis (11), and examined in greater detail the preparation of J5 vaccines.

II. NEUTROPENIC RAT MODEL OF SEPSIS

Although Ziegler and Douglas developed a neutropenic rabbit model of sepsis that mimicked the pathogenesis of sepsis in humans in both the route of infection and inoculum size, the size and cost of rabbits made it difficult to perform experiments with sufficient numbers of animals for statistical validity (12). We previously reported the development of a neutropenic rat model of infection that also employed a modest inoculum typical of human exposure to infection (9). Briefly, Sprague-Dawley rats weighing 200–300 g were pretreated with cefamandole intramuscularly to alter the normal rat gut flora. The rats were given cyclophosphamide at time 0 (150 mg/kg) and at 7 hr (75 mg/kg). The neutropenia thus engendered reached a nadir at day 5 and remained low until day 9, after which the white blood cell counts recovered. Bacteria were fed orally to the rats at time 0 and at 48 and 96 h. The animals were followed for the development of fever with an infrared temperature probe. Treatment was administered intravenously to animals whose temperature was $> 38°C$ (usually day 5). These animals typically had bacteremia with the challenge organism. Animals were followed for 12 days, after which time the white blood cell counts returned to normal and deaths no longer occurred.

III. *ESCHERICHIA COLI* J5 KILLED WHOLE-CELL VACCINE

A. Method of Preparation

While investigators have focused on the source of the J5 isolate used for the preparation of a vaccine, relatively few have carefully examined the manner in which the vaccine is prepared. We originally obtained a culture of *E. coli* O111:B4, J5 mutant from Dr. Elizabeth Ziegler, and kept it frozen at $-70°C$. Since the J5 organism has been described as a "leaky" mutant (13), we streaked the J5 culture for single-colony isolation on Trypticase soy agar. We then selected 5–7 colonies, which were then individually subcultured without shaking on Trypticase soy broth (TSB) overnight at 37°C. On the following day we chose that subculture that had the clearest supernatant, indicative of the isolate with the "roughest" LPS. This subculture was then used to inoculate a 2-L flask containing 1 L of TSB for overnight stationary culture. The following day the bacteria were harvested, washed, and resuspended in saline to a stock optical density (OD) of 2.0, which usually corresponded to a colony count of 1×10^{10} CFU/mL. After samples were obtained to confirm the colony counts, the stock culture was boiled for 1 h, which resulted in complete loss of viability of the culture.

For immunization studies, dilutions of the stock culture were made in saline to achieve a 70% light transmission at 610 nM as was done earlier by Ziegler et al. (12). Alternatively, the boiled vaccine was lyophilized and later administered on a weight basis.

B. Immunization of Rabbits

A suspension of killed *E. coli* J5 whole-cell vaccine at a concentration of 10^{10} CFU/mL was used for immunization of rabbits. Rabbits received a series of primary intravenous immunizations on Mondays, Wednesdays and Fridays for 3 weeks. Doses on the respective days were 0.1, 0.1, and 0.2 mL during the first week; 0.2, 0.2, and 0.4 mL during the second week; and 0.8, 0.8, and 1.6 mL during the third week. Blood samples were collected 10 and 47 days after the primary series of immunizations. Booster injections with 1.0 mL of vaccine were given at approximately 6-week intervals, and about 30 mL of blood was collected 10–14 days after each booster injection. Serum samples were analyzed by enzyme linked immunosorbent assay (ELISA) (14).

ELISA titer of postbleed rabbit serum against J5 LPS 10 days after the primary series of immunizations was 102-fold higher than the prebleed serum (Table 1). The titer of postbleed serum against *E. coli* lipid A was 25-fold higher than the prebleed serum. The ELISA titers dropped to about one-third that level at 47 days post the primary series of immunizations. Booster injection brought the anti-J5 LPS titer close to the 10-day level, but the anti-lipid A titer was about twofold higher than before. Subsequent booster immunizations maintained the high titers against both J5 LPS and lipid A (Table 1).

IV. PURIFIED IMMUNOGLOBULINS AS PROTECTIVE ANTIBODIES

A. Fractionation of Rabbit Sera

The immune rabbit serum was fractionated into purified IgG, IgM, J5 LPS-specific IgG, and non-J5 LPS-specific IgG by affinity chromatography (Fig. 1). In this procedure the whole serum was cycled through protein G-Sepharose immunoadsorbent, which retained most of the IgG present in the serum (Fig. 1, step 1). A small amount of IgG not retained by this column was separated by chromatography on anti-rabbit IgG-Sepharose 4B immunoadsorbent (Fig. 1, step

Table 1 ELISA Titers of Sera from Rabbit #9 (R#9) Immunized with Heat-Killed *E. coli* J5 Whole-Cell Vaccine

	Days after last		Titers in OD units	
Serum description	Primary injection	Booster injection	J5 LPS	Lipid A
Prebleed serum pool	—	—	190	388
Postimmune bleed 1	10	—	19,430	5,900
2	47	—	5,158	2,140
3	68	21	15,628	9,164
4	94	47	10,368	5,491
5	138	14	14,451	15,616
6	151	27	9,676	12,518
7	184	18	14,592	19,040
8	208	10	9,292	11,852

Note: Booster injections were given between bleeds 2 and 3, 4 and 5, 6 and 7, and 7 and 8.
OD = optical density.
Data from Ref. 11.

2). The nonadsorbed serum from step 2 contained IgM and other serum proteins but was free of IgG. Purified IgG was eluted from the protein G-Sepharose column with 0.15 M glycine:HCl buffer pH 2.50 (Fig. 1, step 3). The purified IgG was further fractionated into J5 LPS-specific IgG by chromatography on J5 LPS-EAH-Sepharose 4B immunoadsorbent (Fig. 1, step 4). The IgG not retained by this column is the non-J5 LPS-specific IgG. An alternative scheme for the preparation of purified IgM free of IgG and other serum proteins was successful using size-exclusion chromatography of rabbit serum on a TSK 3000-SW preparative high-performance liquid chromatography (HPLC) column, whereby the IgM elutes at the void volume as the first peak (Fig. 2). A small amount of IgG aggregates co-elutes with IgM and can be removed by affinity chromatography on anti-rabbit IgG-Sepharose 4B as shown in Fig. 1, step 2. Purified IgG was also prepared from the preimmune rabbit serum by affinity chromatography as shown in Fig. 1.

B. Protection of Neutropenic Rats

Protection experiments in neutropenic rats against lethal challenge with a virulent strain of *Pseudomonas aeruginosa* #12:4:4 (Fisher Devlin immunotype 6)

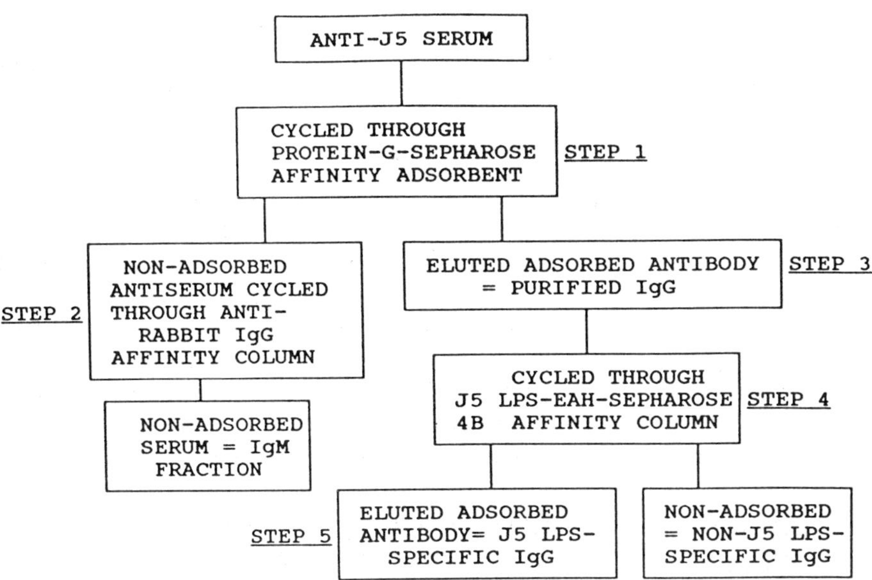

Figure 1 Scheme for the preparation of purified IgG, IgM, and J5 LPS-specific IgG from anti-J5 rabbit serum. The IgM fraction obtained after step 2 was free of IgG but contained other serum proteins. (From Ref. 11.)

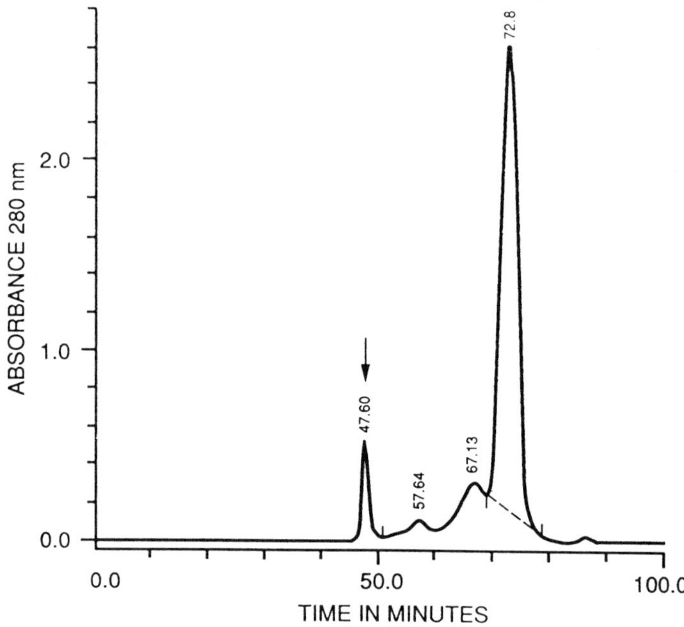

Figure 2 Fractionation of rabbit serum by preparative HPLC on TSK-3000-SW column (22.5 × 600 mm). Elution was performed with 0.01 M Na-phosphate, 0.14 M NaCl, pH 7.4 (PBS) at a flow rate of 2.0 mL/min. The arrow indicates the position of the void volume of this column.

showed that J5 LPS-specific IgG at a dose of 130 μg per rat protected 6 of 8 rats (75%) compared to none of 25 rats treated with IgG (1500 μg per rat) prepared from the preimmune rabbit serum ($p < 0.001$). The unfractionated postimmune IgG at a dose of 2100 μg per rat protected 13 of 20 rats (65%), and the non-J5 LPS-specific IgG at a dose of 2830 μg per rat protected 4 of 13 rats (30%, Fig. 3). These results showed that the J5 LPS-specific IgG was highly protective in this neutropenic rat model of sepsis. In a separate experiment, 9 of 16 rats (56%) were protected when treated with the IgM fraction. This IgM fraction was free of IgG but contained other serum proteins.

V. SUBUNIT VACCINE FORMULATIONS USING PURIFIED *ESCHERICHIA COLI* J5 LIPOPOLYSACCHARIDE

A. Covalent Conjugate with Diphtheria Toxoid

Escherichia coli J5 LPS used alone as vaccine showed only a two- to fourfold rise in anti-J5 LPS antibodies. Therefore, J5 LPS was covalently linked to

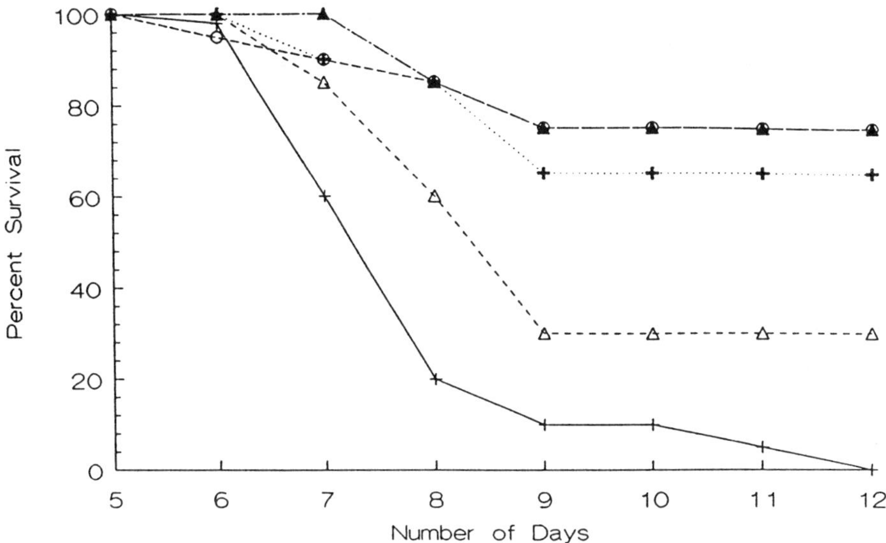

Figure 3 Survival of neutropenic rats against challenge with *Pseudomonas aeruginosa* strain 12:4:4. The antibodies were administered at 9.0 mL/kg. +, IgG from preimmune rabbit serum (1mg/mL); △, non-J5 LPS-specific IgG (1.4 mg/mL); ○, anti-J5 sera; +, purified IgG (1.4 mg/mL); ▲, J5 LPS-specific IgG (96 μg/mL) (From Ref. 11.)

diphtheria toxoid (Dt) by carbodiimide-mediated coupling reaction (15) to give the J5 LPS-Dt covalent conjugate. The molar ratio of J5 LPS:Dt was 5:1. Rabbits were immunized intramuscularly with this vaccine, with and without alum as adjuvant. The conjugate with alum gave only a three- to ninefold rise in titer of anti-J5 LPS antibodies as determined by ELISA. The vaccine given alone in sterile 0.9% NaCl gave a seven- to 16-fold rise in titer against J5 LPS after two doses of vaccine given 4 weeks apart (Table 2). There was only a two- to fourfold rise in titer against *E. coli* lipid A (data not shown). The reason for the vaccine with alum showing weaker anti-J5 antibody response than the J5 LPS-Dt conjugate alone is not clear. In a separate study we found that *Brucella* LPS with alum gave significantly higher antibody response in mice when given subcutaneously than when given intraperitoneally (data not shown).

B.   Noncovalent Complex with *Neisseria meningitidis* group B Outer Membrane Protein

A noncovalent complex vaccine formulation was prepared with purified J5 LPS and *Neisseria meningitidis* group B outer membrane protein (GBOMP) (16).

Table 2 ELISA IgG Titers Versus J5 LPS of Sera from Rabbits Immunized with J5 LPS-Dt Covalent Conjugate

	ELISA titers in OD units			
Rabbit	Prebleed	Post-1	Post-2	Fold rise
56	60	130	172	2.8
57	35	128	324	9.2
58	75	397	527	7.0
59	43	832	697	16.2

Rabbits 56 and 57 were immunized with the vaccine containing alum as adjuvant. Rabbits 58 and 59 were immunized with the vaccine without alum. Post-1 = 4 weeks post primary immunization. Post-2 = 1 week post secondary immunization.

Rabbits immunized with the J5 LPS-GBOMP vaccine in sterile 0.9% NaC1 elicited high-titer anti-J5 LPS antibodies (Table 3). There was a 37- to 142-fold rise in titer 4 weeks after the first injection, and a further three- to sixfold rise in anti-J5 LPS antibody titer 7 days after the second injection. These rabbits did not show any significant rise in anti-lipid A antibodies. The immune rabbit serum protected neutropenic rats against lethal challenge with *Pseudomonas aeruginosa* strain 12:4:4. Six of 10 rats treated with the postimmune whole serum survived, compared to none of 10 rats treated with the preimmune serum from the same rabbit ($p < 0.01$, Fig. 4). *Neisseria meningitidis* GBOMP is a highly hydrophobic protein that is insoluble in aqueous solvents without added detergent (17). In the noncovalent complex formulation with LPS, the detergent is slowly replaced such that the LPS can bind to the protein by hydrophobic interaction. In successful complex formation the hydrophilic parts are exposed, making the complex soluble in aqueous solvents. This process also seem to result in optimal presentation of the protective J5 LPS epitope.

Table 3 ELISA IgG Titers Versus J5 LPS of Sera from Rabbits Immunized with J5 LPS-GBOMP Noncovalent Complex Vaccine

	ELISA titers in OD units			
Rabbit	Prebleed	Post-1	Post-2	Fold rise
62	106	3,995	25,804	240
63	99	4,115	14,873	147
64	32	3,558	N.D.	—
65	32	4,550	16,384	511

Post-1 = 4 weeks post primary immunization. Post-2 = 1 week post secondary immunization. N.D. = not done.

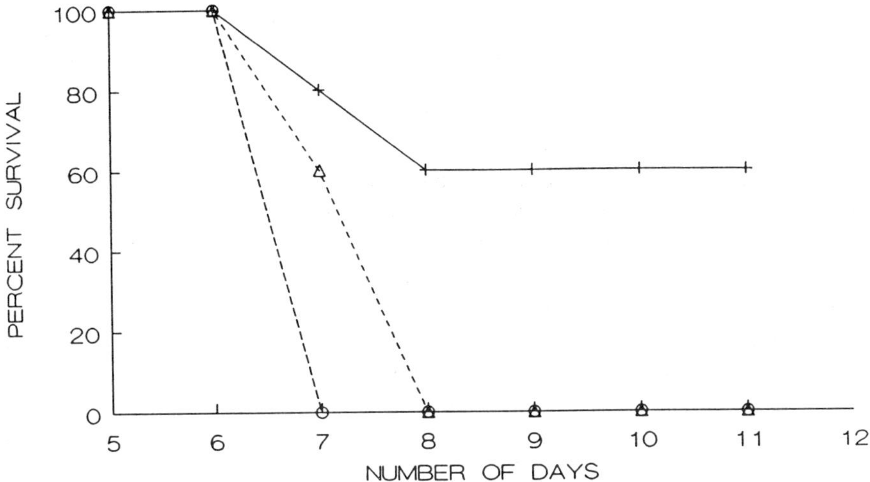

Figure 4 Protection of neutropenic rats against lethal challenge with *Pseudomonas aeruginosa* strain 12:4:4. The antibodies were administered at 9.0 mL/kg. +, postimmune serum of rabbit immunized with J5 LPS-GBOMP vaccine; △, preimmune rabbit serum; ○, PBS control.

VI. CLINICAL SIGNIFICANCE AND FUTURE DIRECTIONS

These data demonstrate that IgG antibody directed toward a J5 epitope, when administered at the onset of fever, is able to protect neutropenic rats from lethal experimental *Pseudomonas* sepsis. The mechanism of this protection is not clear; however, this antibody does not appear to neutralize the biologic activity of endotoxin directly. Preliminary data suggest that it may facilitate the clearance of endotoxin, but this remains to be tested more directly.

It is also necessary to determine the extent to which these anti-J5 antibodies bind to other gram-negative bacteria. When analyzed by flow cytometry, affinity-purified anti-J5 IgG binds to clinical isolates of *E. coli*, *Klebsiella*, and *Enterobacter*, but not to gram-positive cocci (data not shown). IgG prepared from pre-J5 immunization sera did not bind to the gram-negative bacteria. It is necessary to test the protective efficacy of anti-J5 IgG in neutropenic rats that are challenged with gram-negative bacterial pathogens other than *Pseudomonas*.

While our studies in experimental animal models of infection demonstrated the protective efficacy of anti-J5 antibodies, recent clinical studies with J5 antisera and with a J5 hyperimmune IVIG failed to show any benefit (5,6). Before further development of a J5 vaccine, it will be important to resolve the reasons for the failure of anti-J5 therapy in these studies. Our initial studies with the boiled, whole-cell vaccine used sera harvested after booster immunizations for antibody preparation. While the affinity of anti-J5 antibody was not measured, it may be that antibody elicited following booster doses of a J5 vaccine might have a higher affinity than antibody harvested after a primary series. In the two clinical studies, plasma was harvested after the second immunization in a primary series. The plasma of volunteers immunized with a J5 vaccine before preparation of an IVIG had only a two- to threefold increase in anti-J5 antibody. Interestingly, Dale and colleagues found that human anti-J5 antisera, obtained from a volunteer at 9 months after immunization, was more active in vitro than sera from the same individual that was harvested earlier in the course of the immunization (18). Thus, the immunization regimen or the time of harvest of anti-J5 plasma after immunization might be an important variable.

The preparation of the vaccine and primary immunization schedule is another variable that must be evaluated more rigorously. Since there is variability in the degree of rough LPS phenotype among single colonies isolated from a culture of LPS, failure to select a sufficiently rough phenotype may result in a less than optimal presentation of a J5 epitope to the immune system. Even when this is taken into account, we found differences in antibody response to the primary immunization following different immunization regimens and with different concentrations of killed bacteria within the same regimen (data not shown). These factors may have contributed to the differences observed between the efficacy in our experimental studies and the recent clinical studies.

Once lots of J5 LPS vaccine are made under GMP conditions, it will be possible to extend these studies to human subjects and to answer these questions directly.

ACKNOWLEDGMENT

The authors would like to thank Wendell D. Zollinger for a gift of *Neisseria meningitidis* group B outer membrane protein.

REFERENCES

1. Chedid L, Parant M, Parant F, Boyer F. A proposed mechanism for natural immunity to enterobacterial pathogens. J Immunol 1968; 100:292–301.
2. McCabe WR. Immunization with R mutants of *S. minnesota*. I. Protection against challenge with heterologous Gram-negative bacilli. J Immunol 1972; 108:601–610.
3. Braude AI, Ziegler EJ, McCutchan JA, Douglas H. Immunization against nosocomial infection. Am J Med 1981; 70:463–466.
4. Ziegler EJ, McCutchan JA, Fierer J, et al. Treatment of gram negative bacteremia and shock with human antiserum to a mutant *Escherichia coli*. N Engl J Med 1982; 307:1225–1230.
5. Calandra T, Glauser MP, Schellekens J, Verhoef J, Swiss-Dutch. J5 Immunoglobulin Study Group, Treatment of Gram-negative septic shock with human IgG antibody

to *Escherichia coli* J5: a prospective, double-blind, randomized trial. J Infect Dis 1988; 158:312–319.

6. J5 Study Group. Treatment of severe infectious purpura in children with human plasma from donors immunized with *Escherichia coli* J5: a prospective double-blind study. J Infect Dis 1991; 165:695–701.

7. Baumgardner JD. Immunotherapy with antibodies to core lipopolysaccharide: a critical appraisal. Infect Dis Clin North Am 1991; 5: 695–701.

8. Baumgardner JD, Heuman D, Calandra T, Glauser MP. Antibodies to lipopolysaccharides after immunization of humans with the rough mutant *Escherichia coli* J5. J Infect Dis 1991; 163:769–772.

9. Collins HH, Cross AS, Dobeck A, Opal SM, McClain JB, Sadoff JC. Oral ciprofloxacin and a monoclonal antibody to lipopolysaccharide protect leukopenic rats from lethal infection with *Pseudomonas aeruginosa*. J Infect Dis 1989; 159:1073–1082.

10. Cross AS, Opal SM, Palardy JE, Bodmer MW, Sadoff JC. The efficacy of combination immunotherapy in experimental Pseudomonas sepsis. J Infect Dis 1993; 167:112–118.

11. Bhattacharjee AK, Opal SM, Palardy JE, et al. Affinity-purified *Escherichia coli* J5 lipopolysaccharide-specific IgG protects neutropenic rats against gram negative bacterial sepsis. J Inf Dis 1994; 170:622–629.

12. Ziegler EJ, Douglas H, Sherman JE, Davis CE, Braude A. Treatment of *E. coli* and *Klebsiella* bacteremia in granulocytic animals with anti-serum to a UDP-gal epimerase deficient mutant. J Immunol 1973; 111:433–438.

13. Evans ME, Pollack M, Koles NL, Hardegen NJ, Panopoulos D. Lipopolysaccharide heterogeneity in *Escherichia coli* J5 variants: analysis by flow cytometry. J Infect Dis 1992; 166:803–811.

14. Engvall E, Perlmann P. Enzyme-linked immunosorbent assay, ELISA III. Quantitation of specific antibodies by enzyme-labeled anti-immunoglobulin in antigen-coated tubes. J Immunol 1972; 109:129–135.

15. Yamada H, Imoto T, Fujita K, Okazaki K, Motomura M. Selective modification of aspartic acid 101 in lysozyme by carbodiimide reaction. Biochemistry 1981; 20:4836–4842.

16. Zollinger WD, Mandrell RE, Grifiss JM, Altieri P. Complex of meningococcal group B polysaccharide and type 2 outer membrane protein immunogenic in man. J Clin Invest 1979; 63:836–848.

17. Zollinger WD, Boslego J, Moran E, Brandt B, Collins H, Mandrell R, Altieri P, Berman S. Process for the preparation of detoxified polysaccharide-outer membrane protein complexes, and their use as antibacterial vaccines. US Patent 1987; 4,707,543.

18. Dale PA, McQuillen DP, Gulati S, Rice PA. Human vaccination with *Escherichia coli* J5 mutant induces cross-reactive bactericidal antibody against *Neisseria gonorrhoeae* lipopolysaccharide. J Infect Dis 1992; 166:316–325.

2

Monoclonal Antibodies to Endotoxin Core as a New Approach in Endotoxemia Therapy

Franco Di Padova and Hermann Gram
Sandoz Pharma
Basel, Switzerland

G. Robin Barclay
Scottish National Blood Transfusion Service
Edinburgh, Scotland, United Kingdom

Ian R. Poxton
University of Edinburgh Medical School
Edinburgh, Scotland, United Kingdom

Ekke Liehl
Sandoz Research Institute
Vienna, Austria

Ernst th. Rietschel
Forschungsinstitut Borstel
Borstel, Germany

I. INTRODUCTION

Gram-negative sepsis remains one of the most common causes of morbidity and mortality among hospitalized patients, with *Escherichia coli* representing the most common clinical isolate (1–4). Many bacterial components can trigger pathogenic mechanisms, but lipopolysaccharides (LPS) are the major antigenic and toxic components of gram-negative bacteria. The neutralization of LPS-mediated toxic injury has been considered for a long time as a possible therapeutic target in patients with septic shock.

In LPS molecules, three genetically, biochemically, and antigenically distinct regions are present: O-specific polysaccharide chain, the core oligosaccharide, and the lipid A (5). In Enterobacteriaceae, the O-specific side chains are composed of highly variable repeating oligosaccharide units, are immunogenic, and give rise to the high number of known serotypes. When the O-antigen is lost, the core glycolipid is exposed (rough mutant). One core structure accounts for all *Salmonella* spp., while five different chemotypes (R1, R2, R3, R4, and K-12) are known among *E. coli* strains (5,6). These six core types differ in the structural composition of the outer (hexose) region. The inner core is structurally conserved among *E. coli*, *Salmonella*, and *Shigella* (7). Rough chemotypes differing in the length of the core region have also been described. While a *Salmonella* mutant strain of chemotype Ra retains the complete core structure and lipid A and lacks the O side chain, an Rc mutant harbors one hexose in addition to the inner core region and lipid A. Re mutants contain 3-deoxy-D-manno-octulosonic acid and lipid A only. The lipid A component is the endotoxic principle and the most structurally conserved LPS region (5).

The great similarities among core glycolipid and lipid A within the various Enterobacteriaceae supported the hypothesis that antibodies (Ab) to common epitopes in the inner core and lipid A region would be cross-reactive and could be used for immunotherapy in patients with gram-negative septicemia. Several authors have investigated both whether such an approach is feasible and which bacterial epitopes should be targeted, but results have remained controversial. Ab to core antigens such as Rc and Re LPS and lipid A are detected in the serum of healthy human beings (8–11), and both standard intravenous immune globulin and hyperimmune globulin from donors screened for high Ab titers have been used prophylactically or therapeutically, but efficacy was not demonstrated (12,13). However, in these preparations the titers of cross-reactive and cross-neutralizing anti-core Ab are low and difficult to identify, as they are part of a more complex mixture of Ab also comprising serotype-specific Ab.

In other studies, human volunteers have been immunized with J5 vaccines, and their sera or plasma have been used for therapy or passive prophylaxis of septic patients with promising results (14,15). Later on, additional investigations with purified IgG fraction obtained from volunteers immunized with J5 vaccine cast doubts on the neutralizing role of anti-core and anti-lipid A Ab (16). Further analysis of these sera revealed that cross-reactive anti-core or anti-lipid A Ab were not present, and that only a modest and specific Ab response against J5 LPS became evident (17).

More recently, two anti-lipid A monoclonal Ab (MAb) have been used for the treatment of patients with gram-negative sepsis (4,18). The results of these studies have been subjected to widespread criticism, and it was concluded that reduction of mortality rate with use of such Ab had not been conclusively established (19). At the same time, the neutralizing properties of anti-lipid A MAb of IgM class were not confirmed (20).

In conclusion, the controversies about the existence of cross-reactive and cross-neutralizing anti-core or anti-lipid A Ab as well as their potential therapeutic role have not been solved. Recently we have shown that widely cross-reactive Ab can be obtained in mice (21). Here we show that, by using rough mutants expressing the complete core and different immunization protocols, several cross-reactive and cross-neutralizing MAb can be obtained. It is now possible to test the concept that these Ab might be beneficial in patients with endotoxemia and sepsis.

II. MATERIALS AND METHODS

A. Bacterial Strains, LPS, and Lipid A

The *E. coli* strains O4 (E394), O6 (126), O12 (E253), O15 (E568), O16 (E449), O18 (Bort), and O18rf (rough mutant) were kindly provided by Dr. A. S. Cross (Walter Reed Army Institute of Research, Washington DC). The *E. coli* strains F470, F576, F653, F2513, and W3100 were kindly provided by Dr. H. Brade (Forschungsinstitut Borstel, Borstel, Germany). The *Salmonella minnesota* strain R60 was from Dr. I. Poxton (Department of Medical Microbiology, University of Edinburgh, Edinburgh, Scotland).

LPS from *S. abortus equi* (Freiburg strain collection) *E. coli* O4, O6, O12, O15, O16, O18, and O86 were isolated by phenol water extraction (22). LPS from *E. coli* W3100 (K-12), F470 (R1 core), F576 (R2 core), F653 (R3 core), F2513 (R4 core), F515 (Re core), *S. minnesota* R60 (Ra), R345 (Rb$_2$), R5 (RcP-), R7 (Rd$_1$P-), R4 (Rd$_2$), R595 (Re), *S. typhimurium* SL1102 (Rd2), and *Acinetobacter calcoaceticus* (NTCC, London, 10305) were obtained by extraction with phenol/chloroform/petroleum ether (23). LPS from *E. coli* O26:B6, *E. coli* O111:B4, *S. typhimurium* TV119 (Ra), SL684 (Rc), and *Shigella flexneri* (1A) were obtained from Sigma Chemicals (St Louis, MO). LPS from *E. coli* K235, *E. coli* J5 (Rc), *S. minnesota* wild-type, and free lipid A from *E. coli* K-12 (ex-D31m4) and from *S. minnesota* R595 were from List Biological Laboratories, Inc. (Campbell, CA). LPS from *S. typhimurium* SH 4305, SH 4809, SL 3622, *S. enteriditis* SH 1262, *S. newport*, *S. thompson*, and *S. typhi* 253 Ty were obtained from BioCarb Chemicals (Lund, Sweden).

B. MAb

MAb H1 61–2 (IgG1), H5 13–23 (IgG3) and H5 415–6 (IgG2a) were obtained after having fused the spleen cells of two different mice (H1 and H5) with a nonsecreting murine B-cell lymphoma line. Briefly, 8-week-old Balb/c mice were immunized intravenously (i.v.) with 10^8 heat-killed bacteria (*E. coli* F576,

E. coli F653, and *E. coli* W3100). Subsequently, animals were boosted i.v. with the same mixture of heat-killed bacteria on days 7, 13, and 27 (5×10^7 cells) and on day 14 (10^8 cells). On day 71 they received an additional i.v. injection of 10^8 bacteria, i.e., a mixture of *E. coli* F470, *E. coli* F576, *E. coli* F653, and *E. coli* F2513. Four and three days before the fusion (day 80), they received the same amount and mixture of bacteria i.v. and i.p., respectively. MAb WN1 222–5 (IgG2a) and WN1 58–9 (IgG2b) were generated and selected by standard methods after the fusion of spleen cell of one mouse with a nonsecreting murine B-cell lymphoma cell line (24). Twenty-two-week-old NZB mice were immunized i.v. with 10^8 heat-killed bacteria in 0.1 mL. Four immunizations, 1 week apart, were carried out (weeks 1 and 3: *E. coli* F576, *E. coli* F653, and *S. minnesota* R60; weeks 2 and 4: *E. coli* F470, *E. coli* F2513, and *E. coli* 018rf). After 1 month, two injections, 1 day apart, of a mixture of the six strains (10^8 heat-killed bacteria) were given, the first injection i.v., the second i.p. On the fourth day, spleen cells were recovered and fused with a nonsecreting murine B-cell lymphoma cell line, using standard procedures (25).

With minor modifications, supernatants from the different fusions were screened overnight in enzyme linked immunoabsorbent assay (ELISA) with seven different LPS mixtures as described previously (21).

In-vitro experiments were performed with MAb preparations purified on a protein A column from serum- and pyrogen-free cultures. All samples were Limulus amebocyte lysate (LAL) negative.

C. ELISA on Isolated LPS

ELISA was performed as described previously (21). Briefly, LPS or lipid A (2 µg/mL; 50 µL) were coated overnight onto 96-well Microtest III flexible plates (Becton and Dickinson, Oxnard, CA). Fifty microliters of purified MAb (100 ng/mL) diluted in PBS/2% bovine serum albumin (BSA) were added in duplicate overnight to microtiter plates blocked with 250 µL/well of PBS/2% BSA. The reaction was revealed by the subsequent addition of 50 µL/well of biotin-labeled affinity-purified goat anti-mouse isotype Ab (Southern Biotechnology Associates; 3 h at room temperature), and of 50 µl/well of streptavidin alkaline phosphatase conjugate (Jackson Immuno Research Laboratories; 1 h at room temperature). Substrate (PNPP) in diethanolamine buffer was added and absorbance read after 20 min at 405 nm using a Titertek Multiskan ELISA reader (MCC/340, Flowlabs). In all ELISA experiments, the interassay coefficient of variation was less than 5%.

D. Gel Electrophoresis and Blotting

Ten microliters of different LPS solutions (50 µg/mL) were mixed with 10 µL of 0.1 M Tris-HCl buffer (0.1 M, pH 6.8) containing 1% (wt/vol) sodium deoxycholate (DOC), 20% (wt/vol) glycerol, and 0.001% bromophenol blue. The samples were loaded onto electrophoresis gels (4% stacking gel; 14% running gel). A modified Laemmli system (DOC-PAGE) (26) and a Mini Protean II dual-slab cell apparatus (Bio Rad Laboratories) were used. The gels were blotted onto a 0.45-μm nitrocellulose membrane at 60 V for 20 min (Mini transblot electrophoretic transfer cell apparatus, Bio Rad Laboratories). The blots were soaked in Tris buffer saline (TBS: 20 nM Tris-HC1, 0.1 mM NaC1; pH 7.5)/ 1% BSA for 1 h at room temperature (RT). The immunoblots were developed for 2 h at RT with the different MAb (30 ng/mL in TBS/Tween 20 0.05%/1% BSA). The blots were washed twice in TTBS and developed for 45 min at RT with isotype-specific biotin-labeled goat anti-mouse IgG Ab (Southern Biotechnology Associates) and subsequently with streptavidin alkaline phosphatase conjugate (Jackson Immunoresearch Laboratories) and the BCIP/NBT alkaline phosphatase color-development solution (Bio Rad Laboratories). Companion gels were fixed by overnight incubation in a solution containing 40% ethanol and 5% acetic acid and were silver stained according to the method of Tsai and Frasch (27).

E. Sequencing of WN1 222–5 and WN1 58–9

Total RNA was isolated from the hybridoma cells according to the method described by Chomczynski and Sacchi (28). Single-stranded cDNA was synthesized from 3 μg of total RNA using a first-strand cDNA synthesis kit (Pharmacia), and either oligo $(dT)_{18}$ or random hexanucleotides $pd(N)_6$ for priming. First-strand cDNA served as template for the amplification of immunoglobulin variable domains encoding genes by the polymerase chain reaction (PCR). All PCR amplifications were performed on a GeneAmp PCR System 9600 (Perkin Elmer) utilizing standard amplification conditions (reaction volume 50 μL, containing 1.5 mM $MgCl_2$, 2.5 U Taq polymerase, and 50 pMol of the 5′- and 3′-primer, respectively; typically, 25–30 cycles of denaturation at 94°C for 30 s, primer annealing at 50–60°C for 30 s, and elongation at 72°C for 30 s). The following oligonucleotides were designed from a partial amino-terminal amino acid sequence of both the heavy and light chains and utilized for the PCR reactions: 5′AGGTGTCGACTCCGAGGTGAAGCTGGTGGAGTCTGG 3′ and 5′GACC-GATGGGGCTGTTGTTTTGGC 3′ for V_H, and 5′ AGGTACGCGTTGTGA-CATCCAGATGAACCAGTCTCC 3′ and 5′GCACACGACTGAGGCACCTC 3′ for V_L. Both the PCR fragments obtained were cloned into the plasmid pBluescript SKII (Stratagene) digested with EcoRV. Several recombinant clones were picked and sequenced according to Sanger et al. (29).

F. LPS-Induced Monokine Secretion

Freshly collected peritoneal cells (5 × 10^5 cells/ml) from BALB/c mice (BRL, Fullingsdorf, Switzerland) were cultured in 0.2 mL of serum and pyrogen-free medium (IMDM-ATL) in the presence of different *E. coli* LPS (0.05–5 ng/mL) and in the presence or absence of increasing concentrations of the different MAb (20). Culture supernatants were collected after 4 h for IL-6 determinations. Specific biological assays for IL-6 (20) were used. The content of IL-6 in culture supernatants was calculated relative to standard curves. Data are reported as percent inhibition over LPS-stimulated cultures. Background IL-6 levels induced by Ab alone have been subtracted.

G. Mouse Lethality, Galactosamine (D-GalN) Model

Endotoxin shock was induced by i.v. injection of an LD95 dose of *E. coli* O16 LPS (75 ng/kg) in groups of six female C57bl/6 mice, 6 to 8 weeks old (Charles River, Sulzfeld, Germany). D-GalN (800 mg/kg) was administered i.p. at the time of LPS (29). WN1 222–5 (range 62–2000 μg/mouse), diluted in pyrogen-free NaCl solution, was administered i.v. 2 h prior to LPS. Survival was recorded up to 24 h. Animal experiments were performed in accordance with institutional guidelines.

III. RESULTS

A. ELISA Reactivity Pattern

The reactivity of the five anti-core LPS MAb H1 61–2 (IgG1), H5 13–23 (IgG3), H5 415–6 (IgG2a), WN1 222–5 (IgG2a), and WN1 58–9 (IgG2b) for isolated, purified S-form, and R-form LPS and for free lipid A is shown in Table 1. These five MAb were selected in three different fusions and show different isotypes. The five MAb bind to S-form and R-form LPS of *E. coli*, *Salmonella*, and *Shigella* containing the complete core region. In particular, they recognize the five known core types of *E. coli* (R1–R4, K-12). They react with *E. coli* J5 (RcP+ core), but not with *E. coli* F515 (Re) or *E. coli*-free lipid A. In comparison with the other MAb, H5 13–23 and H5 415–6 show lower levels of reactivity with *E. coli* R3. Additional differences are observed in the binding pattern to rough core structures of *Salmonella*. All the MAb recognize *S. minnesota* R60 (Ra), and with the exception of H1 61–2 they also bind to *S. minnesota* R345 (Rb2). WN1 222–5 and WN1 58–9 show some binding to more defective core structures such as *S.minnesota* RcP- and Rd1P-. H5 12–23 and H5 415–6 show a lower degree of reactivity with R-form LPS of *S. typhimurium* and with other *Salmonella* strains. The broad cross-reactivity of these MAb for LPS indicates the existence of common epitopes in the core LPS. Our data suggest that these MAb might actually recognize different epitopes. WN1 222–5 and WN1 58–9 seem to recognize deeper core regions in comparison to H5 13–23, H5 415–6, and H1 61–2. Because none of the MAb shows reactivity with Re structures from *E. coli* or *Salmonella* and with free mono- and bis-phosphoryl lipid A, the epitopes must be localized in the inner outer-core region.

B. Reactivity in Immunoblots

Immunoblots confirmed the cross-reactivity of the MAb for S-form and R-form LPS (data not shown). The ladderlike patterns seen in immunoblots of S-form LPS developed with four different MAb (Fig. 1, A–D) show that these MAb in nanogram amounts react with O-side-chain substituted (slow migrating bands at the top) as well as with unsubstituted LPS species (fast migrating bands at the bottom) of smooth *E. coli*. These data indicate that the MAb bind to LPS-core epitopes which remain accessible on O-side-chain carrying LPS. H5 13–23 and H5 415–6 show a low reactivity with *E. coli* O15 (lanes 14 and 20).

C. Sequencing of WN1 222–5 and WN1 58–9

WN1 222–5 and WN1 58–9 have different isotypes but show very similar binding characteristics in ELISA. Therefore, we analyzed the similarities of these two cell clones at the molecular level. The DNA sequence of the variable regions of heavy and light chains expressed in both cell lines were obtained from the mRNA and found to be highly homologous (Figs. 2 and 3). The sequence analysis did not provide evidence for independent recombination events (V_H-D-J or V_L-J joining) and therefore suggested that the cell lines were of clonal origin and have diverged to different isotype switch variants. The differences observed in the DNA sequences are thought to be due to somatic mutation events which occurred independently in two of the clones originating from the same ancestor.

D. Inhibition of LPS-Induced IL-6 Secretion

These MAb inhibit the secretion of IL-6 by mouse peritoneal cells stimulated with several different R-form and S-form *E. coli* LPS (Figs. 4 and 5). This finding demonstrates that the MAb are able to neutralize LPS in vitro.

As shown in Figs. 4 and 5, WN1 222–5 was the best-neutralizing Ab, as it blocked IL-6 production induced by all R-form and S-form LPS tested. At the lowest concentration used (5 ng/mL), WN1 222–5 inhibited more than 70% the IL-6 production induced by 50 pg/mL of R-form LPS. As expected, higher concentrations of Ab (50–500 ng/mL) were needed to obtain the same level of inhibition with S-form LPS, as these were also used at a higher concentration (0.5–5 ng/mL). The other Ab also showed inhibition of IL-6 secretion. H5

Table 1 Binding of Anti-Core LPS MAb to Isolated LPS and Free Lipid A in ELISA

Type of LPS or lipid A	Serotype or chemotype	OD value for H1 61-2 (0.1 µg/mL)	OD value for H5 13-23 (0.1 µg/mL)	OD value for H5 415-6 (0.1 µg/mL)	OD value for WN1 222-5 (0.1 µg/mL)	OD value for WN1 58-9 (0.1 µg/mL)
E. coli smooth LPS						
E394	O4	1.675	2.437	2.810	2.919	2.837
126	O6	2.692	2.862	2.869	2.914	2.892
E253	O12	2.575	2.665	2.681	2.917	2.851
E449	O16	2.509	2.631	2.649	2.884	2.828
Bort	O18	2.793	2.998	3.011	3.041	2.973
	O26:B6	2.579	2.571	2.661	2.957	2.828
	O111:B4	2.720	1.912	1.735	3.076	2.989
	K235	2.630	2.592	2.697	2.869	2.877
E. coli rough LPS						
F470	R1	2.783	2.868	2.825	2.919	2.956
F576	R2	2.620	2.899	2.828	3.042	3.040
F653	R3	2.501	1.558	1.306	3.089	3.080
F2513	R4	2.873	2.912	2.880	3.143	3.111
W3100	K-12	2.828	2.989	2.932	3.044	3.035
J5	RcP+	1.274	2.051	1.923	2.775	2.693
F515	Re	0.030	0.100	0.130	0.381	0.207
E. coli-free lipid A	K-12	0.319	0.094	0.085	0.165	0.150
S. minnesota smooth LPS	Wild type	2.638	2.364	2.514	2.678	2.730

S. minnesota rough LPS						
R60	Ra	2.939	2.876	2.840	3.024	3.018
R345	Rb2	0.491	2.573	2.592	3.072	3.052
R5	RcP-	0.208	0.058	0.100	1.871	2.063
R7	Rd1P-	0.055	0.041	0.033	0.413	0.406
R4	Rd2P-	0.043	0.118	0.114	0.833	0.783
R595	Re	0.040	0.036	0.022	0.190	0.111
S. minnesota-free lipid A	Re	0.097	0.067	0.094	0.283	0.266
S. typhimurium smooth LPS						
SH 4305		2.657	2.447	2.445	2.761	2.775
SH 4809		2.676	2.922	2.909	3.060	3.013
SL 3622		2.693	2.855	2.737	3.053	3.046
S. typhimurium rough LPS						
TV119	Ra	2.079	1.105	0.480	3.080	3.048
SL684	Rc	2.487	0.229	0.405	2.945	2.881
SL1102	Rd2	0.121	0.093	0.087	0.766	0.504
Other smooth LPS						
S. enteritidis (SH 1262)		1.188	1.077	0.520	2.611	2.456
S. newport		2.508	1.475	0.595	2.887	2.894
S. thompson (ls40)		2.586	2.106	2.005	2.929	2.944
S. typhi (253 Ty)		1.919	1.262	0.898	2.942	2.971
Shigella flexneri	1A	0.748	1.919	2.251	2.552	2.569
A. calcoaceticus		0.039	0.027	0.021	0.125	0.147
Bovine serum albumin		0.019	0.020	0.012	0.029	0.044

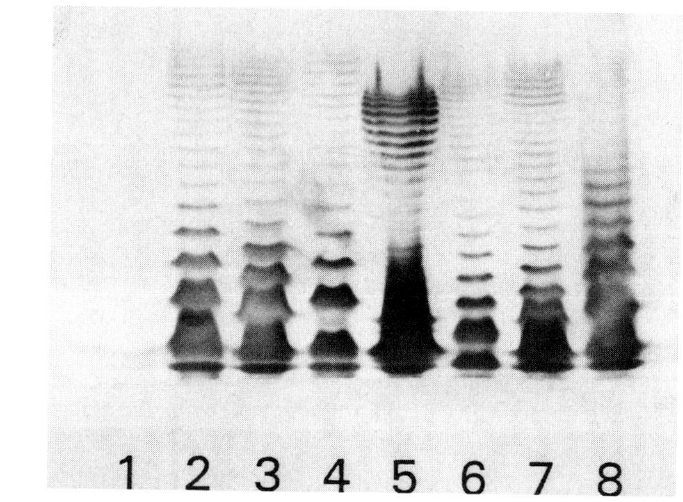

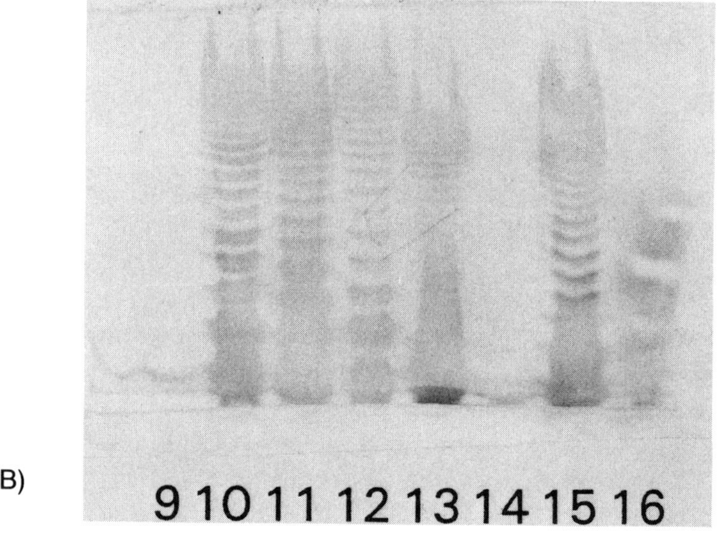

Figure 1 Recognition pattern of S-form *E. coli* and *S. minnesota* LPS after sodium deoxycholate electrophoresis and immunoblot: (A) H1 61-1; (B) H5 13-23; (C) H5 415-6; (D) WN1 222-5. Lanes 1 to 8 and 9 to 16: *S. minnesota* Re, *E. coli* O18K−, O4, O6, O12, O15, O16, O86; lanes 17 to 24: *E. coli* R2, O86, O16, O15, O12, O6, O4, O18rf; lanes 25 to 32: *E. coli* O111, O86, O18, O16, O15, O12, O6, O4.

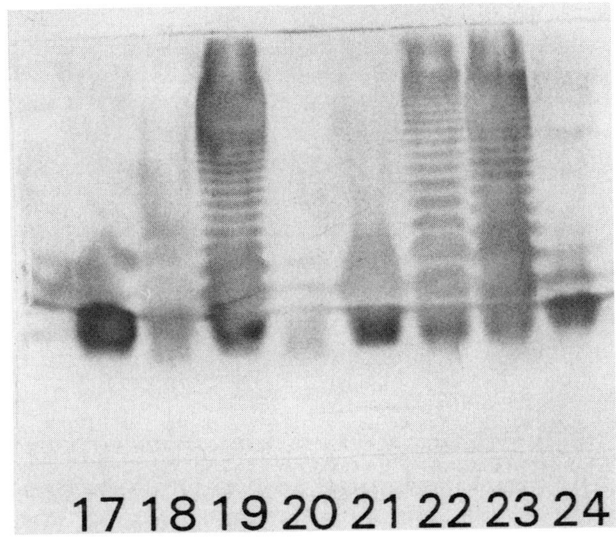
(C)
17 18 19 20 21 22 23 24
(D)
25 26 27 28 29 30 31 32

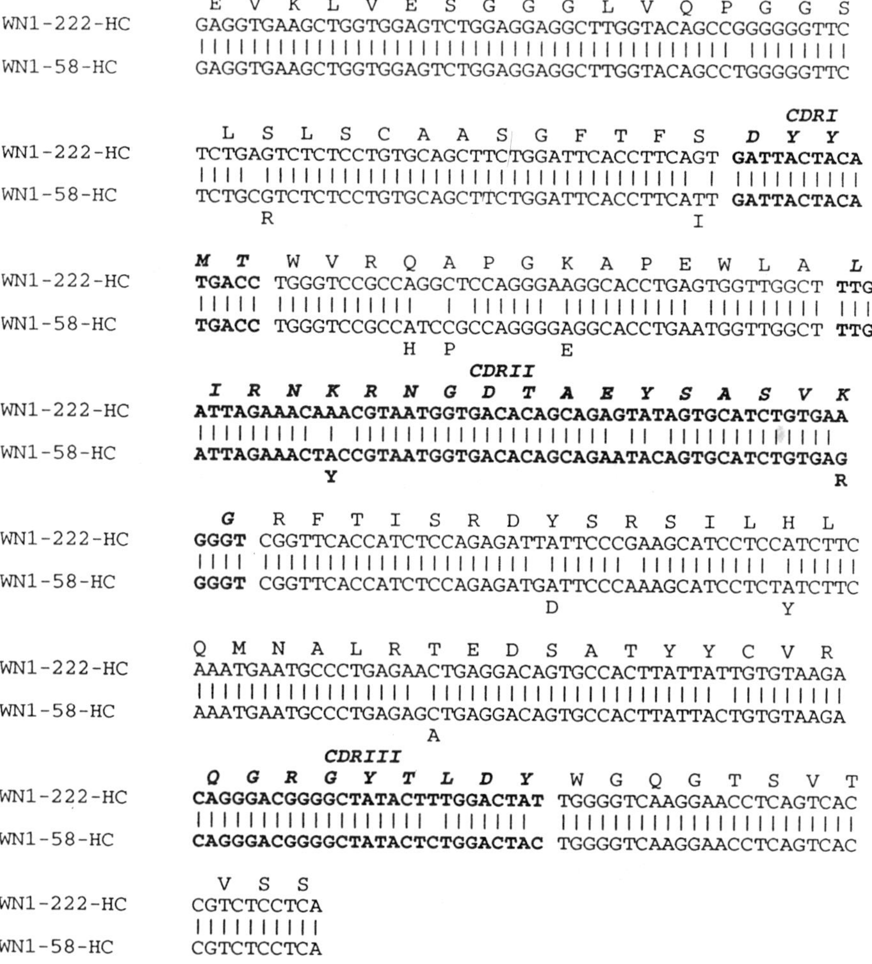

Figure 2 Comparison of the V_H regions of the anti-LPS MAb WN1 222-5 and WN1 58-9. The complementary determining regions (CDR) are printed in bold, and amino acid changes in WN1 58-9 are indicated beneath the DNA sequence.

13–23 and H5 415–6 were particularly effective against *E. coli* R1 and R2 but not against *E. coli* R3 and R4. H1 61–2 showed lower neutralizing activity.

In the absence of LPS, the MAb did not cause any significant release of IL-6, confirming the absence of contaminating LPS in MAb preparations as shown by the LAL assay.

```
             D   I   Q   M   N   Q   S   P   S   S   L   S   A   S   L   G   D
WN1-222-LC   GACATCCAGATGAACCAGTCTCCATCCAGTCTGTCTGCATCCCTCGGAGA
             |||||||||||||||||||||||||||||||||||||||||||||||||
WN1-58-LC    GACATCCAGATGAACCAGTCTCCATCCAGTCTGTCTGCATCCCTCGGAGA


                                                 CDRI
             T   I   S   I   T   C   R   A   S   Q   N   I   N   I   W   L
WN1-222-LC   CACAATTTCCATCACTTGC CGTGCCAGTCAGAACATTAATATT TGGTTAA
             ||||||| ||||||||||| ||||||||| | |||||||||||||| |||||||
WN1-58-LC    CACAATTACCATCACTTGC CGTGCCAGACTGAACATTAATATT TGGTTAA
                                      R   L


             S   W   Y   Q   Q   K   P   G   N   V   P   K   L   L   I   Y   K
WN1-222-LC   GCTGGTATCAGCAAAAACCAGGAAATGTTCCTAAACTTTTAATCTAT AAG
             | ||||| |||||| ||| ||||||||| |||||||||||||| ||||| | |||
WN1-58-LC    GTTGGTACCAGCAGAAAGCAGGAAATATTCCTAAACTTTTGATCTCT AAG
                           A           I                         S

                 CDRII
             A   S   N   L   H   T   G   V   P   S   R   F   S   G   S   G   S
WN1-222-LC   GCTTCCAACTTGCACACA GGCGTCCCATCAAGGTTTAGTGGCAGTGGATC
             |||||||||||||||||| ||||||||||||||||||||||||||||||||||
WN1-58-LC    GCTTCCAACTTGCACACA GGCGTCCCATCAAGGTTTAGTGGCAGTGGATC


             G   T   D   F   T   L   I   I   S   S   L   Q   P   E   D   I
WN1-222-LC   TGGAACAGATTTCACATTAATCATCAGCAGTCTGCAGCCTGAAGACATTG
             |||||||||||||||||||| |||||||||||||| ||||||||||||||
WN1-58-LC    TGGAACAGATTTCACATTAACCATCAGCAGTCTGCGGCCTGAAGACATTG
                                T                 R
                                       CDRIII
             A   T   Y   Y   C   L   Q   G   Q   S   Y   P   R   T   F   G   G
WN1-222-LC   CCACTTACTACTGT CTACAGGGTCAAAGTTATCCTCGTACG TTCGGTGGA
             |||||||||||||| ||||||||||||||||||||||||||| |||||||||
WN1-58-LC    CCACTTACTACTGT CTACAGGGTCAAAGTTATCCTCGTACG TTCGGTGGA


             G   T   K   L   E   I   K
WN1-222-LC   GGCACCAAGCTGGAGATCAAA
             ||||||||||| || ||||||
WN1-58-LC    GGCACCAAGCTTGAAATCAAA
```

Figure 3 Comparison of the V_L regions of the anti-LPS MAb WN1 222-5 and WN1 58-9. The complementary determining regions (CDR) are printed in bold, and amino acid changes in WN1 58-9 are indicated beneath the DNA sequence.

E. Inhibition of LPS-Induced Mouse Lethality (D-GalN Model)

WN1 222–5 was also tested in D-GalN-sensitized mice against *E. coli* O16 LPS (75 ng/kg, i.v.). A representative experiment is shown in Table 2. WN1 222–5 blocked the lethality induced by *E. coli* O16 (100 ng/kg). Protective activity was completely abolished by heat treatment, again confirming that the MAb preparation was not contaminated with LPS and that protection was not due to an independent phenomenon such as endotoxin tolerance.

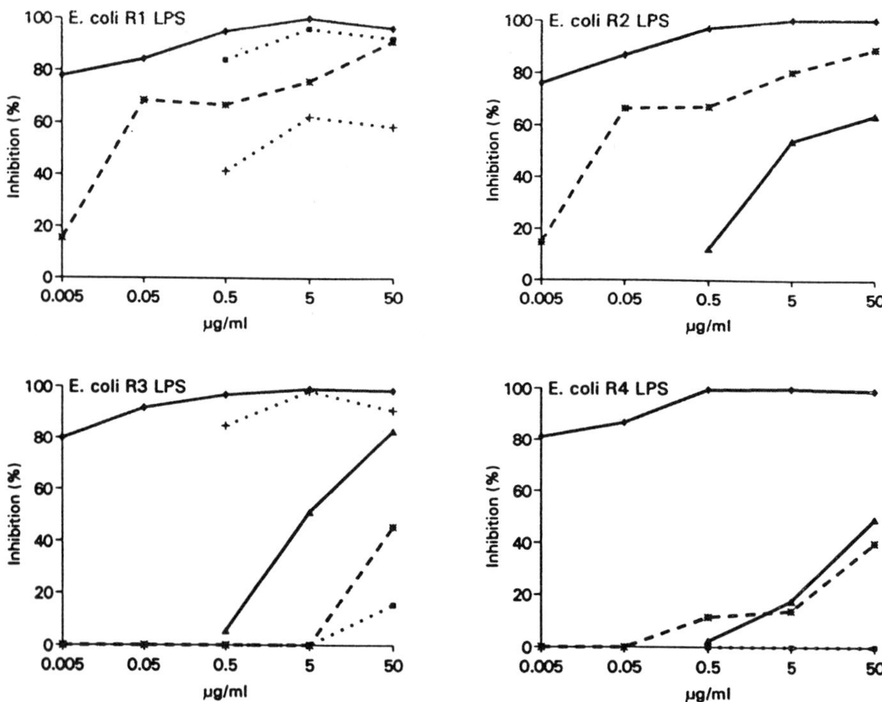

Figure 4 IL-6 secretion by mouse peritoneal cells stimulated with different R-form LPS. *E. coli* R1, R2, R3, and R4 LPS were used at the final concentration of 50 pg/mL. ▲, H1 61-2; *, H5 13-23 ■, H5 415-6; ♦, WN1 222-5; +, WN1 58-9.

Table 2 Neutralizing Activity of WN1 222-5 Against LPS Lethality in D-GalN-Sensitized Mice

WN1 222-5 dose (mg/kg)[a]	No. of survivors/no. of treated animals after administration of *E. coli* O16 LPS (75 ng/kg)
50	7/8
25	8/8
12.5	8/8
6.25	7/8
3.12	8/8
1.56	7/8
Control	0/8

[a]WN1 222-5 was administered i.v. 2 h prior to i.v. administration of LPS and i.p. administration of D-GalN (800 mg/kg).

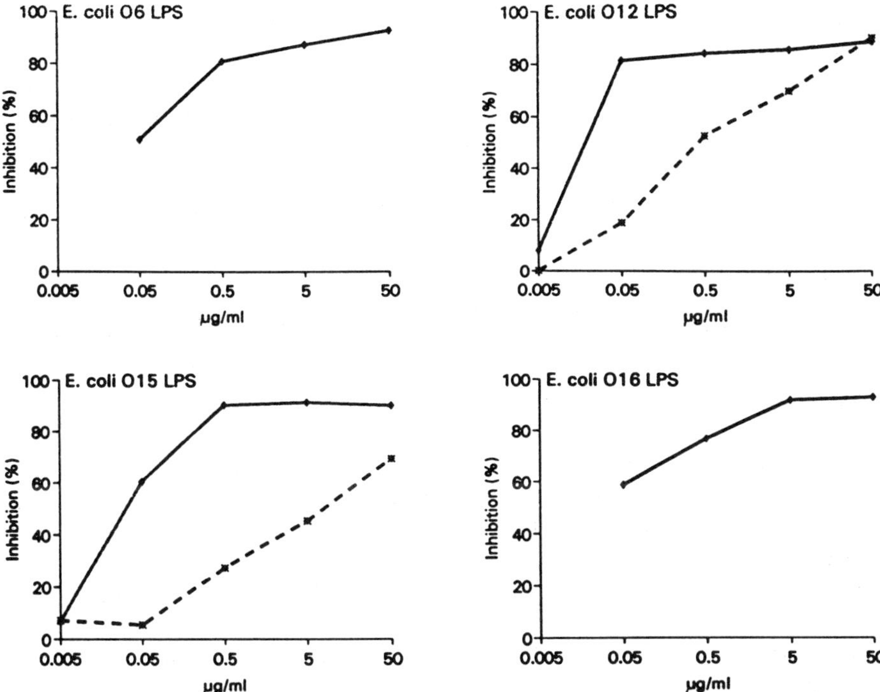

Figure 5 IL-6 secretion by mouse peritoneal cells stimulated with different S-form LPS. *E. coli* O6, O12, and O16 LPS were used at the final concentration of 0.5 ng/mL. *E. coli* O15 LPS was used at 5 ng/mL. ▲, H1 61-2; *, H5 13-23; ■, H5 415-6; ◆, WN1 222-5; +, WN1 58-9.

IV. DISCUSSION

In this study we show that cross-reactive and cross-neutralizing MAb can be obtained in different strains of mice and after different immunization protocols. In our experience, crossreactive Ab are generated only after immunization with rough *E. coli* strains carrying the complete core LPS. Immunization of mice and humans with *E. coli* J5 does not stimulate the development of broadly cross-reactive and cross-protective MAb (17, 31–38). These Ab are specific for the terminal sugars in the core LPS structure of *E. coli* J5, and cross-reactivity is limited or absent. On the contrary, after immunization with rough *E. coli* strains with a complete core region, in addition to Ab recognizing the terminal sugars, several cross-reactive Ab are detected. To optimize the selection of widely cross-reactive Ab, we have used several approaches, including the concomitant use of *E. coli* strains with different core types and boosting with different combinations of bacteria.

As shown in this study, the minimal core structure recognized by the cross-reactive Ab is actually present in *E. coli* J5 which contains the most conserved inner core structure. It is tempting to speculate that the MAb we have selected recognize an epitope located on the lateral side of the LPS molecule. This suggestion is confirmed by DOC-PAGE electrophoresis, which clearly shows that the Ab recognize epitopes which are not covered by the subsequent addition of the O-specific chain.

As suggested by ELISA data, the Ab isolated from different mice seem to recognize different epitopes. On the other hand, the specificity of the Ab selected in the same fusion appear more similar even if the MAb have different isotypes. This observation was confirmed experimentally for WN1 222–5 and WN1 58–9 by analysis of the V_H and V_L regions. The similarities in the sequences of these two Ab indicate that they probably originated from a single cell which through several cycles of division has produced switch variants and point mutations.

These cross-reactive Ab retain the ability to inhibit LPS induced effects. Because all the murine isotypes are represented among these MAb, it is evident that the biological effects are not related to a particular isotype. Moreover, as these Ab do not recognize lipid A, a direct blockade of the toxic moiety of the LPS molecule is not evident. The inhibitory effect could be explained, however, by some form of steric hindrance, disaggregation of supramolecular LPS structure, or a modification of the conformation of the LPS molecule after binding.

In addition, we have reconfirmed previous experiments in which WN1 222–5 was able to vivo to block lethality in galactosamine-sensitized mice (21). The higher neutralizing activity of WN1 222–5 observed in this experiment is probably related to the lower dose of LPS used and to different experimental conditions.

In conclusion, our study demonstrates that different types of cross-reactive and cross-protective Ab against the core region of LPS can be obtained. It is now feasible to evaluate whether this class of widely cross-reactive Ab might be of benefit in blocking the adverse reactions to LPS in patients with endotoxemia and septic shock.

REFERENCES

1. Chamberland S, L'Ecuyer J, Lessard C, et al. Antibiotic susceptibility profiles of 941 gram-negative bacteria isolated from septicemic patients throughout Canada. Clin Infect Dis 1992; 15:615–628.
2. Kreger BE, Craven DE, Carling PC, McCabe WM. Gram-negative bacteremia. III Reassessment of etiology, epidemiology and ecology in 612 patients. Am J Med 1980; 68:332–343.

3. Weinstein MP, Reller LB, Murphy JR, Lichtenstein KA. The clinical significance of positive blood cultures: a comprehensive analysis of 500 episodes of bacteremia and fungemia in adults. I. Laboratory and epidemiologic observation. Rev Infect Dis 1983; 5:35–53.

4. Ziegler EJ, Fischer CJ, Sprung CL, et al. Treatment of gram-negative bacteremia and septic shock with HA-1A human monoclonal antibody against endotoxin. A randomized, double-blind, placebo-controlled trial. N Engl J Med 1991; 324:429–436.

5. Rietschel ETh, Seydel U, Zahringer U, et al. Bacterial endotoxin: molecular relationships between structure and activity. Infect Dis Clin North Am 1991; 5:753–779.

6. Jansson PE, Lindberg AA, Lindberg B, Wollin R. Structural studies on the hexose region of the core in lipopolysaccharides from *Enterobacteriaceae*. Eur J Biochem 1981; 115:571–577.

7. Holst O, Brade H. Chemical structure of the core region of lipopolysaccharides. In: Morrison DC, Ryan JL, eds. Bacterial Endotoxic Lipopolysaccharides. Vol. I. Molecular Biochemistry and Cellular Biology. Boca Raton, FL: CRC Press, 1992:135–170.

8. Schellekens J, Benne CA, De Zeeuw GR, Rozenberg-Arska M, Verhoef J. Natural occurring IgG and IgM antibodies to gram-negative bacteria and lipopolysaccharides in human sera. Serodiag Immunother 1988; 2:433–444.

9. Law BJ, Marks MI. Age-related prevalence of human serum IgG and IgM antibody to the core glycolipid of *Escherichia coli* strain J5, as measured by ELISA. J Infect Dis 1985; 151:988–994.

10. Stoll BJ, Pollack M, Hooper JA. Antibodies to endotoxin core determinants in normal subjects and in immune globulins for intravenous use. Serodiag Immunother 1987; 1:21–31.

11. Mattsby-Baltzer I, Claesson I, Hanson LA, et al. Antibodies to lipid A during urinary tract infection. J Infect Dis 1981; 144:319–328.

12. The Intravenous Immunoglobulin Collaborative Study Group. Prophylactic intravenous administration of standard immune globulin as compared with core-lipopolysaccharide immune globulin in patients at high risk of postsurgical infection. N Engl J Med 1992; 327:234–240.

13. Baumgartner JD, Glauser MP. Controversies in the use of passive immunotherapy for bacterial infections in the critically ill patient. Rev Infect Dis 1987; 9:194–205.

14. Ziegler EJ, McCutchan JA, Fierer J, et al. Treatment of gram-negative bacteremia and shock with human antiserum to a mutant *Escherichia coli*. N Engl J Med 1982; 307:1225–1230.

15. Baumgartner JD, Glauser MP, McCutchan JA, et al. Prevention of gram-negative shock and death in surgical patients by antibody to endotoxin core glycolipid. Lancet 1985; 2:59–63.

16. Calandra T, Glauser MP, Schellekens J, Verhoef J, the Swiss-Dutch J5 Immunoglobulin Study Group. Treatment of gram-negative septic shock with human IgG antibody to *Escherichia coli* J5: a prospective, double blind, randomized trial. J Infect Dis 1988; 158:312–319.

17. Baumgartner JD, Heumann D, Calandra T, Glauser MP. Antibodies to lipopolysaccharides after immunization of humans with the rough mutant *Escherichia coli* J5. J Infect Dis 1991; 163:769–772.

18. Greenman RL, Schein RMH, Martin MA, et al. A controlled clinical trial of E5 murine monoclonal IgM antibody to endotoxin in the treatment of gram-negative sepsis. JAMA 1991; 266:1097–1102.

19. Wenzel RP, Andriole VT, Bartlett JG, et al. Antiendotoxin monoclonal antibodies for gram-negative sepsis: guidelines from IDSA. Clin Infect Dis 1992; 14:973–976.

20. Baumgartner JD, Heumann D, Gerain J, Weinbreck P, Grau GE, Glauser MP. Association between protective efficacy of anti-liopopolysaccharide (LPS) antibodies and suppression of LPS-induced tumor necrosis factor α and interleukin 6. Comparison of O side chain-specific antibodies with core LPS antibodies. J Exp Med 1990; 171:889–896.

21. Di Padova FE, Brade H, Barclay GR, et al. A broadly cross-protective monoclonal antibody binding to *Escherichia coli* and *Salmonella* lipopolysaccharides. Infect Immun 1993; 61:3863–3872.

22. Galanos C, Luderitz O, Westphal O. A new method for the extraction of R lipopolysaccharides. Eur J Biochem 1969; 9:245–249.

23. Westphal O, Jann K. Bacterial lipopolysaccharides: extraction with phenol-water and further application of the procedures. Meth Carbohydr Chem 1965; 5:83–91.

24. Fazekas de St. Groth S, Scheidegger D. Production of monoclonal antibodies: strategy and tactics. J Immunol Meth 1980; 35:1–21.

25. Stahli C, Staehlin T, Miggiano V, Schmidt J, Haring P. High frequencies of antigen-specific hybridomas: dependence on immunization parameters and prediction by spleen cell analysis. J Immunol Meth 1980; 32:297–304.

26. Komuro T, Yomota C, Isaka H. Sodium deoxycholate-polyacrylamide gel electrophoresis of lipopolysaccharides at low temperature. Chem Pharm Bull 1988; 36:1218–1222.

27. Tsai C, Frash CE. A sensitive silver stain for detecting lipopolysaccharides in polyacrylamide gels. Anal Biochem 1982; 119:115–119.

28. Chomczynski P, Sacchi N. Single-step method of RNA isolation by acid guanidinium thiocyanate-phenol-chloroform extraction. Anal Biochem 1987; 162:156–159.

29. Sanger F, Nicklen S, Coulson AR. DNA sequencing with chain-termination inhibitors. Proc Natl Acad Sci USA 1977; 74:5463–5467.

30. Galanos C, Freudenberg MA, Reutter W. Galactosamine-induced sensitization to the lethal effects of endotoxin. Proc Natl Acad Sci USA 1979; 76:5939–5943.

31. Appelmelk BJ, Verweji-Van Vught AM, Maaskant JJ, et al. Production and characterization of mouse monoclonal antibodies reacting with the lipopolysaccharide core region of gram-negative bacilli. J Med Microbiol 1988; 26:107–114.

32. Aydintung MK, Inzana TJ, Letonja T, Davis WC, Corbeil LB. Cross-reactivity of monoclonal antibodies to *Escherichia coli* J5 with heterologous gram-negative bacteria and extracted lipopolysaccharides. J Infect Dis 1989; 160:846–857.

33. Gigliotti F, Shenep JL. Failure of monoclonal antibodies to core glycolipid to bind to intact smooth strains of *Escherichia coli*. J Infect Dis 1985; 151:1005–1011.

34. Miner KM, Manyak CL, Williams E, et al. Characterization of murine monoclonal antibodies to *Escherichia coli* J5. Infect Immun 1986; 52:56–62.
35. Mutharia LM, Crockford G, Bogard WC, Hancock REW. Monoclonal antibodies specific for *Escherichia coli* J5 lipopolysaccharides: cross-reaction with gram-negative bacterial species. Infect Immun 1984: 45:631–636.
36. Nelles MJ, Niswander CA. Mouse monoclonal antibodies reactive with J5 lipopolysaccharide exibit extensive serological cross-reactivity with a variety of gram-negative bacteria. Infect Immun 1984; 46:677–681.
37. Pollack M, Chia JKS, Koles NL, Miller M, Guelde G. Specificity and cross-reactivity of monoclonal antibodies reactive with the core and lipid A regions of bacterial lipopolysaccharides. J Infect Dis 1989; 159:168–188.
38. Salles MF, Mandine E, Zalisz R, Guenounou M, Smets P. Protective effects of murine monoclonal antibodies in experimental septicemia: *E. coli* antibodies protect against different serotypes of *E. coli*. J Infect Dis 1989; 159:641–647.

3

The Use of Bactericidal/Permeability-Increasing Protein and Related Proteins as Potential Therapeutic Agents for the Treatment of Endotoxin-Related Disorders

Marian N. Marra, Randal W. Scott, and Jeffrey J. Seilhamer
Incyte Pharmaceuticals
Palo Alto, California

Steven M. Opal
Brown University School of Medicine
Providence, Rhode Island

I. INTRODUCTION

Bactericidal/permeability increasing protein (BPI) was first discovered by Peter Elsbach and Jerrold Weiss, who identified its unique antibacterial activity, to specifically kill and permeabilize gram-negative bacteria. BPI was purified from human PMN 1978 (1), and was originally isolated from rabbit neutrophils (2). The protein was also isolated at about the same time by John Spitznagel, who named the protein CAP 57, for cationic antibacterial protein of 57,000 m.w. (3). Several papers followed which better characterized the antibiotic properties of BPI, and showed that its specificity for gram-negative bacteria resulted from an avid binding of the protein to a major constituent of the gram-negative bacterial cell wall, bacterial lipopolysaccharide, (LPS) (4–8). The cDNA for BPI was cloned by Gray et al. at Genentech, who reported the full-length sequence in 1989 (9). Our group began working on BPI in 1987, as a result of a collaboration with Carl Nathan's group at Cornell University. These studies were designed to isolate and characterize novel antimicrobial proteins from human neutrophil granules (10). To this end we took a novel approach. Instead of isolating proteins based on their biological activity, our group first isolated azurophil granules, extracted them in weak acid (20 mM glycine, pH 2.0), and ran the extracts over microbore reverse-phase HPLC (RPHPLC). Although this chromatographic method utilizes harsh conditions which are not optimal for recovering maximum biologic activity, this method is highly effective for segregating proteins. The resulting profile from our neutrophil granule extract (shown in Fig. 1), resolved nine discrete peaks, each of which in most cases contained a single protein or, as in the case of the defensins, a family of closely related proteins. These peaks were then subjected directly to N-terminal protein sequencing. Each peak was identified by comparing its N-terminal sequence with known protein sequences. Although the neutrophil had been a well-studied system, we identified several novel proteins, including what was later termed bactericidal/permeability protein (peak 9), azurocidin (peak 6), proteinase 3 (peak 7), as well as a novel member of the defensin family, HNP-4 (peak 2). Each of these was discovered solely based on sequence homology with known proteins. We later termed this process "database discovery," and have continued to develop this method to identify novel proteins and, more recently, genes.

It was not until Ooi published the N-terminal sequence of BPI in 1987 (11) that we were able to correlate our novel peak 9 sequence to that for BPI. Several observations we made about BPI, and its unique physical and biological

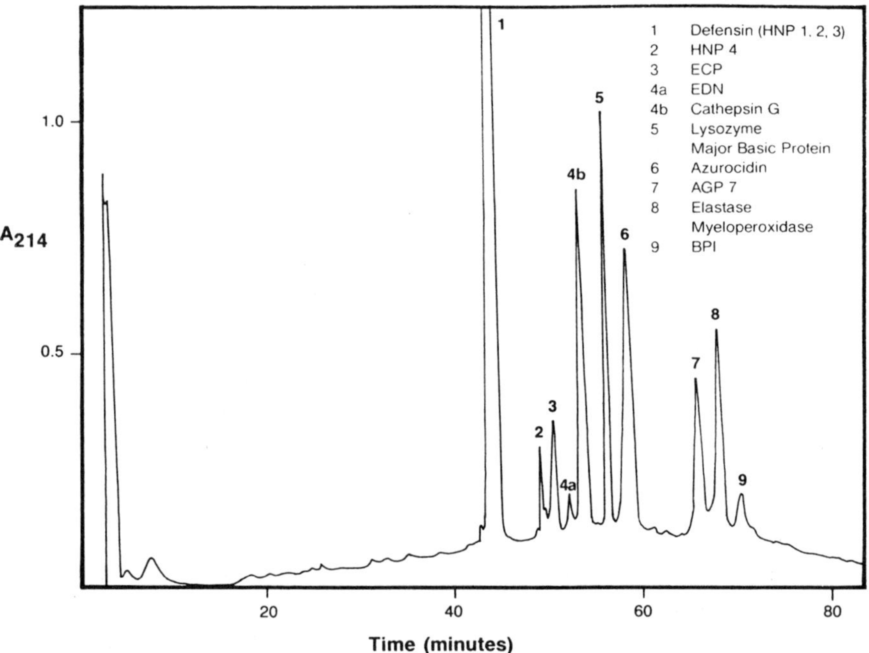

Figure 1 Reverse-phase chromatography of human neutrophil granule extract. Acid extracts of pooled human azurophil granules were prepared and subjected to reverse-phase chromatography as described in (10).

properties contributed to our curiosity about whether bactericidal activity was its sole biological function. First, BPI was the only one of the neutrophil "arsenal" of cationic antimicrobial proteins with potent activity strictly against gram-negative bacteria. Also, it was the only protein which retained its in-vitro bactericidal activity under physiological ionic strength and pH. This contrasted activity of other granule constituents which could only kill microorganisms in hypotonic buffers. Next, BPI is highly soluble in physiological saline without the necessity for detergents, and was easily extracted from whole PMN or isolated granules, suggesting that BPI is not tightly associated with the neutrophil granule membrane, and that it might be released into aqueous solutions when cells lyse or degranulate. Still, although BPI was the only granule protein with antimicrobial activity in physiological pH and salt, antibiotic activity was not comparable to classical antibiotics. When Richard Ulevitch and Peter Tobias at Scripps Institute published their observation of the strong sequence similarity between BPI and lipopolysaccharide-binding protein (LBP) (12), a soluble endotoxin-binding and regulatory protein, it occurred to us that the above-described properties of BPI were also consistent with those of an endotoxin-binding and regulatory molecule, and that perhaps the interaction between BPI and LPS was important for purposes other than bactericidal specificity. In subsequent experiments we were able to show that BPI has potent endotoxin-neutralizing activity in vitro, using inhibition of LPS-mediated neutrophil surface CR upregulation, macrophage cytokine release, and limulus amebocyte lysate assay (LAL) activity as example readout systems (13,14). Subsequent data from our laboratory, along with data from other investigators, have shown that BPI neutralizes LPS-mediated activity in every biological system tested (see below) with a mechanism similar to that of polymyxin B, i.e., by binding to and neutralizing the lipid A moiety of LPS (15,16).

In the following pages we will discuss our experience with human recombinant BPI as a natural LPS antagonist, and explain in detail properties of BPI which are both desirable and deleterious to its use as a therapeutic modality against endotoxin-mediated disease processes in mammalian systems. We will further describe results from testing recombinant BPI along with genetically engineered variants consisting of BPI-LBP fusion proteins which we feel represent promising longer-half-life therapeutics against systemic endotoxin toxicity in humans and animals.

II. ROLE OF ENDOGENOUS BPI IN VIVO

A. Antibiotic Versus Antiendotoxin

As its name suggests, BPI was first described as a potent bactericidal protein—along with other neutrophil granule proteins, a component of the "first line of host defense" against invading microorganisms. Soluble BPI has microbicidal activity in physiological salt and pH, and shows specificity for gram-negative organisms. This specificity results from the high-affinity interaction between BPI and bacterial lipopolysaccharide (LPS), a structural component of the outer bacterial membrane (5–8,15). BPI binds to the bacterial surface and disrupts the integrity of the outer membrane, causing increased permeability to small molecules such as actinomycin D. The N-terminal fragment (BPI-23kDa) is a more potent bactericidal agent than native BPI against smooth bacterial strains (17,18) (see below). BPI and the N-terminal fragment have been shown to kill serum-resistant gram-negative bacteria in human whole blood (19); however, neither protein is as effective as classical antibiotics. We tested the in-vivo antibiotic activity of BPI in vitro in dilution (colony count) assays as well as the more standard MIC assays, and in vivo using lethal live bacterial challenge with a variety of virulent, clinically relevant bacterial strains. While BPI showed potent activity in vitro in a dilution assay for bacterial viability, it had very limited activity in standard MIC assays for antibiotic activity against a panel of bacteria (20). Further, our results showed that, at doses where BPI is highly effective against lethal challenge in mice with isolated LPS, or a lethal dose of live bacteria along with a separate injection of antibiotic (21), we see little protection against live bacterial challenge in models where large numbers of bacteria are delivered intravenously without a coadministered antibiotic (unpublished result). Further experiments were designed to address the possibility that BPI may not have potent in-vivo antibiotic activity by itself, but perhaps synergy occurs if BPI is administered along with classical antibiotics. To test this idea, CD-1 mice were challenged with a serum-resistant, rodent-virulent strain of *K. pneumoniae*, with or without intravenously administered gentamicin. Results showed (21) that animals treated with BPI alone showed no decrease in circulating colony counts relative to saline-treated control animals. Gentamicin treatment alone had marked effects on circulating colony counts, and no further decrease in circulating bacteria was observed in BPI + gentamicin treatment. Thus, in our hands, soluble recombinant BPI is not a very effective antibiotic in vivo.

B. Role of BPI and LBP in Regulating LPS in Vivo

Like other constituents of the azurophil granule, BPI is a cationic antimicrobial protein which is released when neutrophils are stimulated to degranulate (14). Unlike these other granular constituents, BPI shows specificity for gram-negative bacteria, and shares striking homology to another LPS-binding protein, LBP (12,22,23). This homology suggests that BPI, like LBP, is part of the mechanism by which the human host regulates its response to bacterial endotoxin (22,24,25). Structure–functional relationships between BPI and LBP are contrasted in Table 1.

Table 1 Structure–Function Comparison of BPI and LBP

	BPI	LBP
Structure		
Full-length sequence	456 aa	456 aa
Molecular weight	~55 kDa	~60 kDa
Predicted pI	10.6	6.8
Glycosylation sites	2	5
Site of synthesis	Neutrophils	Liver
Effect on LPS		
CD14 binding	Blocks	Catalyzes
Neutrophil activation	Neutralizes	Facilitates
Macrophage activation	Neutralizes	Facilitates
Endothelial cell activation	Neutralizes	Facilitates
Complement activation	Neutralizes	Facilitates
Extrinsic coagulation pathway	Neutralizes	Facilitates
Circulating conc. (normal)	0–10 ng/mL	5–10 μg/mL
Circulating conc. (sepsis)	10–100 ng/mL	10–100 μg/mL
Clearance rate (mice)	13.0 mL/min	0.042 mL/min

Because humans are colonized with commensal enteric bacterial flora, it is easy to imagine the necessity for a physical barrier to entry, namely, the gut wall. However, if this primary defense is breached, the body develops a secondary defense mechanism which uses LPS as a signal. In the presence of LPS, a rapid and vigorous inflammatory response is triggered. Stimulation of cells such as neutrophils and macrophages, along with subsequent release of cytokines and products of complement activation, results in killing and clearance of the invading microorganisms, sometimes at the expense of surrounding "innocent bystander" tissue, before the bacteria can multiply and create a real threat to the host (26,27). In-vitro models of some of these in LPS-mediated in-vivo events can be regulated by BPI and LBP (12,22–25,28–30). The role of LBP is to facilitate the responses of macrophages, neutrophils, and endothelial cells to LPS. In the presence of small amounts of LBP (nanogram-per-milliliter concentrations), cells become more sensitive in vitro to low concentrations of LPS. LBP is thought to act catalytically as a transfer protein to hasten the binding of LPS to the cell surface protein CD14 (31). BPI, on the other hand, blocks access of cells to LPS by binding to LPS with high affinity and preventing LBP-LPS interactions. When inflammatory cells such as neutrophils and macrophages are stimulated with LPS, neutrophils release BPI and prevent further stimulation of macrophages with LBP-LPS. This negative-feedback loop is illustrated in Fig. 2. [adapted from (14)]. How and where this LPS regulation

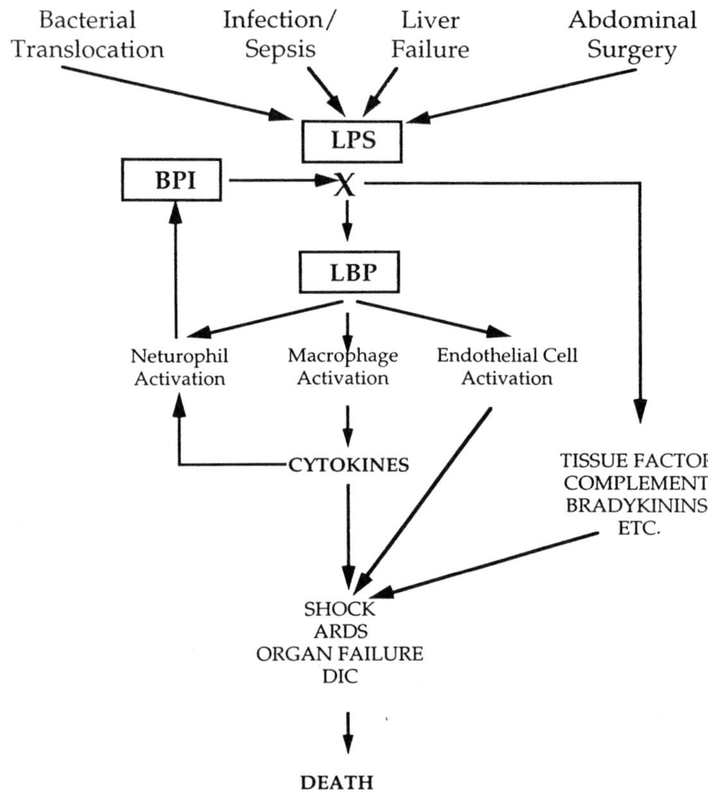

Figure 2   Regulation of the host response to bacterial lipopolysaccharide (LPS) by bactericidal permeability-increasing protein (BPI) and lipopolysaccharide-binding protein (LBP). (Adapted from Ref. 14.)

occurs in vivo is important to understand if we want to optimize our ability to administer exogenous BPI as a therapeutic against endotoxin related disorders in vivo.

We and others have shown that BPI is localized in a specific subset of the primary, or azurophilic granules of mature human neutrophils (32,33). No evidence has been reported for the presence of BPI in any cell type other than neutrophil precursors. A sensitive immunoflourescence assay using an anti-BPI (CAP57) monoclonal antibody was negative with other hematopoeitic cell types (33). BPI is produced during the promyelocyte stage of differentiation and stored in the granule until it is released during degranulation or cellular lysis. Immunofluroescence studies cited above showed that promyelocytes do indeed stain strongly for BPI, and that at this stage of maturity, BPI is present at much higher concentrations than lactoferrin, a specific granule constituent.

It has been suggested that BPI is a membrane-associated protein, or that the carboxyl-terminal domain of the molecule confers membrane-associative properties (9,11,17,34,35). Although some regions of the carboxy-terminal domain of BPI contain hydrophobic amino acids, our experience instructs that BPI may be only loosely associated with azurophil granule membrane, if at all. BPI can be extracted from isolated neutrophil granules in the absence of detergent, and the full-length 55-kDa BPI is stable in physiological saline and pH. Interestingly, full-length BPI is more stable in solution than the N-terminal domain (BPI23kD) and has less tendency to aggregate. The moderately hydrophobic stretches in the carboxy-terminal half do not prevent solubility in water or cause aggregation or micelle formation, which is observed with proteins containing true membrane-spanning domains.

If the above model is correct, and the physiological role of BPI is to compete with LBP for LPS in vivo, then neutrophils must release soluble BPI into physiological fluids in response to stimuli normally encountered in vivo, such as LPS or other bacterial cell wall components. Results from our early work showed that full-length soluble BPI could be detected in the supernatants of isolated neutrophils stimulated with fMLP and cytochalasin B (14). This rather harsh treatment resulted in release of approximately 60% of the total cellular BPI. In later studies, we performed similar experiments using a very sensitive ELISA assay, and measured BPI release in whole blood ex-vivo incubated at 37°C with LPS alone. Results from these experiments (Fig. 3) show that soluble BPI is released in whole blood under these conditions, and that BPI is released in response to lower concentrations of LPS than TNF, and with faster kinetics.

In normal individuals, soluble BPI circulates at very low concentrations, if at all. Initially, our measurements showed BPI present in normal human plasma in amounts up to 20 ng/mL. Subsequent studies have showed that in-vitro neutrophil degranulation occurs under conditions where blood samples are allowed to clot prior to serum collection, and also if anticoagulated samples are collected in tubes contaminated with endotoxin, or are not immediately placed on ice after collection. Optimal conditions for collecting samples for BPI determination are collection in EDTA anticoagulant and immediate chilling the sample prior to centrifugation and plasma separation. An additional high-speed centrifugation of separated plasma further reduces potential neutrophil contamination (unpublished observation).

Under certain physiological conditions, however, it can be demonstrated that circulating BPI levels are elevated. Shindler et al. have shown that dialysis membranes known to stimulate neutrophil degranulation cause release of BPI,

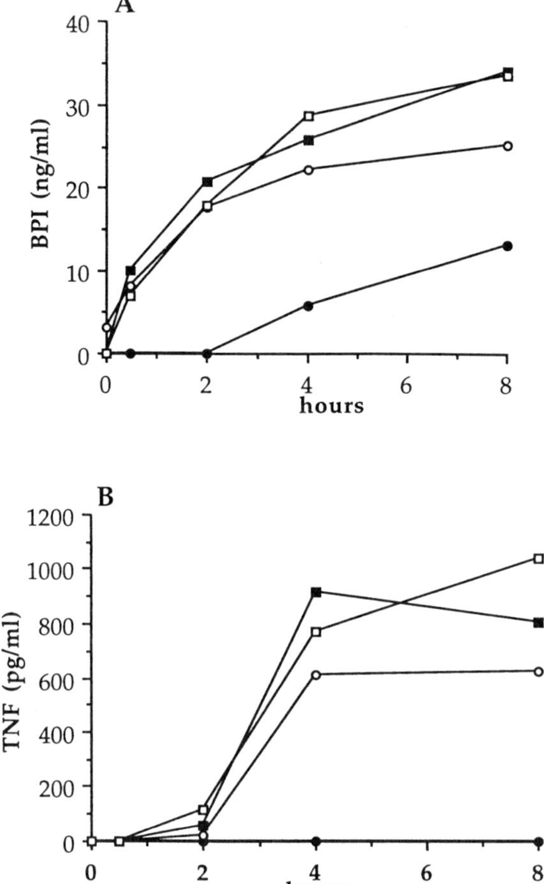

Figure 3   Kinetics of LPS-mediated BPI and TNF release in human whole blood ex vivo. Triplicate 1-mL aliquots of heparinized human whole blood were incubated on a rocking platform in the presence of increasing amounts of *E. coli* O111:B4 LPS. Plasma was collected at the indicated times, and assayed for BPI and TNF by ELISA. Data is from a representative experiment. Filled circles, 0 LPS; open circles 10 pg LPS; filled squares, 100 pg LPS; open squares, 1 ng LPS.

as well as other granule constituents such as elastase, into the dialysate (36). Preliminary studies by Van Deventer (37), in which plasma samples were very carefully collected under endotoxin-free conditions, suggested that BPI levels correlated with survival in sepsis patients. We have also measured BPI in the plasma of a normal volunteers given a low experimental dose of bacterial LPS. In these individuals, soluble circulating BPI levels are increased, and increased amounts of BPI can be detected on the surface of circulating neutrophils (38). These results are consistent with other data which demonstrated that neutrophils stimulated in vitro with LPS, fMLP, or TNF also express elevated surface BPI (14,39). It is not known whether the elevated surface expression of BPI results from soluble released protein being taken up by a putative BPI receptor on the neutrophil cell surface, whether surface expression represents transient cell association prior to release, or true relocalization of BPI to the cell surface where it functions as an LPS-binding and neutralizing protein.

Under conditions where soluble BPI levels are increased, such as in septic patients or LPS-treated volunteers, amounts rarely reach the 100-ng/mL level. The low detectable amounts of BPI may be a consequence of the very rapid clearance of BPI from the circulation. BPI that is released by cells in the vascular compartment may be too transient to be measured reliably. This hypothesis is consistent with the very sporadic peaks and valleys of BPI expression in normal volunteers injected with endotoxin (38). Although, in general BPI levels are elevated following endotoxin challenge, the kinetic profiles vary widely among individuals.

The circulating half-life of recombinant human BPI is remarkably short. In all species tested (including mice, rats, rabbits, and primates), clearance of the protein is so rapid that, following a single bolus injection, circulating BPI levels are reduced by three orders of magnitude after only 30 min. LBP, on the other hand, as a normal plasma protein, is produced constitutively, and circulates at relatively high concentrations. Levels of LBP in normal volunteers are around 5 μg/mL, and in situations where an acute-phase response is elicited, such as sepsis, LBP levels can reach 100 μg/mL. LBP also has a relatively long circulating half-life. Even taking into account that the affinity of BPI for LPS is up to 50- to 100-fold greater than that of LBP (23,40), the vast circulating excess of LBP makes it difficult to postulate that soluble BPI could neutralize LPS in the presence of LBP concentrations which exceed BPI by three orders of magnitude.

The role of endogenous BPI was recently addressed by Opal et al., who examined BPI and LBP levels in extravascular fluids (41). Results from these studies clearly showed that BPI concentrations can and do exceed those of LBP in extravascular fluids. In fluids collected from infected sites, BPI is present in concentrations which would be expected to outcompete LBP for LPS. Examples of BPI and LBP levels from some of these samples are shown in Table 2.

Opal further showed that, as expected, the BPI levels in these fluids correlated

Table 2 BPI and LBP Levels, and BPI/LBP Ratios, in Selected Extravascular Fluid Samples

	μg/mL		BPI/LBP
	BPI	LBP	ratio
Pleural fluid	0.017	4.1	0.004
Synovial aspirate (joint effusion)	0.530	13.1	0.04
Synovial aspirate (septic joint)	8.70	4.6	1.9
Intraabdominal abcess	9.2	4.5	2.0
Pancreatic abcess	2.30	0.07	33.3

Extravascular fluid samples were obtained from the operating room or invasive radiology department in a university-affiliated hospital. Specimens were centrifuged at 4°, the supernatants filtered through a 0.45-μm filter, then frozen at $-70°$ for subsequent analysis. Thawed samples were refiltered immediately before assay. BPI and LBP levels were determined by ELISA.

with the degree of neutrophilic infiltration at the site [$r_s = 0.81$, $p < 0.0001$ (41)]. We can conclude from these studies that, in vivo, BPI probably does not function as a soluble endotoxin-neutralizing protein in the systemic circulation, but rather, BPI is carried by neutrophils to sites of infection or inflammation, where it is released when the cells degranulate or lyse. BPI may function at these sites to prevent release of LPS into the circulation.

We were also interested in determining what form of BPI was present in extravascular biological fluids. When the structure of full-length BPI was determined by Gray et al., certain features of the molecule were revealed. First, the majority of the positive-charged amino acid residues were found in the N-terminal half of the molecule, while the carboxyl-terminal half of the molecule contained stretches of the hydrophobic residues. Ooi et al. had also showed that all of the bactericidal activity of BPI could be recovered from preparations of the N-terminal half of the molecule (11) (see below). Taken together, Gray et al. postulated that perhaps native full-length BPI was anchored by the hydrophobic C-terminal domain to the azurophil granule membrane (9). When the neutrophil engulfed a gram-negative organism, the azurophil granule would fuse with the phagosome. During this process, neutrophil granule proteases such as elastase would become active, and the BPI molecule would be cleaved in half, releasing the antimicrobial N-terminal fragment into the granule lumen, where it would kill the engulfed gram-negative organism contained within. Our previous work indicated that BPI released into the supernatants of isolated human peripheral blood neutrophils in response to stimuli such as LPS, TNF, or fMLP was present only in the 55,000-m.w. form (14). More recently, we subjected pools of extravascular fluids which contained the highest concentrations of BPI from the above study to Western blotting to determine the size of the soluble, extracellular BPI.

Although there was evidence of in-vivo degradation BPI in these samples, we found no evidence for BPI23kD in these blots (42).

The puzzling question of the in-vivo role of LBP still remains. LBP is highly active as an LPS-facilitating molecule in vitro at concentrations of 10 ng/mL. Why, then, does this protein circulate at such high concentrations in normal plasma? Perhaps LBP has another biological role other than regulating LPS, or perhaps nature designed the system so that LBP is never limiting.

III. RECOMBINANT BPI AS A THERAPEUTIC PROTEIN

A. Preclinical Overview

Our studies and others have shown that BPI is a highly effective endotoxin-neutralizing agent in a wide variety of animal model systems. We have tested the effects of BPI on endotoxin challenge using a several different endotoxin chemotypes both in vivo and in vitro, and have found that BPI is effective against all LPS chemotypes tested, including smooth and rough forms. Table 3 shows examples of our preclinical results using recombinant human BPI in some of these animal models.

Table 3 BPI Preclinical Studies

Model	BPI dose	Result	Reference
1. Murine endotoxin challenge (LD_{100} @ 50 mg/kg)	10 mg/kg, i.v.	100% survival	43, 44
2. Murine live bacterial challenge + gentamicin (LD_{100} @ 10^8 organisms)	10 mg/kg, i.v.	80% survival	21
3. Rat endotoxin challenge (LD_{90} @ 7.5 mg/kg)	10 mg/kg, i.v.	80% survival	45
4. *Pseudomonas* sepsis in neutropenic rats (LD_{100})	10 mg/kg, i.v.	75% survival	46
5. Rat hemorrhagic shock (LD_{50})	10 mg/kg	80% survival	47
6. Rabbit dermal Shwartzman	10 mg/kg	Reduced dermal necrosis	21
7. Rabbit endotoxin-induced pyresis	10 mg/kg	Decreased fever response	48
8. Rabbit heat-killed bacterial challenge (LD_{66})	~12 mg/kg total (4-h infusion)	100% survival	48
9. Baboon live bacterial challenge ($2 \times x\ 10^{12}$)	~28 mg/kg total (4-h infusion)	Decreased plasma LPS (no effect on mortality)	49

These studies, and experiments by others, have shown that BPI is a highly effective endotoxin-neutralizing agent in vitro and in vivo. BPI blocks in-vivo effects of endotoxin following lethal and sublethal endotoxin challenge in a variety of model systems, including fever, blood pressure changes, and death. In live bacterial challenge studies, BPI has been shown to be highly effective at reducing the levels of circulating endotoxin, and is effective against lethality in some models. The endotoxin-neutralizing effects of BPI are unlike anti-endotoxin monoclonal antibodies tested to date. While very limited animal model data have shown efficacy of antibodies directed against lipid A, BPI is highly effective. Neither the human- or mouse-derived IgM monoclonal anti-lipid A antibodies (HA-1A and E5, respectively) neutralize LPS biological activity in vitro or in vivo (43). Therefore, an effective anti-endotoxin-neutralizing protein has yet to be tested in a clinical setting in situations where naturally occurring endotoxin may play a role in the pathophysiology of disease.

Cytokine release has been intensively studies as the proximal cause of mortality in animal models and human clinical settings. Anti-cytokine therapeutics such as neutralizing anti-TNF monoclonal antibodies have been shown to increase survival in rodent endotoxin challenge as well as other systems. We have studied circulating cytokine, and particularly TNF, levels in animals challenged with endotoxin with and without BPI administration. Interestingly, in both mouse and rat systems, we found that survival can be uncoupled from circulating TNF levels (21). Further, in our studies of longer-half-life BPI variant proteins (see below), our data show that anti-endotoxin protein administered after circulating TNF levels have peaked still has a marked effect on survival. These models utilize huge bolus injections of endotoxin; for example, in the murine endotoxin challenge experiments, 25–50 mg/kg of LPS are required to give an LD_{100} in 72 h. In models such as the galactosamine- or actinomycin-sensitized mouse, very low doses of LPS are required for lethality, most groups have observed that circulating cytokine levels are decreased in the BPI-treated group, and this decrease is correlated with survival. In unsensitized models, however, circulating endotoxin levels vastly exceed what is observed in human septicemia or SIRS. However, in three separate laboratories it has been observed that circulating TNF levels are not reduced in BPI-treated animals, although mortality is reduced dramatically (21,45,48). From these observations we can conclude that TNF may be necessary, but is certainly not sufficient to cause lethality in these animals under these conditions. Serum IL-6 levels can be markedly reduced by BPI treatment (21,45), indicating also that IL-6 increases are not strictly regulated by TNF. The synergy between TNF and LPS may be a very important component of the lethality observed in these animal systems, and may as well play a role in the pathophysiology of human sepsis. Studies are ongoing to determine whether a combination of BPI and anti-TNF therapies act synergistically in animal models of sepsis.

Perhaps the most clinically relevant animal model we used to test BPI in sepsis is the neutropenic rat model of *Pseudomonas* sepsis (50). In this system, Sprague-Dawley rats are rendered neutropenic with cyclophosphamide, and are given the antibiotic cephamandole to reduce normal flora, allowing *Pseudomonas aeruginosa* organisms delivered via an orogastric tube to colonize the alimentary tract. Sepsis develops at approximately day 5. All animals succumb within 9–11 days in this highly lethal model, and the pathophysiology strongly resembles syndromes observed in humans with sepsis, including ARDS and MOF. As in human sepsis syndrome, circulating colony counts are moderate and cycle during the course of the disease, as does endotoxemia. Antibiotics specific for *P. aeruginosa* (ciprofloxacin/ceftazidime) can cure the animals if given prior to day 5, even though opsonophagocytic antibody activity is reduced in these rats. BPI is highly effective in this model in the absence of coadministered antibiotic, but evidence strongly suggests that efficacy of BPI results from its endotoxin-neutralizing activity, not as a remnant of its antibiotic function. First, other compounds without antibiotic activity, such as neutralizing anti-TNF antibodies, as well as J5 antisera, can prevent lethality in this model (51). Further, in BPI-treated animals, LPS levels fall substantially even without decreases in level of bacteremia. In vitro, BPI is not bactericidal against this strain of *pseudomonas*. We have also utilized a BPI protein variant (see below) which has no intrinsic antibiotic activity, but is highly effective at preventing lethality in this model. What is perhaps most interesting in these studies was that even though BPI is given as a single i.v. bolus injection (10 mg/kg) on day 5, and virtually no circulating BPI could be detected even 1 h after injection (see half-life studies below), the protein was still able to exert a marked effect on survival in this chronic model, where animals succumb 4–6 days after the therapeutic protein is administered.

B. Pharmacokinetics and Mechanism of Action

As mentioned above, the circulating half-life of exogenously administered recombinant BPI has been shown to be remarkably short in all animals tested. We have studied BPI pharmacokinetics in mice, rats, rabbits, and nonhuman primates. A typical pharmacokinetic curve for CD-1 mice is shown in Fig. 4, and illustrates the very rapid initial clearance of BPI. Circulating BPI levels drop three orders of magnitude during the first 30 min postinjection. Imposing standard pharmacoketic analysis on a compound cleared as rapidly as BPI presents difficulties, since during the beta (distribution/clearance) phase, which is usually cited as the ''circulating half-life,'' very little circulating material is detectable. Another characteristic of BPI pharmacokinetics is the very large apparent volume of distribution. Coupled with the fact that the circulating half-life of BPI is not extended in larger animals relative to smaller ones, this suggests an extravascular

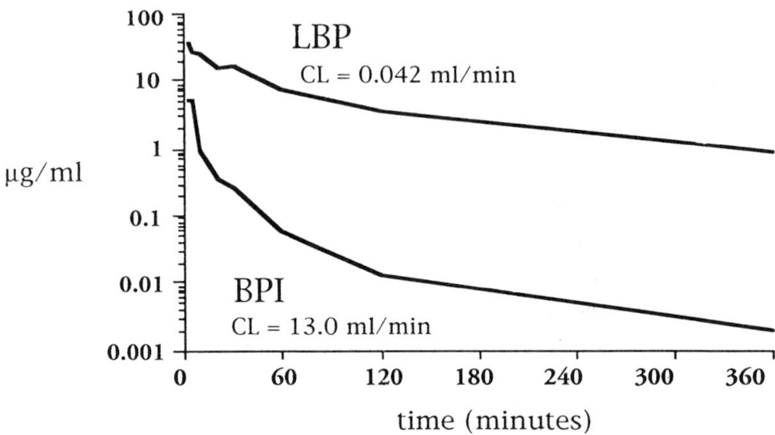

Figure 4 Pharmacokinetics of BPI and LBP. CD-1 mice were given a single bolus injection of 5 mg/kg recombinant protein at time = 0 h. EDTA anticoagulated blood was collected from each of three mice per time point over a 6-h period. Plasma was assayed from each sample separately. Data shown represent mean plasma values for BPI and LBP. Pharmacokinetic analysis was performed using a noncompartmental analysis (PharmK pharmacokinetic software).

binding site for BPI. Disappearance of BPI from the circulation occurs somewhat more rapidly than in-vivo efficacy (see below), further suggesting an extravascular site of action. Radiolabeled BPI clearance studies in rodents indicate that the majority of BPI protein is cleared by the liver (unpublished observation). The liver is the site of clearance and metabolism of LPS. It has thus been suggested that the mechanism of action for BPI is to neutralize LPS in the liver rather than in the circulation.

Therefore, if it is necessary to provide a dose of BPI adequate to maintain high enough circulating levels to compete with LBP for LPS, then effective anti-endotoxin therapy will require very large doses of BPI to be infused over long periods of time. However, if disappearance of BPI from the systemic circulation results from a specific concentration of BPI at its site of action, such as the liver, periodic administration could be effective. To determine the importance of circulating BPI levels in efficacy against lethal endotoxin challenge, BPI was administered to experimental animals at various times prior to lethal endotoxin challenge. When BPI is given within 2 min of LPS (simultaneous administration), 90% of the animals survived at 72 h, compared to 20% survival in the untreated control group. Waiting only 30 min after BPI administration to give LPS resulted in a marked reduction in efficacy (44). Interestingly, we and others have observed a modest effect of preadministered BPI in this model, especially on 24-h survival.

These results indicate that BPI may have an extravascular site of action, but that probably this effect is not long-lived enough to provide therapeutic effect at reasonable doses in a clinical setting. Local delivery of BPI has been investigated by us and others. We have shown that, in the lung, exogenous BPI delivered 20 min before LPS challenge has a dramatic effect on cytokine production detected in BAL fluids (14). Even if the short half-life of BPI makes it unsuitable for systemic delivery, perhaps local administration into the lung would have therapeutic utility against conditions such as ARDS in sepsis, and gram-negative pneumonia.

IV. EXTENDING BPI HALF-LIFE USING BPI-LBP CHIMERIC PROTEINS

There are several mechanisms available for extending circulating half-life of therapeutic proteins. One method which has been successful is to genetically engineer a fusion protein consisting of the therapeutic protein coupled to the constant domain of immunoglobulin (Ig). Since Ig is a normal plasma constituent, with a circulating half-life measured in days, Ig fusion proteins have been shown to extend half-life of their fusion partners. LBP is produced in the liver and circulates at high levels in the plasma. Along with BPI, LBP belongs to a structurally related family of endotoxin-binding proteins. The structure–function relationship between the two proteins is compared in Table 1. The most important differences between BPI and LBP is their divergent roles in regulation of the host response to endotoxin, and their very different circulating half-lives. We took advantage of the structural similarities between these proteins and engineered fusion chimeras containing domains from both proteins with the goal of constructing a potent endotoxin-neutralizing molecule, which did not have LPS-facilitating activity of LBP but which would inherit from LBP the longer circulating half-life necessary for clinical utility. Such BPI-LBP chimeric proteins could also be useful tools to study the functional domains of each molecule.

A. Identification of Functional Domains

In 1987 Ooi reported isolation of a 25-kDa amino-terminal fragment of BPI, which carried all of the in-vitro bactericidal and permeability-increasing properties of the protein (11). Further work by Ooi showed that most of the in-vitro endotoxin-neutralizing activity of BPI could also be found in the N-terminal fragment, although some activity was also observed using the isolated carboxyl-terminal half of the molecule produced by limited proteolysis of the holoprotein isolated from neutrophils (35). No other activity was demonstrated for the C-terminal domain. These results demonstrated that the N-terminal fragment, which also contains the majority of the cationic residues in the protein, in all likelihood contains the LPS-binding site of BPI. Further dissection of the N-terminal domain of BPI was done using overlapping peptides to identify specific domains which were most important for LPS binding and neutralization (52). Based on data showing that the LPS-binding site of BPI resided in the N-terminal domain, we constructed a BPI-LBP chimera which consisted of the N-terminal 199 amino acids of BPI contiguous with the C-terminal region of LBP. We reasoned that adding LBP domains may extend the circulating half-life of the active fragment, thus providing us with a viable anti-endotoxin therapeutic. We also made the alternate construct, one which had the N-terminal acids derived from LBP, and the rest from BPI in order to help us to map endotoxin-enhancing activity of LBP. We also tested the N-terminal fragments of both molecules, as well as the recombinant full-length versions. Table 4 summarizes results we obtained with these chimeric molecules in a panel of assays.

Surprisingly, the two molecules which retained all of the measured activities of BPI did not share the N-terminal fragment, but rather the carboxyl-terminal domain was common. While these results were unexpected, they gave us a substantial amount of insight regarding the structural features of both BPI and LBP. First, probably the N-terminal half of each molecule contains its LPS-binding domain. Comparing regions of sequence identity between BPI and LBP do not make obvious a common LPS-binding site. In fact, sequence alignment

Table 4 Biological Properties of BPI and LBP Holoproteins, N-Terminal Fragments, and Chimeric Proteins

| Protein | LPS-neutralizing activity | | LBP activity[c] | Half-life[d] |
	In vitro[a]	In vivo[b]		
BPI	BPI	BPI	None	Short
BP(11-199)	BPI	None	None	Short
LBP	None	None	LBP	Long
LBP(1-199)	None	None	None	Intermediate
BP(11-199)LBP	None	None	Inconsistent	Short
LBP(1-199)BPI	BPI	BPI	None	Intermediate

[a]In-vitro LPS-neutralizing activity was determined by preincubating recombinant protein with LPS, then measuring residual limulus amebocyte lysate assay activity, or TNF release in human whole blood.
[b]In-vivo LPS-neutralizing activity reflects >70% survival in lethal endotoxin challenge studies using 25 mg/kg *Salmonella abortus equi* LPS challenge in CD-1 mice.
[c]LBP activity was determined by TNF release by human macrophages under serum-free conditions.
[d]Circulating half-life was determined using a 5-mg/kg bolus injection of recombinant protein in CD-1 mice (as in Fig. 4).

between the two proteins shows that regions of identity occur along the entire length of the molecule(s), not just in the N-terminal half. Although the binding affinity of LBP, and its N-terminal 25-kDa domain, in these assays was approximately 50 times lower than that of BPI, when conjugated to the C-terminal domain of BPI, LBP N-terminal fragments take on endotoxin-neutralizing activity, have no LPS-facilitating activity, and are cleared approximately 75 times more slowly than BPI. Apparently, the C-terminal domain exerts a positive influence on LPS-neutralizing activity of this molecule, as well as on full-length BPI. While the N-terminal fragment of BPI blocks in-vitro activity of LPS at similar molar concentrations as BPI, it is ineffective against lethal endotoxin challenge in experiments using very large bolus injections of LPS. This result suggests that BPI-25kDa may be inactivated to some extent in vivo, since in animal studies using galactosamine-sensitized mice and three orders of magnitude less LPS, efficacy can be demonstrated (53). The LPS-facilitating activity of LBP can be mapped to the C-terminal domain of the molecule, since LBP-25kDa had no LPS-facilitating activity. Results from experiments on LBP activity using the BPI-LBP chimeric protein gave equivocal results. This molecule contains the high-affinity binding domain of BPI coupled to the LPS-facilitating domain of LBP. Although binding to LPS-coated microtiter plates was apparently equivalent to BPI, the BPI-LBP chimeric molecule was not LPS neutralizing in assays of LPS-mediated TNF release in blood or in macrophage cultures. Further, although it contains the C-terminal domain of LBP, limited transfer of FITC LPS occurs, even in the presence of very high concentrations of recombinant protein. Since the mechanism of action of LBP is to transfer LPS to CD14 (22,24,25), perhaps this function is hindered by the increased LPS affinity of the BPI domain. Pharmacokinetic studies using a single bolus injection of BPI, LBP, the N-terminal fragments, and chimerics into CD-1 mice also provided several key pieces of information. First, the N-terminal domain of BPI seems to confer short circulating half-life. BPI, the BPI-LBP chimera, and BPI-25kDa all were cleared vary rapidly, while LBP-25kDa N-terminal fragment and the LBP-BPI chimera both had intermediate clearance rates, indicating that the C-terminal end of BPI has no affect the half-life of LBP-25kDa (data not shown).

B. Advantages of Longer-Half-Life Variants

Results from these experiments indicate that both BPI and LBP-BPI are potent endotoxin-neutralizing proteins in vitro and in vivo, and the LBP-BPI chimera has the advantage of longer circulating half-life. The therapeutic advantages of extended half-life are illustrated in two ways. First, the amount of protein required to maintain a 1-μg/mL circulating level over 4 h in nonhuman primates is approximately 10-fold greater for BPI than for the LBP-BPI chimera (42). Also, in similar experiments to those described above for BPI, the fusion protein is effective when given even 4 h prior to endotoxin challenge in CD-1 mice. The LBP-BPI fusion protein was recently also shown to be a highly effective therapeutic against sepsis in the neutropenic rat (54). We are continuing to dissect the BPI and LBP protein domains using the chimeric protein approach in order to determine domains which increase LPS affinity and allow extended circulating half-life.

V. CONCLUSIONS

With the availability of BPI proteins, we can now test the effects of a true anti-endotoxin against lethal gram-negative sepsis, where other anti-endotoxin agents without the neutralizing activity of BPI have failed. It is now possible to evaluate the clinical importance of endotoxin and endotoxemia in a variety of disorders. Questions such as the importance of bacterial or endotoxin translocation following trauma or hemorrhage in animals are now being answered. Further studies will determine the role of endotoxin, if any, in indications such liver disease and surgical outcome following procedures requiring extracorporeal circulation. The creation of long-half-life variants will enable us to give lower doses and provide more cost-efficient therapy for the widening variety of indications. Studies using neutralizing anti-cytokine reagents in combination with BPI proteins will also allow us to explore the role of LPS-cytokine synergies in a number of pathological models and conditions. The potent endotoxin-binding and -neutralizing activities of BPI proteins will, for the first time, permit rigorous tests of the efficacy of antiendotoxin therapy and the role of endotoxin in disease processes.

REFERENCES

1. Weiss J, Elsbach P, Olsson I, Hodberg H. Purification and characterization of a potent bactericidal and membrane active protein from the granules of human polymorphonuclear leukocytes. J Biol Chem 1978; 253:2664–2672.

2. Weiss J, Franson RC, Beckerdite S, Schmeidler K, Elsbach P. Partial characterization and purification of a rabbit granulocyte factor that increases permeability of *Escherichia coli*. J Clin Invest 1975; 55:33–42.

3. Shafer WM, Martin LE, Spitznagel JK. Cationic antimicrobial proteins isolated from human neutrophil granulocytes in the presence of diisopropyl fluorophosphate. Infect Immun 1984; 45:29–35.

4. Hovde CJ, Gray GH. Physiological effects of a bactericidal protein from human polymorphonuclear leukocytes on *Pseudomonas aeruginosa*. Infect Immun 1986; 54:142–148.

5. Weiss J, Muello K, Victor M, Elsbach P. The role of lipopolysaccharide in the action of the bactericidal/permeability-increasing neutrophil protein on the bacterial envelope. J Immunol 1984; 132:3109–3115.

6. Weiss J, Beckerdite-Quagliata S, Elsbach P. Resistance of gram-negative bacteria to purified bactericidal leukocyte proteins: relation to binding and bacterial lipopolysaccharide structure. J Clin Invest 1980; 65:619–628.

7. Farley MM, Shafer WM, Spitznagel JK. Lipopolysaccharide structure determines ionic and hydrophobic binding of a cationic antimicrobial neutrophil granule protein. Infect Immun 1988; 56:1589–1592.

8. Weiss J, Hutzler M, Kao L. Environmental modulation of lipopolysaccharide chain length alters the sensitivity of *Escherichia coli* to the neutrophil bactericidal/permeability-increasing protein. Infect Immun 1986; 51:594–599.

9. Gray PW, Falggs G, Leong SR, et al. Cloning of the cDNA of a human neutrophil bactericidal protein. J Biol Chem 1989; 264:9505–9509.

10. Gabay JE, Scott RW, Campanelli D, et al. Antibiotic proteins of human polymorphonuclear leukocytes. Proc Natl Acad Sci USA 1989; 86:5610–5614.

11. Ooi CE, Weiss J, Elsbach P, Frangione B, Mannion B. A 25kDa NH2-terminal fragment carries all the anti-bacterial activities of the human neutrophil 60kDa bactericidal/permeability-increasing protein. J Biol Chem 1987; 262:14891–14894.

12. Tobias PS, Mathison JC, Ulevitch RJ. A family of lipopolysaccharide binding proteins involved in responses to gram-negative sepsis. J Biol Chem 1988; 263:13479–13481.

13. Marra MN, Wilde CG, Griffith JE, Snable JL, Scott RW. Bactericidal/permeability-increasing protein has endotoxin neutralizing activity. J Immunol 1990; 144:662–666.

14. Marra MN, Wilde CG, Collins MS, Snable JL, Thornton MB, Scott RW. The role of bactericidal/permeability-increasing protein as a natural inhibitor of bacterial endotoxin. J Immunol 1992; 148:532–537.

15. Gazzano-Santoro H, Parent JB, Grinna L, et al. High affinity binding of the bactericidal/permeability-increasing protein and a recombinant amino-terminal fragment to the lipid A region of lipopolysaccharide. Infect Immun 1992; 60:4754–4761.

16. Morrison DC, Jacobs DM. Binding of polymyxin B to the lipid A portion of bacterial lipopolysaccharides. Immunochemistry 1976; 13:813–818.

17. Elsbach P, Weiss J. The bactericidal/permeability-increasing protein (BPI), a potent element in host-defense against gram-negative bacteria and lipopolysaccharide. Immunobiology 1993; 187:417–429.

18. Capodici C, Chen S, Sidorczyk Z, Elsbach P, Weiss J. Effect of lipopolysaccharide (LPS) chain length on interactions of bactericidal/permeability-increasing protein and its bioactive 23-kilodalton NH2-terminal fragment with isolated LPS and intact *Proteus mirabilis* and *Escherichia coli*. Infect Immun 1994; 62:259–265.

19. Weiss J. Elsbach P, Shu C, et al. Human bactericidal/permeability-increasing protein and a recombinant NH2-terminal fragment cause killing of serum-resistant gram-negative bacteria in whole blood and inhibit tumor necrosis factor release induced by the bacteria. J Clin Invest 1992; 90:1122–1130.

20. Scott RW, Wilde CG, Lane JC, Snable JL, Marra MN. Antimicrobial and antiendotoxin activities of bactericidal/permeability-increasing protein in vitro and *in vivo*. In: Levin J. Alving CR, Munford RS, Stutz PL, eds. Bacterial Endotoxin: Recognition and Effector Mechanisms. Amsterdam: Elsevier, 1993: 373–378.

21. Opal SM, Palardy JE, Romulo RLC, et al. Bactericidal/permeability increasing protein lowers endotoxin levels and improves survival in experimental gram-negative bacteremia. Manuscript submitted.

22. Schumann RR, Leong SR, Flaggs GW, et al. Structure and function of lipopolysaccharide binding protein. Science 1990; 249:1429–1431.

23. Wilde CG, Seilhamer JJ, McGrogan M, et al. Bactericidal/permeability-increasing protein and lipopolysaccharide (LPS)-binding protein: LPS binding properties and effects on LPS-mediated cell activation. J Biol Chem 1994; 269:17411–17416.

24. Mathison JC, Tobias PS, Wolfson E, Ulevitch RJ. Plasma lipopolysaccharide (LPS)-binding protein. A key component in macrophage recognition of gram-negative LPS. J Immunol 1992; 149:200–206.

25. Tobias PS, Soldau K, Ulevitch RJ. Identification of a lipid A binding site in the acute phase reactant lipopolysaccharide binding protein. J Biol Chem 1989; 264:10867–10871.

26. Morrison DC, Ulevitch RJ. Endotoxins and disease mechanisms. Annu Rev Med 1987; 38:417–432.

27. Morrison DC, Ulevitch RJ. The effects of bacterial endotoxins on host mediation systems. Am J Pathol 1978; 93:526–617.

28. Marra MN, Thornton MB, Snable JL, et al. Regulation of the response to bacterial lipopolysaccharide by endogenous and exogenous lipopolysaccharide binding proteins. Blood Purif 1993; 11:134–140.

27. Heumann D, Galley P, Betz-Corradin S, Barras C, Baumgartner J-D, Glauser MP. Competition between bactericidal/permeability-increasing protein and lipopolysaccharide-binding protein for lipopolysaccharide binding to monocytes. J Infect Dis 1993; 176:1351–1357.

30. Dentener MA, Won Asmuth EJU, Fancot GJM, Marra MN, Buurman WA. Antagonistic effects of lipopolysaccharide binding protein and bactericidal/permeability-increasing protein on lipopolysaccharide-induced cytokine release by mononuclear phagocytes. J Immunol 1993; 151:4258–4265.

31. Wright SD, Ramos RA, Tobias PS, Ulevitch RJ, Mathison JC. CD14, a receptor for complexes of lipopolysaccharide (LPS) and LPS-binding protein. Science 1990; 249:1431–1433.

32. Pereira HA, Spitznagel JK, Winton EF, et al. The ontogeny of a 57Kd cationic antimicrobial protein of human polymorphonuclear leukocytes: localization of a novel granule population. Blood 1990; 76:825–834.

33. Weiss J, Olsson I. Cellular and subcellular localization of the bactericidal/permeability-increasing protein of neutrophils. Blood 1987; 69:652–659.

34. Ooi CE, Weiss J, Elsbach P. Structural and functional organization of the human neutrophil 60kDa bactericidal/permeability-increasing protein. Agents and Actions 1991; 34:274–277.

35. Ooi CE, Weiss J, Doerfler ME, Elsbach P. Endotoxin-neutralizing properties of the 25kD N-terminal fragment and a newly isolated 30kD C-terminal fragment of the 55–60 kD bactericidal/permeability-increasing protein of human neutrophils. J Exp Med 1991; 174:649–655.

36. Schindler R, Marra MN, McKelligon BM, et al. Plasma levels of bactericidal/

permeability-increasing protein (BPI) and lipopolysaccharide binding protein (LBP) during hemodialysis. Clin Nephrol 1993; 40:346–351.

37. von der Mohlen MAM, Marra MN, Wortel CH, ten Cate JW, van Deventer SJH. Bactericidal permeability increasing protein levels predict survival in patients with gram-negative sepsis. 13th International Symposium on Intensive Care and Emergency Medicine, Brussels, Belgium, Mar 23–26, 1993.

38. Calvano SE, Thompson WA, Marra MN, et al. Changes in polymorphonuclear leukocyte surface and plasma bactericidal/permeability-increasing protein and plasma lipopolysaccharide binding protein during endotoxemia or sepsis. Arch Surg 1994; 129:220–226.

39. Weersink AJL, van Kessel KPM, van den Tol JE, et al. Human granulocytes express a 55kDa lipopolysaccharide-binding protein on the cell surface that is identical to the bactericidal/permeability-increasing protein. J Immunol 1993; 150:253–263.

40. Gazzano-Santoro H, Meszaros K, Birr C, et al. Competition between rBPI23, a fragment of bactericidal/permeability-increasing protein and lipopolysaccharide (LPS)-binding protein for binding to LPS and gram-negative bacteria. Infect Immun 1994; 62:1185–1191.

41. Opal SM, Palardy JE, Marra MN, Fisher CJ Jr., McKelligon BM, Scott RW. Relative concentrations of endotoxin-binding proteins in body fluids during infection. Lancet 1994; 344:429–431.

42. Marra NM, Scott RW, McKelligon BM, Opal SM. Bactericidal/permeability-increasing protein (BPI) levels exceed lipopolysaccharide binding protein (LBP) levels in fluids at infected sites. American Federation of Clinical Research Meeting, Baltimore, MD, Apr 29–May 2, 1994.

43. Marra MN, Thornton MB, Snable JL, Wilde CG, Scott RW. Endotoxin-binding and -neutralizing properties of recombinant bactericidal/permeability-increasing protein and monoclonal antibodies HA-1A and E5. Crit Care Med 1994; 22(4):559–565.

44. Fisher CJ Jr., Marra MN, Palardy JE, Marchbanks CR, Scott RW, Opal SM. Human neutrophil bactericidal/permeability-increasing protein reduces mortality rate from endotoxin challenge: a placebo-controlled study. Crit Care Med 1994; 22:553–558.

45. Jin H, Yang R, Bunting S, Marra MN, Scott RW, Baker J. Protection against endotoxic shock by bactericidal/permeability-increasing protein in rats. Manuscript submitted.

46. Fisher CJ Jr., Opal SM, Marra MN, Palardy JE, Scott, RW. Bactericidal/permeability-increasing protein reduces mortality in experimental sepsis. 2nd International Conference on Shock, Vienna, Austria, June 2–6, 1991.

47. Bahrami S, Redl H, Yu Y, Jiang JX, Leichtfried G, Schlag G. Bactericidal/permeability-increasing protein (BPI) reduces lipopolysaccharide (LPS)-induced cytokine formation and mortality in rats. 3rd International Conference on Shock, Vienna, Austria, May 9–13, 1993.

48. Porat R, Paddock HN, Cominelli F, et al. Effects of bactericidal/permeability-increasing protein on endotoxin-induced fever and *Escherichia coli*-induced shock in rabbits. Manuscript submitted.

49. Rogy MA, Moldawer LL, Oldenburg HSA, et al. Anti-endotoxin therapy in primate bacteremia with HA-1A and BPI. Ann Surg 1994; 220:77–85.
50. Opal SM, Cross AS, Kelly NM, et al. Efficacy of a monoclonal antibody directed against tumor necrosis factor in protecting neutropenic rats from lethal infection with *Pseudomonas aeruginosa*. J Infect Dis 1990; 161:1148–1152.
51. Cross AS, Opal SM, Palardy JE, Bodmer MW, Sadoff JC. The efficacy of combination immunotherapy in experimental pseudomonas sepsis. J Infect Dis 1993; 167:112–118.
52. Little RG, Kelner DN, Lim E, Burke DJ, Conlon, PJ. Functional domains of recombinant bactericidal/permeability-increasing protein (rBPI^{23}). J Biol Chem 1994; 269:1865–1872.
53. Kohn FR, Ammons WS, Horwitz A, et al. Protective effect of a recombinant amino-terminal fragment of bactericidal/permeability-increasing protein in experimental endotoxemia. J Infect Dis 1993; 168:1307–1310.
54. Opal SM, Palardy JE, Donsky C, Romulo RLC, Parejo N, Marra MN. The activity of a chimeric LBP-BPI fusion molecule in experimental gram negative sepsis. 34th Interscience Conference on Anti-microbial Agents and Chemotherapy, Orlando, FL, October 4–7, 1994.

4

Protective Effects of an N-Terminal Fragment of Bactericidal/Permeability-Increasing Protein in Endotoxemia and Gram-Negative Sepsis

W. Steve Ammons, Fred R. Kohn, and Yue Lin
XOMA Corporation
Berkeley, California

Ada H. C. Kung
Skyline Technology Consulting Group
San Francisco, California

I. INTRODUCTION

Polymorphonuclear leukocytes produce a number of molecules with bactericidal or endotoxin-neutralizing activities [for review, see (1)]. The most potent of these substances is a cationic, 55-kDa protein contained within azurophilic granules called bactericidal/permeability-increasing protein (BPI). This protein was first purified by Weiss et al. in 1978 (2) and has been isolated from human and rabbit neutrophils (2,3). Its primary structure has been established (4) and is now known to have considerable sequence homology with lipopolysaccharide (LPS)-binding protein (5).

BPI kills a variety of gram-negative bacteria. Killing is associated with high-affinity binding of BPI to the lipid A moiety of LPS in the outer membrane (6–8). BPI also binds to isolated LPS of both rough and smooth forms (6). Binding of BPI to LPS on gram-negative bacteria increases as LPS chain length decreases (9,10) and is followed rapidly by an increase in permeability to small hydrophobic molecules (11–13) and selective activation of enzymes that hydrolyze phospholipids and peptidoglycans (2,3,14,15). If binding is sustained, irreversible structural damage to the inner cytoplasmic membrane occurs and death ensues (11). The mechanisms involved in this irreversable lethal damage remain undefined.

Isolated BPI inhibits LPS-mediated responses in vitro including expression of neutrophil cell surface receptors for complement (16), and secretion of tumor necrosis factor (TNF) from human mononuclear cells (17) and in whole human blood (18). It also inhibits fever in rabbits (17). Recently it was reported that BPI increases survival in mice challenged with LPS (19).

Ooi et al. (18,20) demonstrated that the 25-kDa N-terminal portion of BPI possesses essentially all of its LPS-neutralizing and bactericidal properties. The role of the C-terminal portion is not yet clearly identified, although it may have some endotoxin-neutralizing activity (18). A recombinant 23-kDa N-terminal fragment of BPI, $rBPI_{23}$, binds with the same high affinity to LPS as the holoprotein (6). $rBPI_{23}$ inhibits LPS-induced cytokine release and oxygen free-radical generation in whole human blood (21), nitric oxide production in macrophages (22), adherence of neutrophils to endothelial cells (23), and induction of procoagulant tissue factor in monocytes (24). Furthermore, $rBPI_{23}$ prevents death and cytokine elevation in endotoxemic mice (25); prevents hemodynamic responses, TNF elevation, and changes in glucose and lactate in endotoxemic rats (26,27); and inhibits pulmonary dysfunction in endotoxemic pigs (28). $rBPI_{23}$ may have more potent bactericidal activity than the holoprotein (29), perhaps because it is less sensitive to the inhibitory effect of increased LPS chain length (20,29). Consistent with its gram-negative antibacterial properties, $rBPI_{23}$ prevents death and enhances bacterial clearance in a mouse model of gram-negative pneumonia (30).

This chapter will focus on the activity of another recombinant N-terminal fragment of BPI, $rBPI_{21}$, which has been developed for evaluation in animal models. $rBPI_{21}$ has equivalent activity as $rBPI_{23}$ in in-vitro assays and has the same LPS binding kinetics (Parent et al., manuscript in preparation). The studies described below indicate that $rBPI_{21}$ also is protective in animals challenged with either LPS or gram-negative bacteria.

II. MATERIALS AND METHODS

A. Bacteria

Experiments were performed with three strains of gram-negative bacteria, *Escherichia coli* O7:K1 (ATCC 23503), *Escherichia coli* O111:B4, provided by L. R. Young (Medical Research Institute, San Francisco, CA); and a clinical isolate of *Pseudomonas aeruginosa* (strain 12.4.4) provided by S. M. Opal (Brown University, Providence, RI) (31). Suspensions of the bacteria in log phase were prepared in phosphate-buffered saline and diluted until a spectrophotometric reading was obtained that corresponded to the necessary CFU/mL based on a standard curve.

B. Reagents

LPS from *E. coli* O111:B4 or *E. coli* O113 was dissolved in phosphate-buffered saline by sonication and vigorous vortexing. $rBPI_{21}$ is a cysteine substitution analog of rBPI$_{23}$ encoding amino acid residues 1–193 of BPI. An alanine substitution was made for the cysteine residue at position 132. rBPI$_{21}$ was cloned and expressed in CHO-K1 cells and purified (at least 97%) by cation-exchange chromatography. The vehicle for rBPI$_{21}$ was a solution of 20 mM citrate and 150 mM sodium chloride (pH 5.0) with stabilizers. Cefamandole nafate (Mandol; Eli Lilly, Indianapolis, IN) was prepared in phosphate-buffered saline.

C. Mouse Lethal Endotoxemia Model

Male ICR mice, 6–8 weeks old, were housed in polycarbonate cages and allowed access to food and water ad libitum. Each mouse received an intravenous injection of 20 mg/kg of LPS (*E. coli* O111:B4) followed by a second intravenous injection of either rBPI$_{21}$ (20–30 mg/kg) or vehicle. Treatment was delayed for as long as 3 h after LPS challenge. Mortality was recorded for a 7-day period.

D. Conscious Rabbit Endotoxemia Model

Adult male New Zealand White rabbits (1.8–2.3 kg; Charles River, St. Constant, Canada) were anesthetized with an intramuscular injection of ketamine (80 mg/ kg) and xylazine (4 mg/kg). A catheter was placed in the left femoral artery for blood pressure measurements and for blood samples. A second catheter was implanted in the right jugular vein with the tip adjacent to the right atrium for administration of saline for cardiac output determinations. A 3.5-French thermistor-tipped catheter (Columbus Instruments, Columbus, OH) was advanced into the aortic arch by way of the right carotid artery. All catheters were then exteriorized at the base of the neck. LPS was administered through a 20-gauge × 1.25-in. angiocath (Bectin Dickinson Vascular Access, Sandy, UT) placed in the marginal ear vein. rBPI$_{21}$ or vehicle was administered through the jugular-vein catheter.

After complete recovery from anesthesia, i.e., when all recorded parameters were in the normal range, the rabbits were injected with 6 µg/kg LPS (*E. coli* O113) in 1 mL over 1 min and treated with vehicle (LPS/vehicle group, $N = 9$) or 4 mg/kg of rBPI$_{21}$ (LPS/rBPI$_{21}$ group, $N = 5$). The vehicle and rBPI$_{21}$ were given in the same volume over 2 min beginning 30 s before initiation of the LPS injection. A third group of rabbits, not challenged with LPS, served as controls and received saline and vehicle (saline/vehicle group, $N = 7$). Hemodynamics and pulmonary function were measured over a 3-h period following LPS injection.

E. Rat Intravenous Bacterial Challenge Model

Rats were challenged intravenously with 3×10^8 CFU of *E. coli* O7:K1 bacteria in 0.5 mL. Immediately after bacterial challenge, the rats were treated intravenously with 10–20 mg/kg of $rBPI_{21}$ or an equal volume of vehicle. Blood was obtained from the retro-orbital sinus at various time points for measurement of bacterial counts and TNFα.

F. Mouse Intraperitoneal Bacterial Challenge Model

Mice received an intraperitoneal injection of 2×10^7 CFU of *E. coli* O7:K1 or 3×10^6 CFU of *P. aeruginosa* in 0.5 mL. Immediately after bacterial challenge, the animals received an intraperitoneal injection of 1 mL of vehicle or $rBPI_{21}$ in doses of 10–500 µg per mouse (0.33–18 mg/kg). $rBPI_{21}$ alone, when administered to unchallenged mice at doses up to 500 µg, had no observable effect. Survival was monitored for 7 days. In separate experiments, blood from the retro-orbital sinus and peritoneal lavage fluid were collected following bacterial challenge for measurement of TNFα and interleukin-6 (IL-6) or for bacterial cultures (4–8 mice per time point). For cytokine assays, millip-filtered (0.2 µm) serum or peritoneal lavage fluid was stored at -70°C until assay. Bacterial counts were determined by plating 10-fold dilutions of blood or peritoneal lavage samples on Trypticase soy agar and incubating overnight at 37°C.

G. Cytokine Assays

TNFα was quantified using an L929 cytolytic assay as described (32). Mouse recombinant TNFα (Genzyme Corporation, Cambridge, MA) was used to generate a standard curve. The specific activity of the TNFα standard was approximately 500 units/ng, where 1 unit is defined as the quantity of TNFα required to kill 50% of L929 cells. Mouse IL-6 was quantified using a standard alkaline phosphatase-based sandwich ELISA (anti-IL-6 capture and detection antibodies were obtained from Pharmingen, San Diego, CA).

H. Data Analysis

All values are expressed as mean ± SE. Survival of different groups was compared with the chi-square statistic. Statistical comparisons of other data was performed with the analysis of variance. When F ratios exceeded the critical value ($p < 0.05$), individual means were compared with the Newman-Keuls test.

III. RESULTS

A. Mouse Lethal Endotoxemia Model

LPS administration resulted in death within 3 days of all 15 mice that were treated with the vehicle. $rBPI_{21}$, when injected immediately after LPS challenge, resulted in a dose-dependent increase in survival; 8 of 15 mice treated with 20 mg/kg and all 15 treated with 30 mg/kg survived. Furthermore, all mice survived when treatment was delayed for 1 h after LPS challenge (Fig. 1). A significant effect of $rBPI_{21}$ was still observed when treatment was delayed for as long as 3 h after LPS challenge, a time when the mice were lethargic and exhibited piloerection.

B. Conscious Rabbit Endotoxemia Model

1. Pulmonary Function

The first observable symptom in the LPS/vehicle group was an increase in respiration rate (Fig. 2A). Within 40 min of LPS injection, respiration rate was nearly twice the level observed in the control saline/vehicle group of rabbits. In contrast, $rBPI_{21}$-treated rabbits never exhibited significant tachypnea.

LPS administration resulted in a decrease in arterial oxygen tension (pO_2) and an increase in alveolar-arterial oxygen gradient ($AaDO_2$) in the LPS/vehicle

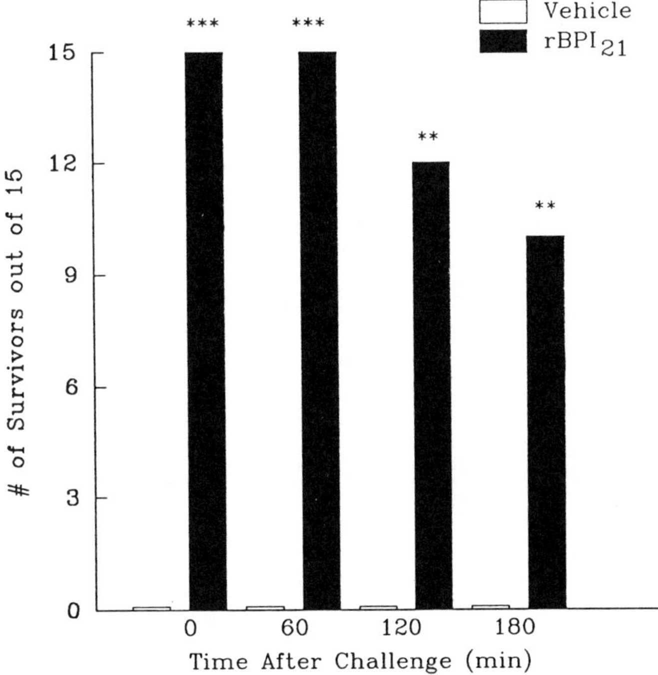

Figure 1 Effect of $rBPI_{21}$ on survival in the mouse endotoxemia model. Mice were injected i.v. with 20 mg/kg of LPS and then treated with an i.v. injection of 30 mg/kg of $rBPI_{21}$ either immediately after (time 0) or from 1 to 3 h. after LPS challenge. Survival was monitored for 7 days. **, $p < 0.01$ vs vehicle; ***, $p < 0.001$.

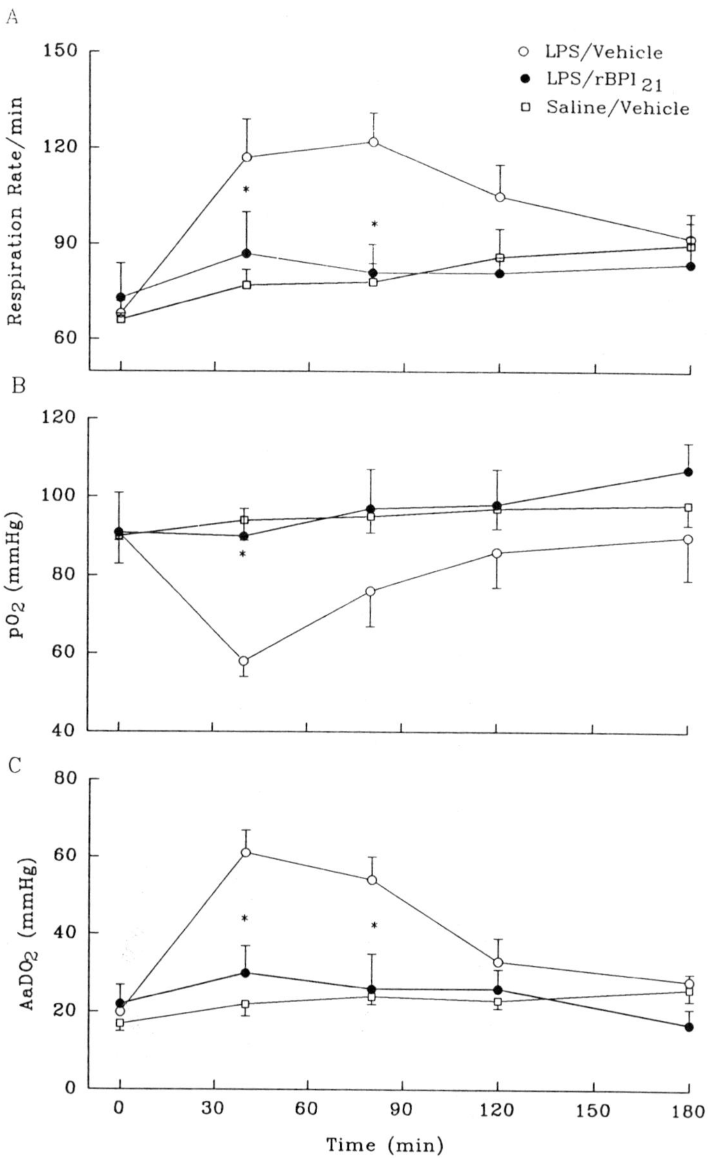

Figure 2   Protective effect of rBPI$_{21}$ on respiration rate (A), arterial oxygen tension (B), and alveolar-arterial oxygen gradient (C) in the conscious rabbit endotoxemia model. Rabbits were challenged with 6 μ/kg of LPS and treated with vehicle or 4 mg/kg of rBPI$_{21}$.pO$_2$, partial pressure of oxygen in arterial blood; AaDO$_2$, difference in partial pressure of oxygen in alveoli and arterial blood.*, $p < 0.05$ versus LPS/vehicle group.

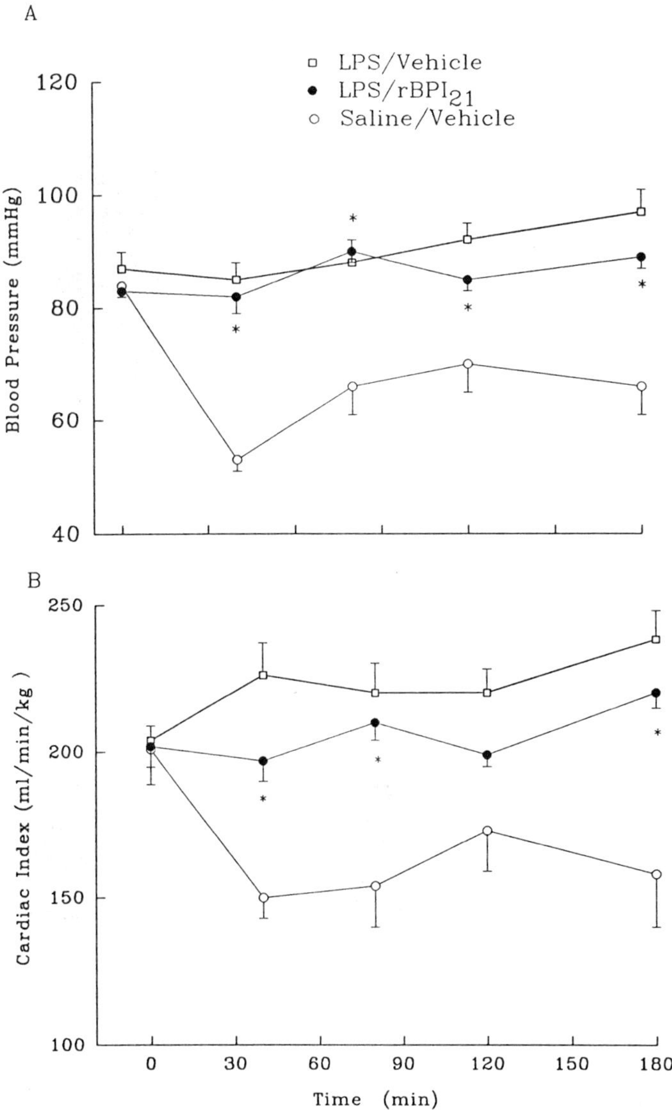

Figure 3 Protective effect of rBPI$_{21}$ on blood pressure (A) and cardiac index (B) in the conscious rabbit endotoxemia model.*, $p < 0.01$ versus LPS/vehicle group.

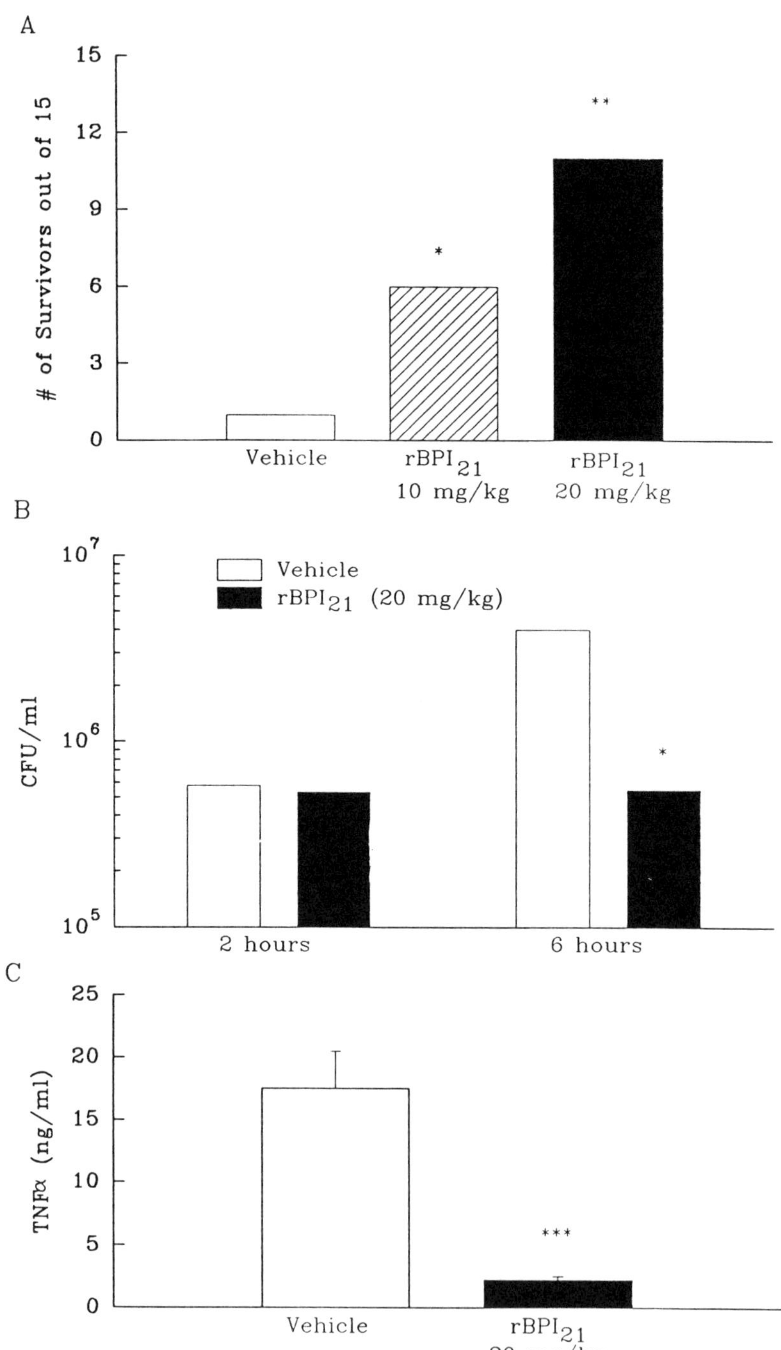
A
# of Survivors out of 15
15
12
9
6
3
0
*
**
Vehicle
rBPI$_{21}$
10 mg/kg
rBPI$_{21}$
20 mg/kg
B
CFU/ml
10^7
10^6
10^5
Vehicle
rBPI$_{21}$ (20 mg/kg)
2 hours
6 hours
*
C
TNFα (ng/ml)
25
20
15
10
5
0
***
Vehicle
rBPI$_{21}$
20 mg/kg

group (Figs. 2B and 2C). pO_2 and $AaDO_2$ of rabbits treated with $rBPI_{21}$ did not vary significantly at any time from levels observed in the unchallenged vehicle/ saline group.

2. Cardiovascular Function

LPS challenge resulted in a sustained and profound hypotension and a decrease in cardiac index in the LPS/vehicle rabbits within 20–40 min (Fig. 3A). Treatment with $rBPI_{21}$ eliminated the LPS-induced hypotension and the decrease in cardiac index. Cardiovascular functions of $rBPI_{21}$-treated rabbits were stable throughout the experiment and did not differ from those of the saline/vehicle control group.

C. Rat Intravenous Bacterial Challenge Model

1. Survival

All but one of 15 rats challenged with *E. coli* O7:K1 bacteria died within 6 days of infection (Fig. 4A). Significant protection was associated with $rBPI_{21}$ treatment; 6 of 15 rats treated with 10 mg/kg and 11 of 15 treated with 20 mg/ kg of $rBPI_{21}$ survived.

2. Bacteremia and TNFα

Levels of *E. coli* O7:K1 bacteria in the blood of rats treated with vehicle rose during the first 6 h after bacterial challenge (Fig. 4B). In contrast, bacterial counts in $rBPI_{21}$-treated rats did not rise significantly during this period and were significantly less than in vehicle-treated rats at 6 h.

In vehicle-treated rats, TNFα levels were significantly elevated 90 min after the challenge and then returned to baseline within 3 h. There was significantly less TNFα in the sera of $rBPI_{21}$-treated rats at 90 min (Fig. 4C).

D. Mouse Intraperitoneal Bacterial Challenge Model

1. Survival

$rBPI_{21}$ treatment resulted in a dose-dependent increase in survival of mice challenged with *E. coli* O7:K1 bacteria (Fig. 5A). Significant protection was associated with a dose of 10 μg/mouse, and complete protection was observed with 100 μg/mouse. $rBPI_{21}$ also protected mice challenged with *P. aeruginosa* bacteria, although higher doses were required (Fig. 5B).

Figure 4 Effect of $rBPI_{21}$ treatment in the rat intravenous bacterial challenge model. Rats were challenged with 3×10^8 CFU of *E. coli* O7:K1 bacteria i.v. and treated with vehicle or $rBPI_{21}$ i.v. (A) Effect of $rBPI_{21}$ on survival after 7 days. (B) Bacterial levels in blood 2 and 6 h after challenge. (C) TNFα levels in serum, measured by bioassay, 90 min after challenge.*, $p < 0.05$ versus vehicle; **, $p < 0.01$; ***, $p < 0.001$.

2. Bacterial Counts and Cytokines

After intraperitoneal injection of *E. coli* O7:K1, bacterial levels in peritoneal lavage fluid and blood increased rapidly in animals treated with vehicle, peaked in 4–6 h, and remained stable for at least 24 h. Treatment with 50 μg/mouse of $rBPI_{21}$ resulted in a significant reduction in bacterial counts determined after 24 h (Fig. 5C). $rBPI_{21}$ treatment also significantly reduced bacterial levels in peritoneal lavage fluid and blood of mice challenged with *P. aeruginosa* (Fig. 5D).

$rBPI_{21}$ (50 μg/mouse) significantly inhibited the rise in serum TNFα and IL-6 resulting from injection of *E. coli* O7:K1 bacteria (data not shown).

3. Combination Treatment with $rBPI_{21}$ and Cefamandole

$rBPI_{21}$ treatment alone (500 μg/mouse) did not increase survival of mice challenged with 2.5×10^9 CFU of *E. coli* O111:B4 (Fig. 6A). Since a large number of bacteria were required to achieve an LD_{90}, we conducted separate experiments with lower doses of the same bacterial strain. $rBPI_{21}$ (500 μg/mouse) remained ineffective in mice challenged with 10^9 or 3×10^8 (LD_{60}) CFU of the same bacterial strain (data not shown). However, when the same dose of $rBPI_{21}$ was administered after an intraperitoneal injection of 100 mg/kg of cefamandole, there was a significant increase in survival above that achieved by either treatment alone. Furthermore, $rBPI_{21}$, when combined with cefamandole, reduced bacterial counts in peritoneal lavage fluid and blood significantly below those achieved by the antibiotic alone, despite its failure to affect bacterial levels in the absence of the antibiotic (Fig. 6B and C).

IV. DISCUSSION

Data from in-vivo and in-vitro studies have demonstrated that BPI and $rBPI_{23}$ are potent endotoxin-neutralizing agents (16,17,19,21–28). Other studies have established that these proteins are also bactericidal toward gram-negative bacteria (1,29). These results are the first to indicate that $rBPI_{21}$, like $rBPI_{23}$, is capable of inhibiting the biological responses to both LPS and bacteria in vivo.

Results from the two endotoxemia models provide insights into some of the important pathological mechanisms associated with LPS administration that are blocked by $rBPI_{21}$ therapy. The lethal mouse endotoxemia model establishes that $rBPI_{21}$ increases survival even when administered as long as 3 h after challenge with a high dose of LPS. $rBPI_{21}$ is therefore therapeutic even after animals are lethargic, exhibit evidence of catecholamine release (piloerection), and are known to have elevated cytokine levels (33). Despite considerable exposure to LPS, the ability of $rBPI_{21}$ to neutralize residual LPS is beneficial.

The pulmonary distress observed in our rabbit experiments is typical of pa-

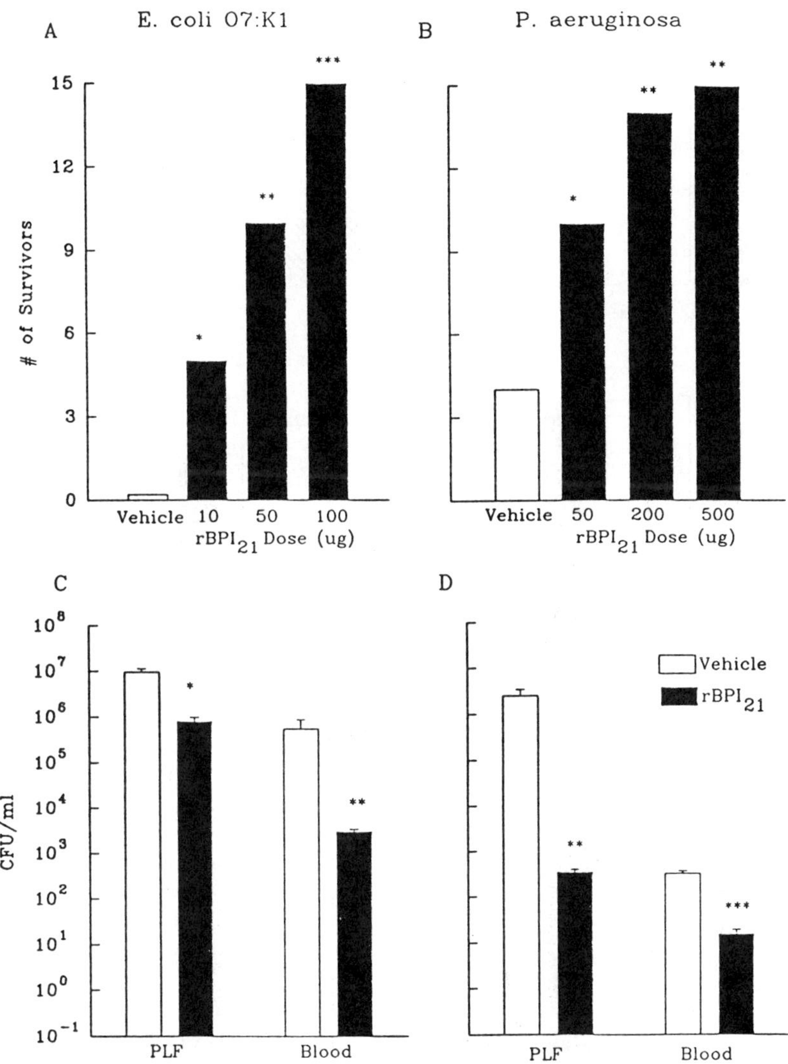

Figure 5   Protective effects of rBPI$_{21}$ in the mouse in the mouse intraperitoneal bacterial challenge model. Mice were challenged with intraperitoneal injections of 2×10^7 CFU of *E. coli* O7:K1 or 3×10^6 CFU of *P. aeruginosa* bacteria and treated with intraperitoneal injections of rBPI$_{21}$. A and B, dose-dependent increase in survival of mice treated with rBPI$_{21}$ (groups of 15 for *E. coli* and 20 for *P. aeruginosa*). C and D, Reductions in bacterial levels in blood and peritoneal lavage fluid (PFL) at 24 h in mice (4–6 per group) treated with 50 µg/mouse of rBPI$_{21}$.

Ammons et al.

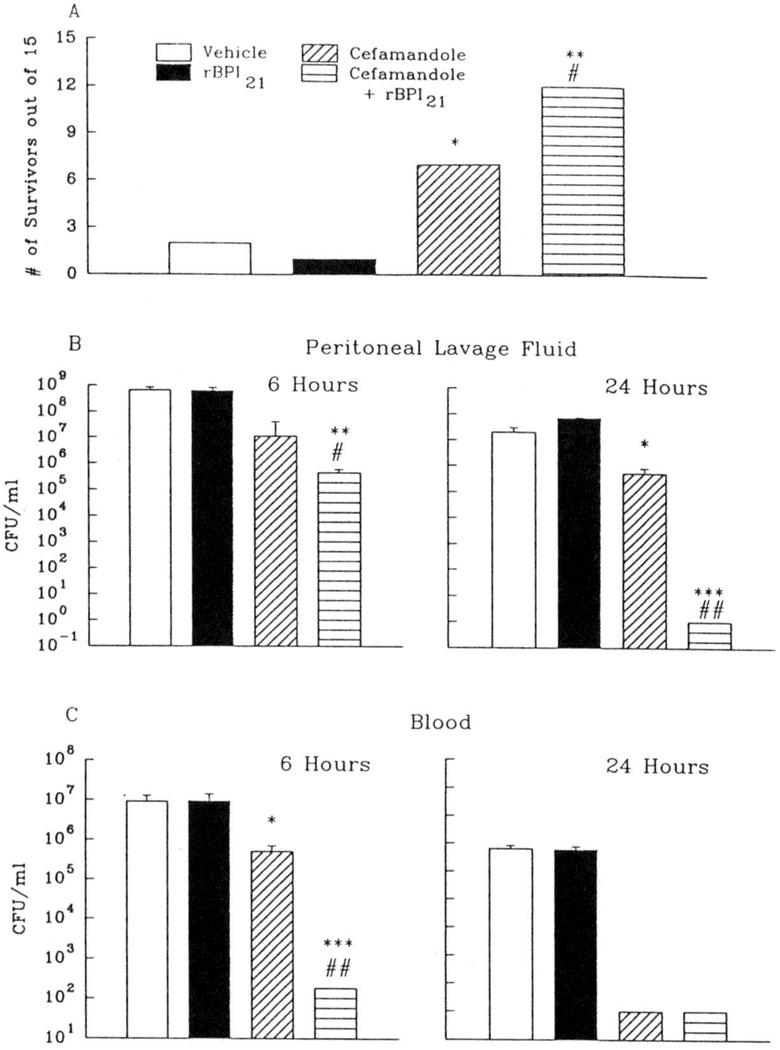

Figure 6 Effect of rBPI$_{21}$ on survival (A), and bacterial counts in peritoneal lavage fluid (B) and blood (C). Mice were challenged with 2.5 × 10^9 CFU of *E. coli* O111:B4 and treated with vehicle, 500 μg/mouse of RBPI$_{21}$, 100 mg/kg of cefamandole, or both rBPI$_{21}$ and cefamandole in the above doses.*,$p < 0.05$ versus vehicle;**, $p < 0.01$; ***,$p < 0.001$; #, $p < 0.05$ versus cefamandole; ##, $p < 0.01$.

tients with the adult respiratory distress syndrome that is often a complication of sepsis (34). The accompanying shock state that we observed also makes this model useful for studying mechanisms that are relevant to the sepsis syndrome. The ability of $rBPI_{21}$ to inhibit pulmonary and cardiovascular responses to LPS in conscious rabbits provides evidence that $rBPI_{21}$ will be useful in clinically relevant endotoxemic states that follow gram-negative infections. We have observed qualitatively similar effects with $rBPI_{23}$ (35).

Our two bacterial challenge models provide evidence for the efficacy of $rBPI_{21}$ in gram-negative infections. In particular, the intravenous challenge model indicates that $rBPI_{21}$ may be therapeutic in states of bacteremia. The efficacy of $rBPI_{21}$, in both the intravenous and the intraperitoneal challenge models, was associated with enhanced clearance of bacteria as well as reduced production of serum cytokine levels. The ability of $rBPI_{21}$ to enhance bacterial clearance may be an important therapeutic property. The mechanisms underlying this effect are unclear but could represent the bactericidal activity of this molecule.

The most intriguing finding of these studies is the ability of the antibiotic cefamandole to potentiate the protective effects of $rBPI_{21}$. In the presence of the antibiotic, $rBPI_{21}$ increased survival and enhanced clearance of bacteria in animals challenged with *E. coli* O111:B4. This occurred despite the inability of $rBPI_{21}$ to protect on its own. One interpretation of these results is that *E. coli* O111:B4 was converted from insensitive to sensitive to $rBPI_{21}$ by the antibiotic. Thus $rBPI_{21}$ dramatically increased the clearance of bacteria and presumably was bactericidal in combination with the antibiotic but not alone. Alternatively, it is possible that $rBPI_{21}$ amplified the activity of the antibiotic. Although the mechanism of the potentiating effects associated with the combination therapy is unclear, synergism between $rBPI_{21}$ and antibiotics in vitro has been reported previously (36).

V. CONCLUSIONS

These studies support the concept that $rBPI_{21}$, like $rBPI_{23}$, may be a clinically useful therapeutic agent for treating gram-negative bacterial infections as well as the endotoxemia that accompanies such infections. The endotoxin-neutralizing activity of $rBPI_{21}$ is an important function that should be of therapeutic benefit. In addition, these studies also support the concept that the ability of $rBPI_{21}$ to enhance clearance of bacteria, possibly as a result of its bactericidal actions, provides a second important therapeutic benefit. This activity may be more potent in combination with antibiotic therapy.

ACKNOWLEDGMENTS

The authors gratefully acknowledge the technical assistance of Will Leach, Juergen Pfeiffer, Virginia Mohler, Craig Fujii, Gregg Prawdzik, Robert Peterson, and Richard Fleisher. We also thank Drs. Károly Mészáros, Patrick Trown, and Pat Scannon for reviewing the manuscript. The assistance of Beth Lacerna and Carroll Hess is also appreciated.

REFERENCES

1. Elsbach P, Weiss J. Phagocytic cells: oxygen-independent antimicrobial systems. In: Gallin JI, Goldstein IM, Snyderman R, eds. Inflammation: Basic Principles and Clinical Correlates. New York: Raven Press, 1992:603–636.

2. Weiss J, Elsbach P, Olsson I, Odeberg H. Purification and characterization of a potent bactericidal membrane active protein from the granules of human polymorphonuclear leukocytes. J Biol Chem 1978; 253:2664–2672.

3. Elsbach P, Weiss J, Franson R, Beckerdite-Quagliata S, Schneider A, Harris L. Separation and purification of a potent bactericidal/permeability-increasing protein and a closely associated phospholipase A2 from rabbit polymorphonuclear leukocytes. J Biol Chem 1979; 254:11000–11009.

4. Gray PW, Flaggs G, Leong SR, et al. Cloning of the cDNA of a human neutrophil bactericidal protein. J Biol Chem 1989; 264:9505–9509.

5. Tobias PS, Mathison JC, Ulevitch RJ. A family of lipopolysaccharide binding proteins involved in responses to gram-negative sepsis. J Biol Chem 1988; 263:13479–13481.

6. Gazzano-Santoro H, Parent JB, Grinna L, et al. High affinity binding of the bactericidal/permeability increasing protein (nBPI55) and a recombinant amino terminal fragment (rBPI23) to the lipid A region of LPS. Infect Immun 1993; 60:4754–4761.

7. Mannion BA, Kalatzi ES, Weiss J, Elsbach P. Preferential binding of the neutrophil cytoplasmic granule-derived bactericidal/permeability increasing protein to target bacteria. J Immunol 1989; 142:2807–2812.

8. Weiss J, Muello K, Victor M, Elsbach P. The role of lipopolysaccharides in the action of the bactericidal/permeability increasing neutrophil protein. J Immunol 1984; 132:3109–3115.

9. Weiss J, Hutzler M, Kao L. Environmental modulation of lipopolysaccharide chain length alters the sensitivity of *Escherichia coli* to the neutrophil bactericidal/permeability increasing protein. Infect Immun 1986; 51:594–599.

10. Capodici C, Chen S, Sidorczyk Z, Elsbach P, Weiss J. Effect of lipopolysaccharide (LPS) chain length on interactions of bactericidal/permeability-increasing protein and its bioactive 23-kilodalton NH_2-terminal fragment with isolated LPS and intact *Proteus mirabilis* and *Escherichia coli*. Infect Immun 1994; 62:259–265.

11. Mannion BA, Weiss, J, Elsbach P. Separation of sublethal and lethal effects of polymorphonuclear leukocytes on *Escherichia coli*. J Clin Invest 1990; 86:631–641.

12. Weiss J, Muello K, Victor M, Elsbach P. The role of lipopolysaccharides in the action of the bactericidal/permeability-increasing protein of neutrophils on the bacterial envelope. J Immunol 1984; 132:3109–3115.

13. Weiss J, Victor M, Elsbach P. Role of charge and hydrophobic interactions in the action of the bactericidal/permeability-increasing protein of neutrophils on gram negative bacteria. J Clin Invest 1993; 71:540–549.

14. Wright GC, Weiss J, Kim SK, Verheij J, Elsbach P. Bacterial phospholipid hydrolysis enhances the destructionof *Escherichia coli* ingested by rabbit neutrophils. J Clin Invest 1990; 85:1925–1935.
15. Weiss J, Beckerdite-Quagliata S, Elsbach P. Determinants of the action of phospholipases A on the envelope phospholipids of *Escherichia coli*. J Biol. Chem 1979; 154:11010–11014.
16. Marra MN, Wilde CG, Griffith JE, Snable JL, Scott RW. Bactericidal/permeability-increasing protein has endotoxin-neutralizing activity. J Immunol 1990; 144:662–666.
17. Marra M, Wilde CG, Collins MS, Snable JL, Thornton MB, Scott RW. The role of bactericidal/permeability-increasing protein as a natural inhibitor of bacterial endotoxin. J Immunol 1992; 148:532–537.
18. Ooi CE, Weiss J, Doerfler ME, Elsbach P. Endotoxin-neutralizing properties of the 25 kD N-terminal fragment and a newly isolated 30 kD C-terminal fragment of the 55–60 kD bactericidal/permeability- increasing protein of human neutrophils. Exp Med 1991; 174:649–655.
19. Fisher CJ, Marra MN, Palardy JE, Marchbanks CR, Scott RW, Opal SM. Human neutrophil bactericidal/permeability-increasing protein reduces mortality rate from endotoxin challenge: a placebo-controlled study. Crit Care Med 1994; 22:553–558.
20. Ooi CE, Weiss J, Elsbach P, Frangione B, Mannion B. A 25-kDa NH2-terminal fragment carries all the antibacterial activities of the human neutrophil 60-kDa bactericidal/permeability-increasing protein. Biol Chem 1987; 262:14891–14894, 1987.
21. Meszaros K, Parent JB, Gazzano-Santoro H, et al. A recombinant amino terminal fragment of bactericidal/permeability increasing protein inhibits the induction of leukocyte responses by LPS. J Leukocyte Biol 1993; 54:558–563.
22. Betz-Corradin SB, Heumann D, Gallay P, Glauser MP. Bactericidal/permeability-increasing protein inhibits induction of macrophage nitric oxide production by lipopolysaccharide. J Infect Dis 1994; 169:105–111.
23. Huang K, Conlon PJ, Fishwild DM. A recombinant amino terminal fragment of bactericidal/permeability increasing protein (rBPI$_{23}$) inhibits soluble CD14-mediated LPS-induced endothelial adherence for human neutrophils. Shock 1994; 81–88.
24. Meszaros K, Aberle S, Dedrick R, et al. Monocyte tissue factor induction by lipopolysaccharide [LPS]: dependence on LPS-binding protein and CD14, and inhibition by a recombinant fragment of bactericidal/permeability increasing protein. Blood 1994; 83:2516–2525.
25. Kohn FR, Ammons WS, Horwitz A, et al. Protective effect of a recombinant amino-terminal fragment of bactericidal/permeability increasing protein in experimental endotoxemia. J Infect Dis 1993; 168:1307–1310.
26. Ammons WS, Kung AHC. Recombinant amino terminal fragment of bactericidal/permeability increasing protein prevents hemodynamic responses to endotoxin. Circ Shock 1993; 41:176–184.
27. Lin Y, Kohn FR, Kung AHC, Ammons WS. Protective effect of a recombinant fragment of bactericidal/permeability increasing protein against carbohydrate dyshomeostasis and tumor necrosis factor-α elevation in rat endotoxemia. J Biochem Pharmacol 1994; 43:1553–1559.

28. VanderMeer TJ, Menconi MJ, O'Sullivan BP, et al. Bactericidal/permeability increasing protein ameliorates acute lung injury and neutrophil activation in porcine endotoxemia. J Appl Physiol 1994; 76:2006–2014.

29. Weiss J, Elsbach P, Shu C, et al. Human bactericidal/permeability-increasing protein and a recombinant NH_2-terminal fragment cause killing of serum-resistant gram-negative bacteria in whole blood and inhibit tumor necrosis factor release induced by bacteria. J Clin Invest 1992: 90:1122–1130.

30. Kelly CJ, Cech AC, Argenteanu M, et al. Role of bactericidal permeability increasing protein in the treatment of gram-negative pneumonia. Surgery 1993; 114:140–146.

31. Cross AS, Opal SM, Palardy JE, Bodmer MW, Sadoff JC. The efficacy of combination immunotherapy in experimental *Pseudomonas* therapy. J Infect Dis 1993; 167:112–118.

32. Kohn FR, Philips GL, Klingemann HG. Regulation of tumor necrosis factor-α production and gene expression in monocytes. Bone Marrow Transplant 1992; 9:369–376.

33. Evans GF, Snyder YM, Butler LD, Zuckerman SH. Differential expression of interleukin-1 and tumor necrosis factor in murine septic shock models. Circ Shock 1989; 29:279–290.

34. Martin MA, Silverman HJ. Gram-negative sepsis and the adult respiratory distress syndrome. Clin Infect Dis 1992; 6:1213–1228.

35. Lin Y, Leach W, Ammons WS, Kung AHC. Protective effect of a recombinant N-terminal fragment of bactericidal/permeability increasing protein (rBPI[23]) in a conscious rabbit model of endotoxin shock. FASEB J 1994; 8:A797.

36. Saunders N, Cohen J. Interactions between bactericidal/permeability increasing protein (BPI) and gentamicin. In: Proceedings and Abstracts of the 33rd International Conference on Antimicrobial Agents and Chemotherapy, New Orleans, LA, October 3–7, 1993, abstr. 316, p. 177.

5

CAP18: A Novel LPS-Binding/Antimicrobial Protein

James W. Larrick
Palo Alto Institute of Molecular Medicine
Mountain View, California

Michimasa Hirata
Iwate Medical University
Morioka, Japan

Robert F. Balint
Palo Alto Institute of Molecular Medicine
Mountain View, California

Tai-huang Huang and Chinpan Chen
Academia Sinica
Nankang, Taipei, Taiwan, Republic of China

Jian Zhong and Susan C. Wright
Palo Alto Institute of Molecular Medicine
Mountain View, California

I. INTRODUCTION

A rational approach to the control of inflammation caused by gram-negative bacteria is to counteract the deleterious effects of LPS (1). Although antibiotics kill bacteria, they do not neutralize LPS, and many potentiate bacterial release of LPS that can accelerate the inflammatory process (2). LPS activates macrophages and endothelial cells, stimulating release of potent inflammatory mediators such as tumor necrosis factor (TNF) (3) and free radicals. Cationic antibiotics such as polymyxin B bind to and neutralize some types of LPS; however, clinical use is limited by toxicity (4,5), despite efforts to generate nontoxic molecules (6). Polyclonal antisera raised against the lipid-containing inner core structure of lipopolysaccharides, exposed on the outer membranes of rough mutant strains, exhibit cross-reactive anti-endotoxin and protective activities (7,8). Generation of neutralizing monoclonal antibodies (MABs) recognizing various types of LPS is another therapeutic approach; however, the large numbers of serologically unique gram-negative bacteria limit this approach. Antibodies made to the conserved regions of LPS such as the lipid A or core glycolipid appear to be ineffective against smooth forms of LPS, possibly due to steric effects of the O-antigen-specific polysaccharides. In-vitro studies, animal models, and clinical trials of various monoclonal and polyclonal antibodies have yielded equivocal or negative results (9–13).

Another therapeutic approach is to identify protein other than antibodies that bind to and neutralize LPS, such as proteins derived from the horseshoe crab, *Limulus* (14). The limulus anti-LPS factors (LALF) are isolated from the amebocytes of *Limulus polyphemus* (15) and *Tachypleus tridentatus* (16). These proteins are 70% homologous and have a molecular weight of 11,800. Recent studies suggest that the *L. polyphemus* protein partially protects rabbits from meningococcal septic shock (17). It is likely, however, that these proteins are highly immunogenic, thus limiting their potential therapeutic utility.

Several LPS-binding human proteins have been described, including an acute-phase protein produced by the liver called LPS-binding protein (LBP) (18–20) and a PMN granule protein called bactericidal permeability-increasing protein (BPI, CAP57) (21,22). Although recent studies demonstrate homologies between the sequences of LBP and BPI, the effects of these proteins on cellular responses appear to be opposite. High levels of LBP are produced in response to LPS. Furthermore, LPS complexed to LBP binds to the macrophage surface protein CD14 (23,24) and is 100-fold more potent than LPS alone in triggering various monocyte responses such as synthesis of TNF. Therefore, LBP may contribute to the pathogenesis of sepsis by augmenting macrophage activation in response to the complex of LBP and LPS. In contrast, BPI appears to function as part of the neutrophil's arsenal of antibacterial peptides. When granulocytes are attracted to sites of infection, they engulf gram-negative bacteria. BPI is located membrane bound inside the azurophilic granules and is therefore well situated to bind LPS released from phagocytosed bacteria. Furthermore, recent studies demonstrate that BPI binding to lipid A (25) inhibits many of the cellular responses to LPS. Accordingly, recombinant BPI (26) and the 23-kDa N-terminal fragment of BPI (27), which binds to LPS, are under clinical evaluation for treatment of sepsis.

Rabbit granulocytes contain an 18-kDa cationic protein with antimicrobial properties. We have purified this protein, called CAP18, using as an assay its capacity to agglutinate sheep red cells sensitized with LPS (28,29). This is a nonspecific assay, and we have corroborated the LPS-binding and antimicrobial activity of the molecule in several other systems (30–32). We have cloned human CAP18 and demonstrated that the C-terminal portion of human CAP18 also binds to LPS, neutralizes LPS-mediated activation of monocytes, and protects mice injected with lethal quantities of LPS.

II. MATERIALS AND METHODS

A. Endotoxins

LPS was from List Biologicals (Campbell, CA) unless indicated otherwise. *Escherichia coli* 0113 LPS and the *Pseudomonas aeruginosa* type 6 (12.4.4) were prepared by hot phenol extraction described by Rudbach et al. (33).

B. RBC Agglutination Assay

One milliliter of 1% erythrocytes (human O type, C3H/HeN mouse or sheep) was sensitized by incubating with 0.2 mL of Re-LPS solution [100 µg/mL] at 37°C for 30 min, followed by washing with PBS. Fifty microliters of 1.0% suspension of sensitized erythrocytes was mixed with 50 µL of a two-fold serial dilution of CAP18 or CAP18 peptides in a U-bottom microtiter plate and incubated at 37°C for 1 h. Activity of CAP18 was expressed as minimum agglutinating concentration (MAC).

C. Cloning of Human CAP18 cDNA

1.   Rabbit CAP18 cDNA

Details of the cDNA cloning of rabbit CAP18 have been published (34). The sequence is listed in GENBANK accession #M73998. The cDNA encodes a mature protein of 142 amino acids with a conventional 29-amino acid signal sequence (see Fig. 1). The sequence and hydropathic profile of this novel protein distinguishes it from other LPS-binding proteins such as LBP or BPI. The predicted m.w. is 16.6 kDa. The predicted pI is 10. There are no asparagine-linked carbohydrate attachment sites.

2. Human CAP18 cDNA

Numerous attempts to identify human CAP18 using PCR primers designed from C-terminal 37 amino acids of rabbit CAP18 were unsuccessful. Subsequently, duplicate filters were prepared from a million plaques and controls of a lambda gt11 human bone marrow cDNA library (purchased from Clontech Laboratories,

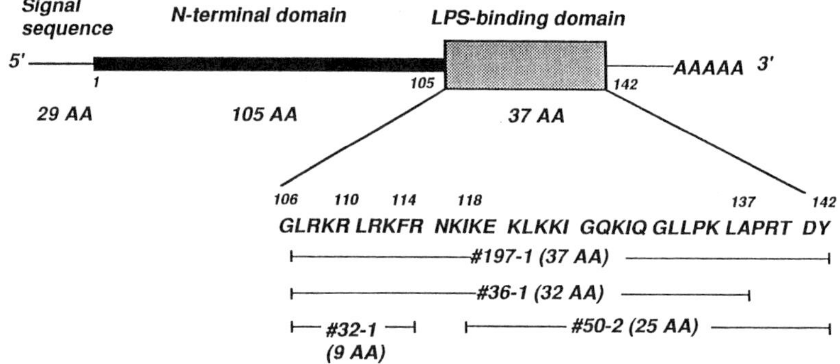

Peptides		LPS-binding	LPS-neutralizing	Anti-bacterial	Anti-coagulant
#197-1	CAP-18106-142	+	+	+	+
# 36-1	CAP-18106-137	+	+	+	+
# 32-1	CAP-18106-114	-	-	-	-
# 50-2	CAP-18118-142	-	-	-	-

Figure 1 Schematic presentation of the rabbit CAP18 cDNA. The protein is comprised of a 29-amino acid signal sequence, a conserved 105-amino acid N-terminal domain, and an LPS-binding 37-amino acid domain. The sequences and positions of the LPS-binding peptides used in this study are shown. Relative activities of the peptides in LPS binding, LPS neutralizing, antimicrobial, and anticoagulant assays are shown.

Palo Alto, CA). One set of filters was screened with the rabbit CAP18 cDNA and the other was screened with a $CAP_{104-140}$ probe. Both probes were labeled with ^{32}P using PCR. No positives were identified from a total of 500,000 plaques screened at standard stringency using the probe. However, using the CAP18 probe, 14 putative positives were identified from a total of 500,000 plaques screened under reduced stringency. In this case temperature and salt were kept constant and formamide was reduced from 50% to 30% during prehybridization and hybridization with washing at 50°C instead of 65°C. Six of the most intense positives were chosen for a second round of screening, and four of these yielded unequivocal individual positive plaques. Lambda DNA was purified and the inserts cloned into TA sequencing vectors. One of these was a false positive, whereas three were bona-fide CAP18 cDNAs of slightly different lengths.

D. Assay of Reactive Nitrogen Intermediates

The murine macrophage cell line RAW 264.7 (obtained from ATCC) and thiogly-collate-elicited murine peritoneal exudate cells were used to produce RNI. Cells were cultured at 1×10^6/mL in RPMI-1640 + 2.5% FCS in 24 well plates in the presence or absence of different concentrations of LPS or murine rIFNγ. After 24 h of incubation at 37°C, the cell-free supernatant was collected and tested for the presence of reactive nitrogen intermediates (RNI). Accumulation of nitrite in the medium was measured by a colorimetric assay based on the Griess reaction (35) using sodium nitrite standards. Sample (50 μL) was mixed with 50 μL of Griess reagent (1% sulfanilamide, 0.1% naphthalene diamine dihydrochloride, 2.5% H_3PO_4) and, after 10 min at room temperature, absorbance was read at 570 nm.

E. Tissue Factor Assay

Salmonella minnesota smooth LPS was incubated with indicated concentrations of each peptide for 5 min, then the mixture was added to peritoneal murine macrophages obtained 4 days after thioglycollate stimulation. Cells were cultured with LPS +/-CAP18 peptides for 6 h at 37°C in a 5% CO_2 incubator. The cell suspension was centrifuged and the cell pellet was frozen at -80°C until clotting assays were run. Tissue factor activity was tested in modified unactivated partial thromboplastin time. Cell lysate (1×10^6 cells, 100 μL) was preincubated with 100 μL of mouse plasma at 37°C for 3 min. Then 100 μL of 25 mM $CaCl_2$ containing phospholipid was added to the mixture and clotting time was measured using a Fibrometer (BioQuest Division, Becton Dickinson, Cokeysville, NC).

F. Preparation of Peptides

1. General

Peptide synthesis was carried out on either an Applied Biosystems model 430A or 431A peptide synthesizer. High-performance liquid chromatography (HPLC) was performed on an LDC apparatus equipped with two Constametric pumps, a Gradient Master solvent programmer and mixer, and a Spectromonitor III variable-wavelength ultraviolent detector. Analytical HPLC was performed in reversed-phase mode on a Waters mBondapak C_{18} column (0.4 $\times$ 30 cm) using linear gradients of buffer A (0.022% TFA/H_2O) and buffer B (0.022% TFA/CH^3CN) at 2.0-mL/min flow rate. Preparative HPLC separations were run on a Whatman Magnum 20 partisil 10 ODS-3 column (2 $\times$ 50 cm) equipped with a Waters Guard-Pak C_{18} precolumn. For amino acid composition analyses, peptides were hydrolyzed in 6 N HCI, containing 1 mg of phenol, at 115°C for 22 h in sealed, evacuated hydrolysis tubes. Analyses were performed on a Waters HPLC-based amino acid analysis system using either a Waters Cat Ex resin or a Pierce AA511 column and ninhydrin detection. HF cleavage reactions were performed in a Peninsula Teflon HF apparatus. Fast-atom bombardment mass spectra (FAB-MS) were obtained on a VG 70E-HF mass spectrometer.

2. Reagents

Unless otherwise stated, all reagents and solvents were obtained commercially as reagent grade and used without further purification. DIPEA was purchased from PPG Industries (Natrium, WV) and distilled from CaO and ninhydrin. TFA was purchased from Halocarbon (North Augusta, SC). Water for HPLC was prepared from doubly deionized, filtered water and purified on a Hydro Services purification unit. t-Boc and Fmoc protected amino acids were purchased from Bachem (Torrance, CA) or Advanced ChemTech (Louisville, KY). BHA resin (100–200 mesh) was obtained from Bachem. Boc-Tyr(Br-Z)-OCH$_2$-Pam resin and HMP resin were obtained from Applied Biosystems (Foster City, CA).

3. Preparation of Peptides

Rabbit CAP18 is comprised of 142 amino acids; human CAP18 is comprised of 140 amino acids. Peptide fragments of CAP18 are numbered accordingly. Peptide synthesis was carried out on either an Applied Biosystems model 430A or 431A peptide synthesizer. HPLC chromatography was performed on an LDC apparatus equipped with two Constametric pumps, a Gradient Master solvent programmer and mixer, and a Spectromonitor III variable-wavelength UV detector. Fast-atom bombardment mass spectra (FAB-MS) were obtained on a VG 70E-HF mass spectrometer. Final purification was carried out by preparative HPLC. The peptides were applied to the column in a minimum volume of either 10–20% AcOH or 0.1% TFA. Gradient elutions were performed using linear gradients of buffer A (0.1% TFA/H$_2$O) and buffer B (0.1% TFA/CH$_3$CN) at a flow rate of 8.0 mL/min with UV detection at 220 nm. Fractions were collected at 1.5- to 2.5 to -min intervals and inspected by analytical HPLC in the reversed-phase mode as stated above. Fractions judged to be of high purity were pooled and lyophilized. The final products were characterized by analytical HPLC and amino acid analysis. The purified peptides were also subjected to fast-atom bombardment mass spectrometry (FAB-MS) and yielded the expected parent M + H ions within acceptable limits (± 1 mass unit).

CAP 18$_{104-140}$-derived peptides were prepared using solid-phase synthesis procedures as generally described by Barany and Merrifield (36). All amino acids were protected either as the N^a-Boc or N^a-Fmoc derivatives. The protecting groups for the amino acid side chains were as follows: Boc chemistry: Arg(tosyl), Asp (cyclohexyl ester), Glu (benzyl ester), Tyr (2,6-dichlorobenzyl ether), Lys (2-chloro-benzyloxycarbonyl), and Thr (benzyl ether); Fmoc chemistry: Arg(Pmc), Asp and Glu (t-butyl ester), Asn and Gln (trityl), Lys (Boc), and Thr and Tyr (t-butyl ether). For the synthesis of C-terminal amides using Boc or Fmoc chemistry, BHA resin or Fmoc-Linker-Bha resin (37) was used, respectively. For the synthesis of C-terminal acids using Boc or Fmoc chemistry, Boc-Tyr(Br-Z)-OCH$_2$-Pam resin or HMP resin was used, respectively. Solid-phase synthesis was performed on the Applied Biosystems synthesizers using standard protocols. For Boc chemistry, all amino acids were coupled as the preformed symmetrical anhydrides (2:1 equivalent, protected amino acid/DCC) except for Asn, Gln, and Arg, which were incorporated as performed HOBT esters. For Fmoc chemistry, all amino acids were coupled using the HBTU/HOBT "FastMoc" protocol.

Peptides were deblocked and cleaved from the resin by either of two methods. For Boc/Bzl chemistry, the peptide resins (0.5 g) were treated with 50 mL of ethanedithiol, 0.5 mL of anisole, and 4.5 mL of liquid hydrogen fluoride at 0°C for 45 min. Volatile reagents were removed under vacuum at ice-bath temperature. The residues were washed with three 20-mL volumes of Et_2O and filtered. The peptides were extracted from the resin by washing with three 20-mL volumes of 10% AcOH and filtered. The combined aqueous filtrates were lyophilized to yield the crude product. For Fmoc/tBu chemistry, the peptide resins (0.5 g) were treated with 50 mL of dimethylsulfide, 50 mL of ethanedithiol, 150 mL of anisole, and 5.0 mL of trifluoroacetic acid at room temperature for 2 h. The reaction mixture was filtered and the spent resin washed with three 1-mL volumes of trifluoroacetic acid. The combined filtrates were precipitated from 200 mL of Et_2O. The precipitated solid was filtered off, washed with three 20-mL volumes of Et_2O, redissolved in 10% AcOH, and filtered. The combined aqueous filtrates were lyophilized to yield the crude product.

Final purification was carried out by preparative HPLC. The peptides were applied to the column in a minimum volume of either 10–20% AcOH or 0.1% TFA. Gradient elutions were performed using linear gradients of buffer A (0.1% TFA/H_2O) and buffer B (0.1% TFA/CH_3CN) at a flow rate of 8.0 mL/min with UV detection at 220 nm. Fractions were collected at 1.5- to 2.5-min intervals and inspected by analytical HPLC in the reversed-phase mode as stated above. Fractions judged to be of high purity were pooled and lyophilized.

The final products were characterized by analytical HPLC and amino acid analysis. The composition values obtained were within acceptable limits. The purified peptides were also subjected to fast-atom bombardment mass spectrometry (FAB-MS) and yielded the expected parent M + H ions within acceptable limits ($\pm$1 mass unit).

G. Mouse LPS-Induced Lethality Assays

1. Galactosamine-Sensitized Mouse Model

This assay was performed as described by Galanos et al. (38). C57BL/6 mice (males, 8–12 weeks of age) were injected i.p. with 15 mg of galactosamine alone or 15 mg of galactosamine plus 0.1 μg of smooth LPS from *S. minnesota*. Equal volumes of 100 μL of LPS or CAP 18 peptides were mixed and incubated for 30 min at 37°C prior to injection. Survival at 1 week was recorded.

2. Actinomycin D-Sensitized Mouse Model

This assay was performed as described by Pieroni et al. (39). Briefly, 10-fold dilutions of *E. coli* O111:B4 LPS in pyrogen-free saline or saline alone were incubated 1:1 with 20 μ/mL of CAP18$_{104-140}$ for 30 min at 37°C. One hundred microliters of this solution together with 100 μL of a solution of 250 μmL actinomycin D were injected i.p. into groups of 7–11 ddY mice (male, 10–12 weeks of age). Thus, all mice received 1.0 μg of CAP18 peptides, 25 μg of actinomycin D, and dilutions of LPS or saline. Results were recorded as survivors/total mice at 1 week.

H. Antibacterial Activity

1. Bacterial Strains

S. typhimurium LT2(S), *S. minnesota* R595 (Re), *E. coli* O9:K39 (K$^+$, K$^-$), *E. coli* O111:B4, *Streptococcus pneumoniae*, *S. pyogenes*, *P. aeruginosa*, *Klebsiella pneumoniae*, *Staphylococcus aureus* (methicillin sensitive = MSSA and resistant = MRSA), and *Candida albicans* were used. The latter five strains were clinical isolates.

2. Bactericidal Assay

All strains were grown in Tryptosoy broth (Eiken Co., Tokyo, Japan). *S. typhimurium* LT2(S), *S. minnesota* R595(Re), *E. coli* O9:K39(K$^+$, K^{K-}), *E. coli* O111:B4, and *K. pneumoniae* were plated on nutrient agar (Eiken Co.). *P. aeruginosa* and *C. albicans* were plated on NAC agar and GS (Guanofracin-Sabouraud) agar plates, respectively. Bacterial cultures were collected at logarithmic phase and washed twice with phosphate-buffered saline pH 7.2, and adjusted to a final concentration of $5 \times 10^3 - 1 \times 10^4$ cells/mL. To 450 μL of bacterial suspension, 50 μL of peptide was added and incubated at 37°C for 1 h, and 100 μL of the reaction mixture was plated on the agar plate. After 24-hincubation at 37°C, colony-forming units (CFU) were counted. As a control experiment, PBS was added to bacterial suspension and incubated for 1 h, plated on agar, and cultured. For some experiments the percent of control CFU was determined.

I. ^{3}H-Thymindine-Incorporation Bacterial Proliferation Assay

Bacteria were grown in Trypticase broth overnight. The following day, bacteria were suspended at 10^5/mL in RPMI with 10% fetal calf serum (FCS). The assay was set up in a 96-well plate containing 50μL of bacteria plus 50 μL of peptides and incubated at 37°C for 1 h, then 1 μCi of [^{3}H]-thymidine (Amersham) was added to each well and incubated with the bacteria overnight. The assay was terminated by addition of 10% TCA, and cells were harvested and counted on a Matrix 96 Packard beta counter.

J. Statistical Analysis

Results are expressed as mean $\pm$ SD of at least three or four samples. Student's *t* test for unpaired data was used to determine statistical significance. A two-tailed *p* value of <0.05 was considered significant. IC_{50} values were determined by least-squares linear regression.

III. RESULTS

A. Identification and Structure of CAP18

Rabbit CAP18 was identified and cloned as previously described (34). The protein was shown to have two domains, a highly conserved N-terminal domain of 105 amino acids and a less conserved LPS-binding domain. Figure 1 presents a schematic diagram of the rabbit CAP18 cDNA and summarizes the activity of the C-terminal domain-derived peptides.

The human CAP18 cDNA was identified and sequenced as described under "Materials and Methods" (see Fig. 1). Translation of the cDNA reveals a protein with a conventional 30-amino acid signal sequence. Like rabbit CAP18, the mature protein has two domains: an amino-terminal domain with high homology to other known members of the CAP18 gene family and a carboxy-terminal endotoxin-binding domain with less homology. The amino acid identities of human, cow, pig, and rabbit CAP18s are shown in Fig. 2. Tables 1 and 2 indicates the amino acid and base composition homologies of the rabbit and human CAP18 proteins. There is a much higher level of nucleic acid and amino acid conservation in the N-terminal domain compared to the carboxy-terminal LPS-binding domain. The overall nucleic acid identity between domains is similar, 73–74%, but the N-terminal domains share 63% amino acid whereas the C-terminal domains share only 38% identity.

B. Anti-LPS Activities of CAP18 Peptides

1. Synthetic CAP18$_{104-140}$ Peptides Inhibit Bioactivities of LPS in vitro

a. Agglutination of LPS-Sensitized Erythrocytes by Synthetic CAP18 Peptides; LPS-Binding Activity.   Previous studies showed that rabbit CAP18 was comprised of two domains: a highly conserved N-terminal domain of unknown

Table 1 Human and Rabbit CAP 18 Amino Acid Identity

Domain	Nucleic acid	Amino acid
N-terminal domain	74%	63%
LPS-binding domain	73%	38%

CAP18 Family

Cysteine Rich Domain

```
CAP18    (Hum)       QVLSYKEAVLRAIDGINQRSSDANLYRLLDLDPRPTMDGDPDTPNPV
CAP18    (Rab)       QDLTYREAVLRAVDAFNQQSSEAHLYRLLSMDPQQLEDAKPYTPQPV

Cathelin (Pig)        LRYREAVLRAVDRLNEQSSEANLYRLLELDQPPKADEDPGTPKPV
PMAP-36              QALSYREAVLRAVDRLNEQSSEANLYRLLELDQPPKADEDPGTPKPV
PMAP-23              QALSYREAVLRAVDRLNEQSSEANLYRLLELDQPPKADEDPGTPKPV
PG-2                 QALSYREAVLRAVDRLNEQSSEANLYRLLELDQPPKADEDPGTPKPV
PR-39               QALSYREAVLRAVDRLNEQSSEANLYRLLELDQPPKADEDPGTPKPV
Indol    (Cow)       QALSYREAVLRAVDQLNELSSEANLYRLLELDPPPKDNEDLGTRKPV
p15hα    (Hu)       IPHRRLRYEEVVAQALAFYNEGQQGQPLYRLLEATPPPSLNSKS..RIPL
p15hβ               --R-----------------------------------------------

CAP18    (Hum)       SFTVKETVCPRTTQQSPEDCDFKKDGLVNRCMGTVTLNQARGSFDISCDN
CAP18    (Rab)       SFTVKETECPRTTWKLPEQCDFKEDGLVKRCVGTVTRYQAWDSFDIRCNR

Cathelin (Pig)       SFTVKETVCPRPTRQPPELCDFKE....KQCVGTVTLNPSIHSLDISCNE
PMAP-36             SFTVKETVCPRPTWPPPELCDFKENGRVKQCVGTVTLNPSNDPLDINCDE
PMAP-23             SFTVKETVCPRPTRQPPELCDFKENGRVKQCVGTVTLKEIRGNFDITCNQ
PG-2                SFTVKETVCPRPTRQPPELCDFKENGRVKQCVGTVTLDQIKDPLDITCNB
PR-39               SFTVKETVCPRPTRQPPELCDFKENGRVKQCVGTVTLNPSIHSLDISCNE
Indol    (Cow)       SFTVKETVCPRTIQQPAEQCDFKEKGRVKQCVGTVTLDPSNDQFDLNCNE
p15H     (Hum)       NFRIKETVCIFTLDRQPGNCAFREGGEERICRGAFVRRRRVRALTLRCDR
p15hβ               -----------------------------------------W-------------
```

Antimicrobial Domain

```
CAP18    (Hum)       DNKRFA      LLGDFFRKSNEKIGNEFKRIVQRIKDFLRQLVPRTES
CAP18    (Rab)       AQESPEPT    GLRKRLRKFRNKIKEKLKKIGQKIQGLLPKLAPRTDY

Cathelin (Pig)       IQSV
PMAP-36             IQSV        GRFRRLRKKTRKRLKKIGKVLKWIPPIVGSIPIGCG
PMAP-23             LQSV        RIIDLLWRVRRPQKPKFVTVWVR
PG-2                VQGV        RGGRLCYCRRRFCICVG
PR-39               IQSV        RRRPRPPYLPRPRPPFFPPRLPPRIPPGFPPRFPPRFPGKT
Indol    (Cow)       LQSV        ILPWKWPWWPWRRG
p15H     (Hum)       DQRR        QPEFPRVTRPAGPTA
p15hβ               --------------------
```

Figure 2 Comparison of amino acid sequences of CAP18 family members, human, pig, rabbit, cow.

function and a much less conserved C-terminal domain with anti-LPS and antimicrobial function (see Fig. 1). These studies also identified a more active fragment corresponding to rabbit CAP18$_{106-137}$. Therefore we studied the full-length C-terminal fragment of human CAP18, CAP18$_{104-140}$, and a truncated version, human CAP18$_{104-135}$. The capacity of these human and rabbit peptides to agglutinate LPS-sensitized erythrocytes is compared in Table 3. As was the case for the rabbit peptides, the truncated human peptide (CAP18$_{104-135}$) is more active than the full-length human peptide CAP18$_{104-140}$. The activities of these two peptides were compared in several of the assays described below.

Table 2 Identical Amino Acids in the N-Terminal Domains of CAP18 Family Members

	Human	Pig	Cow	Rabbit	p15H
Human	100%				
Pig	61.6%	100%			
Cow	58.4%	78.9%	100%		
Rabbit	63.1%	64.2%	59.4%	100%	
p15H	31.3%	34.4%	33.3%	31.3%	100%

Table 3 LPS-Binding Activities of Synthetic Human and Rabbit CAP18-Derived Amino-Terminal Peptides

	Sequence	LPS-binding activity (MAC; μg/mL)
Rabbit	$CAP18_{106\text{-}142}$	4.2
	$CAP18_{106\text{-}137}$	2.1
Human	$CAP18_{104\text{-}140}$	12.1
	$CAP18_{104\text{-}135}$	1.6

MAC, minimal agglutinating concentration of *S. minnesota* Re-LPS-sensitized sheep erythrocytes. Average of two experiments.

b. Synthetic Human $CAP18_{104-140}$ Inhibits LPS-Induced RNI Production. Low concentrations of lipopolysaccharide stimulate mouse macrophage RAW 264.7 cells to produce substantial quantities of reactive nitrogen intermediates (RNI). An LPS dose-response is shown in Fig.3 (upper). Figure 3 (lower) demonstrates the capacity of synthetic rabbit $CAP18_{106-137}$ and human $CAP18_{104-140}$ to inhibit RNI release from RAW 264.7 cells stimulated with 2.5 ng/mL LPS. The IC_{50} is approximately 50 nM. Control experiments demonstrated that one of the inactive cationic fragments of rabbit $CAP18_{104-140}$ ($CAP18_{122-142}$) did not block LPS-induced nitric oxide release (data not shown), and addition of CAP18 or CAP18 peptides to supernatants from LPS-stimulated RAW264.7 cells did not interfere with the ability to detect RNI in the Griess reaction (data not shown).

c. $CAP18_{104-140}$ Peptides Inhibit LPS-Induced Tissue Factor Generation by Macrophages. Previous studies demonstrated that unpurified CAP inhibited LPS-induced tissue factor expression by murine macrophages. After the identification of rabbit $CAP18_{106-142}$ as the active LPS-binding portion of CAP18, these

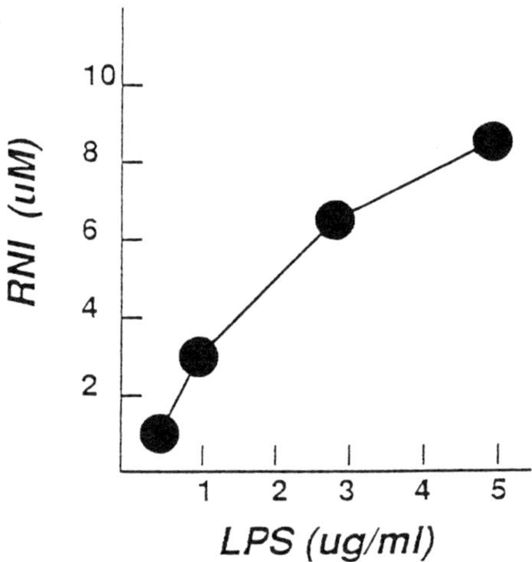

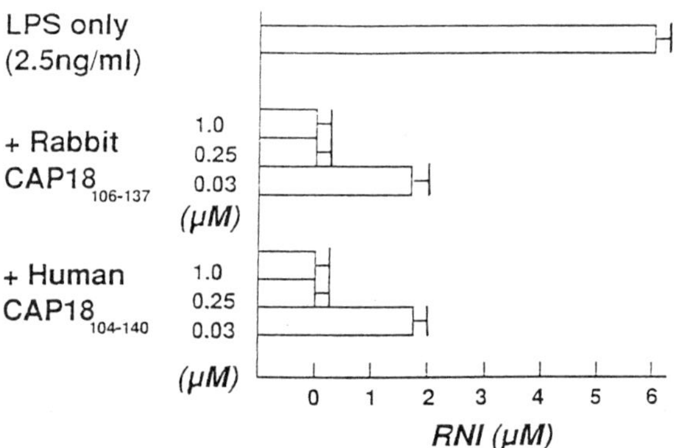

Figure 3 Synthetic human CAP18$_{104-140}$ and rabbit CAP18$_{106-137}$ inhibit LPS-stimulated release of nitrogen radicals by murine RAW 64.7 macrophages: upper, LPS dose response; lower, inhibition of RNI released in response to 2.5 ng/mL of LPS by CAP18 peptides.

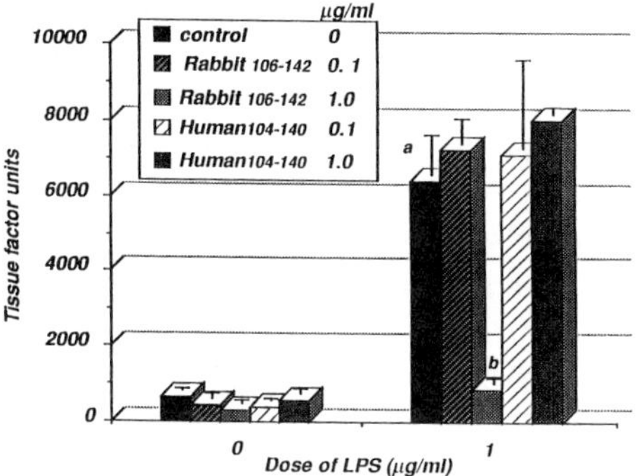

S-LPS was incubated with each peptide at 37 °C for 5 min, then the mixture was added to cell suspension and cultured for 6 hours.
a) $p < 0.05$ compared with medium control.
b) $p < 0.05$ compared with LPS control.

(A)

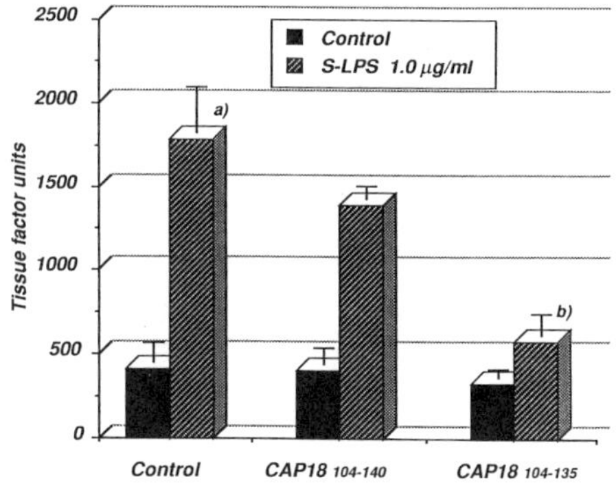

S-LPS was incubated with each peptide (1.0 µg/ml) at 37°C for 5 min, then the mixture was added to cell suspension and cultured for 6 hours.
a) $p < 0.05$ compared with medium control.
b) $p < 0.05$ compared with LPS control.

(B)

Figure 4 Effect of human and rabbit CAP18 peptides on LPS-induced tissue factor generation. (A) Full-length rabbit $CAP18_{106-142}$ peptide but not full-length human $CAP18_{104-140}$ peptide is active. (B) Truncated human CAP18 peptide $CAP18_{104-135}$ attenuated LPS-induced generation of tissue factor.

findings were confirmed using synthetic $CAP18_{106-142}$ and derivative peptides (Hirata, in prep.). The activities of human $CAP18_{104-140}$ and the truncated $CAP18_{104-135}$ were compared to the rabbit peptides. Various concentrations of *S. minnesota* smooth LPS were incubated with each peptide at 37°C for 5 min prior to mixing with thioglycollate-stimulated murine peritoneal macrophages.

Production of tissue factor after 6 h was measured by clotting assay. Figure 5 shows that the tissue factor induced in response to 0.1 and 1μg/mL LPS was inhibited by full-length rabbit but not full-length human CAP18 peptides. Previous work demonstrated that the non-LPS-binding peptides $CAP18_{105-114}$ and $CAP18_{117-142}$ do not inhibit LPS-induced tissue factor (Hirata), and in the absence of LPS no tissue factor is synthesized by these cells. The truncated human CAP18 peptide ($CAP18_{104-135}$) demonstrated activity comparable to that of the rabbit peptide (see Fig. 5).

In summary, the truncated human peptide $CAP18_{104-135}$ inhibits LPS induction of tissue factor at concentrations similar to those previously observed for the rabbit CAP18 peptides. Related cationic peptides without LPS-binding activity do not inhibit LPS induction of tissue factor.

2.   Synthetic $CAP18_{104-140}$ Fragment Inhibits LPS Lethality in Mice

Murine models of endotoxemia were tested to evaluate the ability of CAP18 peptides to neutralized LPS in vivo. Although rodents are relatively resistant to the lethal effects of LPS, pretreatment with galactosamine or actinomycin D will augment their sensitivity. $CAP18_{104-135}$ attentuates the lethality of LPS to

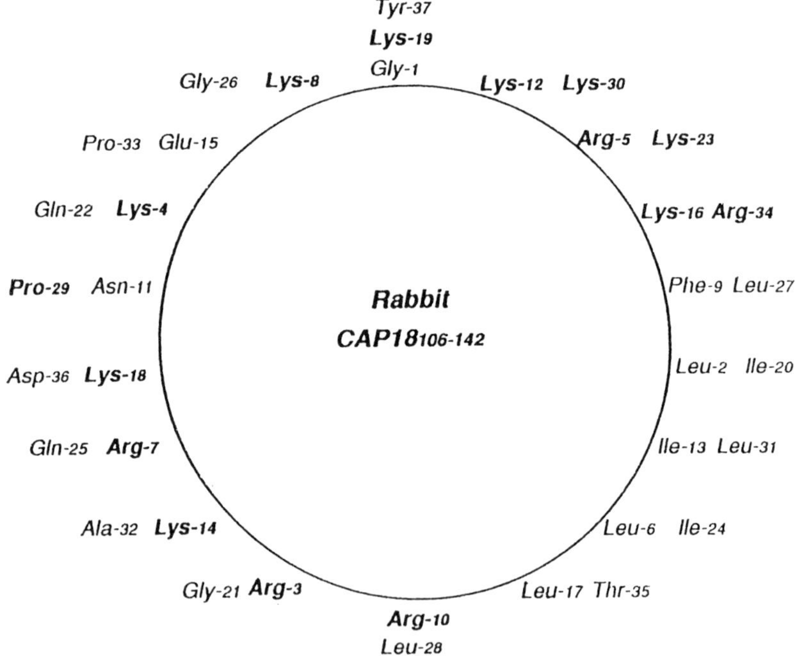

Figure 5   Alpha-helical presentation of rabbit $CAP18_{106-142}$.

actinomycin D-sensitized (Table 4A) and galactosamine-sensitized mice (Table 4B), but $CAP18_{104-140}$ was not protective in these models, which is consistent with its relatively weaker anti-LPS activity in vitro (data not shown).

C. Antimicrobial Activity of CAP18 Peptides

1. Activity of Rabbit CAP18 Peptides

Previously we showed that rabbit CAP18 peptides have antimicrobial activity versus gram-positive bacteria, suggesting that their activity is not limited to interaction with LPS. Table 5 summarizes the antimicrobial activity of full-length C-terminal rabbit $CAP18_{106-142}$ compared to a more active 5-amino acid truncated version of this peptide, $CAP18_{106-137}$, and two non-LPS-binding, non-microbial fragments of rabbit CAP18.

Table 4A Human $CAP18_{104-135}$ Blocks LPS Lethality in Actinomycin D-Treated Mice

Peptide (μg/mouse)	S-LPS (μg/mouse)	No. of mice dead/total	Survival (%)
—	—	0/7	100
—	1.0	10/11	9.1
$CAP18_{104-140}$ 1.0	1.0	7/7	0
$CAP18_{104-135}$ 1.0	1.0	2/7	71.4[a]

S-LPS (10 μg/mL) was incubated with equal volume of each peptide (10 μg/mL) at 37°BC for 30 min, then the mixture (0.2 mL) was injected i.p. Actinomycin D was injected i.p. (25 μg/ mouse).
[a]$p < 0.05$ compared with LPS control.

Table 4B Human $CAP18_{104-135}$ Blocks LPS Lethality in Galactosamine-Treated C57BL/6 Mice

$CAP18_{104-135}$ (μg/mouse)	S-LPS (μg/mouse)	No. of mice dead/total	Survival (%)
—	—	0/7	100
1	—	0/7	100
—	0.1	13/16	18.8
0.1	0.1	8/12	33.3
1	0.1	4/12	66.7[a]

S-LPS (1 μg/mL) was incubated with equal volume of each peptide (10 or 1 μmg/mL) at 37°BBC for 30 min, then the mixture (0.2 mL) was injected i.p. Galactosamine was injected i.p. (15 mg/mouse).
[a]$p < 0.05$ compared with LPS control.

Table 5 Antibacterial Activity of Rabbit CAP18 Peptides

		CAP18$_{106-142}$ IC$_{50}$(μg/mL)	CAP18$_{106-137}$ IC$_{50}$(μg/mL)	CAP18$_{106-114}$ IC$_{50}$(μg/mL)	CAP18$_{118-142}$ IC$_{50}$(μg/mL)
Gram negative	*S. typhimurium* LT2(S)	0.22–0.28	0.14–0.25	>20	>20
	S. minnesota Re	<0.25	<0.25	>20	>20
	E. coli O111:B4	0.50	0.20	20	>20
	E. coli O9:K39 K$^+$	0.14	0.58	—	—
	K$^-$	0.68	0.90	—	—
	P. aeruginosa	<0.25	<0.25	>20	>20
	K. pneumoniae	0.44	0.54	—	—
Gram positive	*S. aureus* MSSA*	0.94	0.58	—	—
	MRSA**	1.00	0.72	—	—
	C. albicans	>20	>20	—	—

*Methicillin sensitive; **methicillin resistant.

2. Human CAP18 Peptides Inhibit Growth of Diverse Strains of Gram-Negative and Gram-Positive Bacteria

The antimicrobial activity of the human peptides was measured in standard CFU assays. Table 6 summarizes the IC_{50} for both gram-negative and gram-positive bacteria. The full-length human peptide is less active and the truncated human peptide is more active than their rabbit homologs. The antimicrobial activity of the human peptides was evaluated versus clinical isolates of *S. aureus*. The truncated human $CAP18_{104-135}$ is more active versus both methicillin-sensitive and methicillin-resistant *S. aureus* (respective $IC_{50} = 2.8$ μg/mL versus 7.2–9.0 μg/mL, see Table 6). The truncated human peptide $CAP18_{104-135}$ is more actively antimicrobial versus almost all of the strains tested.

Lipoteichoic acid (LTA) is a component of the cell wall of most gram-positive bacteria and can bind to mammalian cells and elicit a variety of responses. LTA from *S. aureus* induces macrophage tissue factor. Preliminary dose-response studies demonstrated that 1.0 μg/mL of *S. aureus* LTA gave optimal stimulation (data not shown). Human $CAP18_{104-135}$ peptide does not inhibit lipoteichoic acid–induced generation of tissue factor (data not shown).

Finally, the effect of serum on killing was studied becuase other antimicrobial peptides require nonphysiological conditions [e.g., hypotonic buffers and acidic pH (5.0–5.5)] to exhibit activity. The addition of 10% fetal calf serum to the proliferation assay performed in RPMI-1640 results in only a modest decrease in antibacterial activity (13–17%, data not shown).

The highly active antibacterial peptides human and rabbit CAP18 peptides were inactive versus *C. albicans* (IC_{50} >20 μg/mL). The most active rabbit

Table 6 Antibacterial Activity of Human CAP18 Peptides

		$CAP18_{104-140}$ IC_{50} (μg/mL)	$CAP18_{104-135}$ IC_{50} (μg/mL)
Gram negative	*S. typhimurium* LT2(S)	3.5	3.7
	S. minnesota Re	0.2	<0.1
	E. coli	1.6	2.2
	E. coli O9:K39 K^+	0.9	0.5
	K^-	1.3	2.1
	P. aeruginosa	1.3	0.6
	K. pneumoniae	4.2	4.0
Gram positive	*S. aurens* MSSA*	7.2	2.8
	MRSA**	9.0	2.8
	C. albicans	>20	>20
LPS-binding activity, MAC (μg/mL)		12.5	1.6

*methicillin sensitive; **methicillin resistant.

peptide was inactive versus multiple drug-resistant *M. tuberculosis* and two strains of *Mycobacterium avium* (Dr. Heifets, National Jewish Center for Immunology and Respiratory Medicine, Denver, CO; data not shown).

IV. DISCUSSION

CAP18 was originally described as a cationic antimicrobial protein of molecular weight 18 kDa that agglutinated Re-LPS-coated erythrocytes and mediated bacterial cytolysis in vitro. Using as an assay the agglutination of Re-LPS-coated erythrocytes, we purified rabbit CAP18 and cloned the cDNA (34). To our surprise, the sequence of the purified protein corresponded to the C-terminal 37 amino acids of the protein. Subsequent experiments confirmed that the C-terminal domain of CAP18 neutralized various activities of LPS. Recently we cloned the human CAP18 cDNA. Using the translation of this cDNA, we have identified the corresponding C-terminal domain, $CAP18_{104-140}$.

Since the publication of our original paper describing the cDNA for CAP18, several interesting sequences have been added to the databases, suggesting that CAP18 is a member of a novel multigene family comprised of two functional domains (see Fig. 2). We hypothesized that the LPS domain would be highly conserved and designed our initial cloning strategy accordingly. Unexpectedly, this domain shares less than 40% amino acid identity among CAP18 family members versus the N-terminal domain, which shares 60–70% homology. A more distant relative of the family (about 30% identity) was cloned by Levy et al. (40). This protein, also isolated from human leukocytes, potentiates the antimicrobial activity of BPI. An interesting paper from the group of Ritonja et al. (41), suggesting that porcine CAP18 was a cysteine protease inhibitor, proved to be incorrect when this group subsequently reported identification of a stefinlike protease inhibitor active in the low picomolar range from pig leukocytes that probably contaminated their preparation of porcine CAP18. Thus, at the present time the function of the more highly conserved N-termainal domain of CAP18 is not known.

Several other families of granulocyte proteins exhibit LPS binding and antimicrobial activity. These include the 13-amino acid C-terminal peptide of bovine indolicidin, the 30- to 35-amino acid family of defensins (42,43), and azurocidin (CAP37) (33). The indolicidin peptides (42) and the defensins inhibit the growth of gram-positive and gram-negative bacteria only in hypotonic media, thus distinguishing them from $CAP18_{104-140}$ (JWL, unpublished). A recent publication describes peptides derived from CAP37 which are active at a concentration approximately 2–3 logs higher than the peptides derived from CAP18 described herein (43). Future studies will be required to investigate the relative roles of this diverse group of proteins in host defense.

Human $CAP18_{104-135}$ binds to and inhibits LPS activity in several in-vitro assays. These include the capacity to inhibit LPS-induced generation of nitric oxide and tissue factor. Binding to LPS and inhibition of multiple LPS activities appears to be a major function of the C-terminal domain of CAP18, $CAP18_{104-140}$. The truncated 32-amino acid peptide, $CAP18_{104-135}$, is more active than the native peptide. $CAP18_{104-140}$ was originally defined by its inhibition of LPS induction of nitric oxide synthetase. Uncontrolled synthesis of nitric oxide "reactive nitrogen intermediates" by monocytes and macrophages is a key step in the systemic vascular response in sepsis. Although RNI produced by macrophages play a beneficial and important role in the antimicrobial and antitumor activities of monocytes, they also mediate carcinogenic and tissue-destructive activities of inflammatory cells (44–49). Activated macrophages metabolize L-arginine to citrulline and NO^{2-}/NO^{3-}. Cellular injury from induction of this pathway results from NO inhibition of several important enzymes, including the tricarboxylic acid cycle enzyme aconitase, complex I and complex II of the electron transport chain, and ribonucleotide reductase. In addition, nitric oxide is released by endothelial cells and accounts for the activity of endothelium-derived relaxing factor (EDRF) (50,51). Recent studies indicate that EDRF may mediate TNF-induced hypotension (52). Native rabbit $CAP18_{104-140}$ inhibits the synergistic activity of LPS and interferon gamma to stimulate macrophage RNI production. Thus LPS directly induces substances such as TNF and other cytokines, nitric oxide, etc., that mediate deleterious effects on microvascular cells that contribute to capillary leak, tissue injury, and ultimately to multiple organ failure. Thus attenuation of these LPS-induced mediators by $CAP18_{104-135}$ may be a crucial event in decreasing the in-vivo toxicity of LPS.

In the direct inhibition of LPS-induced nitric oxide production, approximately 1μg/mL of $CAP18_{104-135}$ was required to block the activity of 1–5 ng/mL of purified LPS. It is not clear why a large molar excess of the peptide is required to block activity in vitro (e.g., in the LPS-induced RNI assays), whereas a smaller molar excess is required in vivo. One possibility is that the peptide does not neutralize LPS directly in vivo but rather acts to clear LPS. Another possibility is that the peptide has other activities such as modulation of blood coagulation (Hirata et al., unpublished). Finally, it should be noted that the plasma of septic humans seldom contains >1 ng/ml of LPS (53). Because limited toxicology studies indicated that $CAP18_{104-135}$ does not exhibit acute toxicity in mice when given at doses up to 20 mg/kg, it is likely that LPS released during sepsis in humans can be neutralized by achievable concentrations of CAP18 peptides. These findings and the fact that $CAP_{104-135}$ given by a different route can block the lethality of LPS in mice suggests that this peptide may have utility in attenuating LPS toxicity in humans.

Many questions remain to be addressed regarding $CAP18/CAP18_{104-140}$. For example, is CAP18 proteolytically cleaved to $CAP18_{104-140}$ and/or other fragments in vivo, or is $CAP18_{104-140}$ an in-vitro artifact of the original purification scheme? When Ritonja et al (45) purified pig CAP18 homolog, cathelin, no other fragments corresponding to CAP18$_{104-140}$ were identified. Under what conditions is CAP18$_{104-140}$ released, and what is the role of CAP18/CAP18$_{104-140}$ in the inflammatory response to septic injury? Do CAP18/CAP18$_{104-140}$ have other activities? How does CAP18$_{104-140}$ ''neutralize'' LPS? Are there other proteins that modulate the LPS-CAP18 binding and neutralization?

Earlier we reported that rabbit CAP18-derived peptides have potent antimicrobial activity. The data presented above demonstrate that human CAP18 peptides exhibit potent antimicrobial activity versus both gram-positive and gram-negative bacteria.

Although more in-depth structure activity and mechanism of killing studies are in progress, at least two characteristics of the CAP18 peptides merit comment. The first of these is the cationic charge. The outer membrane of gram-negative bacteria provides an effective permeability barrier against external noxious agents, including antibiotics. Numerous studies have shown that antibacterial agents such as polycations and chelators weaken the molecular interactions of the LPS with the outer membrane (54). Polycations can under certain conditions bind to the anionic sites of lipopolysaccharide. Many molecules disorganize and cross the outer membrane and render it leaky to drugs that normally permeate the intact outer membrane very poorly. Such polycations include polymyxins and their derivatives, protamine, polymers of basic amino acids, compound 48/80, insect cecropins, reptilian magainins, various cationic leukocyte peptides (defensins, bactenecins, bactericidal/permeability-increasing protein, and others), aminoglycosides, etc. We hypothesize that part of the growth-inhibitory activity of CAP proteins is mediated by binding to cell wall components bearing a negative charge. The fact that the cell wall of yeast is comprised of mannans and other neutral sugars may partially explain the resistance of fungi to CAP proteins. However, in the present studies and in previous work it is clear that the cationic nature of these agents is not the sole determinant required for the antimicrobial activity.

A second characteristic is structure. An alpha-helical presentation of rabbit CAP18 peptide shown in Fig. 5 demonstrates the amphipathic character of the peptide. The left side of the schematic is comprised largely of cationic residues, whereas the right side is comprised of hydrophobic residues. Tossi et al. (55) correlated the alpha-helical structure (by measuring CD spectra) with the antimicrobial activity of various derivatives of the first 20 amino acids of rabbit CAP18. These studies indicated that substitutions (such as proline for one of the hydrophobic amino acids) destroyed the alpha-helical structure of the peptide, destroyed the antibacterial activity of the peptide, and destroyed the capacity of the peptide to permeabilize the bacterial inner membrane. Recent NMR studies demonstrate the alpha-helical nature of the truncated rabbit CAP18 peptide (see Fig. 6) (Huang et al., in press).

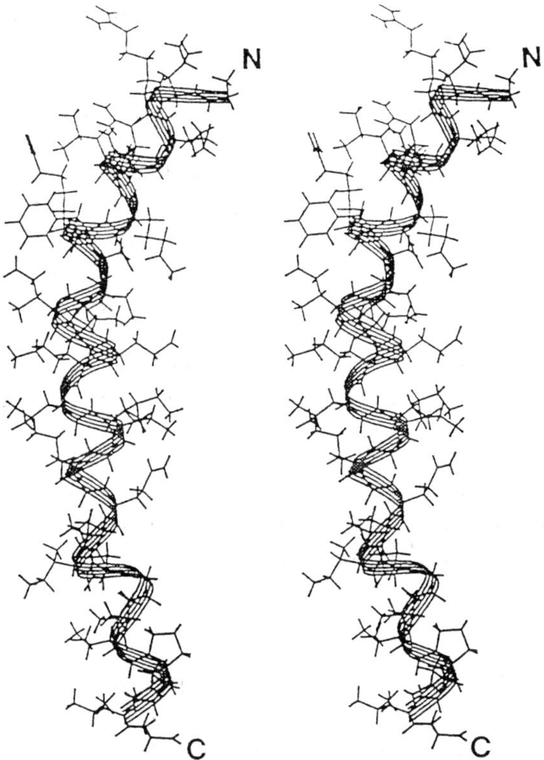

Figure 6 NMR structure of rabbit peptide CAP18$_{106-137}$ (Huang et al. In press).

Several other families of granulocyte proteins exhibit LPS-binding and antimicrobial activity. These include BPI, the 13-amino acid C-terminal peptide of bovine indolicidin (56), the 30- to 35-amino acid family of defensins (57), and azurocidin (CAP37). The indolicidin peptide and the defensins inhibit the growth of gram-positive and gram-negative bacteria only in hypotonic media, thus distinguishing them from the human and rabbit CAP18 peptides. A recent publication described peptides derived from CAP37 which are active at a concentration approximately 2–3 logs higher than those derived from CAP18 (43).

The activity of CAP18 is to be contrasted with that of BPI, which was originally shown to have antibacterial activity versus a variety of gram-negative bacteria, with no activity versus gram-positive or fungal organisms. BPI demonstrates high-affinity binding to LPS and can apparently inhibit the activity of LPS in vitro. Both the amino-terminal fragment (rBPI$_{23}$) and the holoprotein (BPI$_{55}$) inhibit encapsulated *E. coli*. While both BPI$_{55}$ and rBPI$_{23}$ inhibited the growth of a rough mutant strain of *Proteus mirabilis*, only the rBPI$_{23}$ inhibited growth of the wild-type smooth organism. Neither rBPI$_{23}$ nor holoprotein BPI$_{55}$ inhibits the growth of gram-positive *S. aureus.*

Future work will address several important questions. For example, what target structures are recognized by CAP18 peptides on the surface of gram-positive bacteria, and how do CAP18 peptides mediate cytotoxicity to these microorganisms? Although the present studies do not address these questions directly, it is clear that the antimicrobial effect is highly selective because no activity is observed versus *Mycobacterium* spp. or *Candida albicans.* Like gram-negative bacteria, the cell walls of gram-positive bacteria contain negatively charged molecules such as lipoteichoic acids. Interestingly, a serum protein has been identified that binds LPS and lipoteichoic acids in serum (58). However, recent studies from this laboratory indicate that the CAP18 peptides do not inhibit lipoteichoic acid-induced activation of macrophage tissue factor (Hirata et al., unpublished data).

In summary, CAP18 contains a C-terminal peptide with anti-LPS and antimicrobial activities. These activities are stereospecific and may depend on an amphipathic alpha-helical structure. The clinical potential of these peptides awaits further evaluation in relevant animal models.

ACKNOWLEDGMENT

Excellent technical support was provided by R. Hyman and I. Plooy. Secretarial help was generously supplied by Wolfgang Arlo Scatman and Elham Elahi. Parts of this work were supported by NIH grant RO1-GM47720 and a Grant-in-Aid for Scientific Research from the Ministry of Education of Japan.

REFERENCES

1. Morrison DC, Ryan JL. Endotoxins and disease mechanisms. Annu Rev Med 1987; 38:417.
2. Shenep JL, Barton RP, Mogan KA. Role of antibiotic class in the rate of liberation of endotoxin during therapy for experimental Gram-negative bacterial sepsis. J Infect Dis 1985; 151:1012.
3. Beutler B, Cerami A. Tumor necrosis, cachexia, shock and inflammation: a common mediator. Annu Rev Biochem 1987; 57:505.
4. Storm DR, Rosenthal SL, Swanson PE. Polymyxin and related peptide antibiotics. Annu Rev Biochem 1977; 46:723.
5. Vaara M. Agents that increase the permeability of the outer membrane. Microbiol Rev 1992; 56:395.
6. Vaara M, Vaara T. Sensitization of Gram-negative bacteria to antibiotics and complement by a nontoxic oligopeptide. Nature 1983; 303:526.
7. Chedid L, Parant M, Parant F, Boyer F. A proposed mechanism for natural immunity to enterobacterial pathogens. J Immunol 1968; 100:292.

8. Zeigler EJ, McCutchan JA, Fierer J, MP, et al. Treatment of Gram-negative bacteremia and shock with human antiserum to mutant *E. coli*. N Engl J Med 1982; 307:1225.

9. Ziegler EJ. Protective antibody to endotoxin: the emperor's new clothes. J Infect Dis 1988; 158:312.

10. Calandra T, Glauser MP, Schelleken JJ, Verhoef Swiss-Dutch J5 Immunoglobulin Study Group. Treatment of Gram-negative septic shock with human IgG antibody to *E. coli* J5: a prospective, double-blind, randomized trial. J Inf Dis 1988; 158:312.

11. Zeigler, EJ, Fisher CJ, Sprung CL, et al. Treatment of Gram-negative bacteremia and septic shock with HA-1A human monoclonal antibody against endotoxin. N Engl J Med 1991; 324:429.

12. Greenman RL, Schei RMH, Martin MA. A controlled clinical trial of E5 murine monoclonal antibody to endotoxin in the treatment of Gram-negative sepsis. JAMA 1991; 266:1097.

13. Warren HS, Danner L, Munford RS. Anti-endotoxin monoclonal antibodies. N Engl J Med 1992; 3; 26:1152.

14. Aketagawa J, Miyata T, Ohtsubo S, et al Primary structure of limulus anti-LPS factor. J Biol Chem 1986; 261:7357.

15. Muta T, Miyata T, Tokunaga F, et al. Primary structure of anti-lipopolysaccharide factor from American horseshoe crab, *L. polyphemus*. J Biochem 1987; 101:1321.

16. Tanaka S, Nakamura T, Morita T, Iwanaga S. Limulus anti-LPS factor: an anticoagulant which inhibits the endotoxin-mediated activation of limulus coagulation system. Biochem Biophys Res Commun 1982; 105:717.

17. Alpert G, Baldwin G, Thompson C, et al. Limulus antilipopolysaccharide factor protects rabbits from meningococcal endotoxin shock. J Infect Dis 1991; 165:494.

18. Tobias PS, Soldau K, Ulevitch RJ. Isolation of a LPS-binding acute phase reactant from rabbit serum. J Exp Med 1986; 164:777.

19. Tobias PS, Mathison JC, Ulevitch RJ. A family of LPS binding proteins involved in responses to Gram-negative sepsis. J Biol Chem 1988; 263:13479.

20. Schumann RR, Leong SR, Flaggs GW, et al. Structure and function of LPS binding protein. Science 1990; 249:1429.

21. Elsbach P, Weiss J, Franson RC, Beckerdite-Quagliata A, Schneider A, Harris L. Separation and purification of a potent bactericidal/permeability increasing protein and a closely related phospholipase A2 from rabbit PMNs. Observations on their relationship. J Biol Chem 1979; 254:11000.

22. Farley MM, Shafer WM, Spitznagel JK. Antimicrobial binding of a radiolabeled cationic neutrophil granule protein. Infect Immun 1987; 55:1536.

23. Wright SD, Ramos R, Tobias PS, Ulevitch RJ, Mathison JC. CD14, a receptor for complexes of LPS and LPS binding protein. Science 1990; 249:1431.

24. Wright SD, Ramos R.D Hermanowski-Vosatka A, Rockwell P, Dimers PA. Activation of the adhesive capacity of CR3 on neutrophils by endotoxin: dependence on LPS binding protein and CD14. J Exp Med 1991; 173:1281.

25. Gazzano-Santoro H, Parent JB, Grinnal L, et al. High-affinity binding of BPI and a recombinant amino-terminal fragment to the lipid A region of LPS. Infect Immun 1992; 60:4754.

26. Marra MN, Wilde CG, Collins MS, Snable JL, Thornton MB, Scott RW. The role of BPI as a natural inhibitor of bacterial endotoxin. J Immunol 1992; 148:532.

27. Weiss J, Elsbach P, Shu C, et al. Human BPI and a recombinant NH_2-terminal fragment cause killing of serum-resistant Gram-negative bacteria in whole blood and inhibit TNF release induced by the bacteria. J Clin Invest 1992; 90:1122.

28. Hirata M, Larrick JW, Shimomura Y, Yoshida M. Modification of LPS activity by LPS-binding protein CAP-18. 1st Congress of the International Endotoxin Society, San Diego, CA, 1990.

29. Hirata M, Yoshida M, Inada K, Kirikae T. Investigation of endotoxin binding cationic proteins from granulocytes. Agglutination of erythrocytes sensitized with Re-LPS. Adv Exp Biol Med 1990; 256:287.

30. Larrick JW, Hirata M, Zheng H, et al. A novel granulocyte-derived peptide with LPS neutralizing activity. *J Immunol* 1993; 152:231.

31. Hirata M, Shimomura Y, Yoshida M, et al. Characterization of a rabbit cationic protein (CAP18) with lipopolysaccharide-inhibitory activity. *Infect Immun* 1993; 62:1421.

32. Larrick JW, Hirata M, Shimomura Y, et al. Antimicrobial activity of rabbit CAP18-derived peptides. Antimicrob Agents Chemother 1993; 37:2534.

33. Rudbach JA, Akiya Fl, Elin RJ, et al. Preparation and properties of a national reference endotoxin. J Clin Microbiol 1976; 3:21.

34. Larrick JW, Hirata M, Morgan JG, Yen M. Cloning of a cDNA for CAP18, a cationic lipopolysaccharide binding protein. Biochem Biophys Res Commun 1991; 179:170.

35. Green LC, Wagner DA, Glogowski J, Skipper PL, Wishnok JS, Tannenbaum SR. Analysis of nitrate, nitrite, and [^{15}N15N]nitrate in biological fluids. Anal Biochem 1982; 126:131.

36. Barany G, Merrifield RB. In: Gross E, Meienhofer J, eds. The Peptides, Vol. 2. New York: Academic Press, 1980:1–284.

37. Bernatowicz MS, Daniels SB, Koster H. Tetrahedron Lett 1989; 30:4645.

38. Galanos C, Freudenberg MA, Reutter W. Galactosamine-induced sensitization to the lethal effects of endotoxin. Proc Natl Acad Sci USA 1979; 76:5939.

39. Pieroni RE, Broderick EJ, Bundeally A, Levine L. A simple method for the quantitation of submicrogram amounts of bacterial endotoxin. Proc Soc Exp Biol Med 1970; 133:790.

40. Levy O, Weiss J, Zarember K, Ooi CE, Elsbach P. Antibacterial 15 kDa protein isoforms (p15s) are members of a novel family of leukocyte proteins. J Biol Chem 1993; 268:6058.

41. Ritonja A, Kopitar M, Jerala R, Turk V. Primary structure of a new cysteine proteinase inhibitor from pig leucocytes. FEBS Lett 1989; 255:211.

42. Selsted ME, Brown DM, DeLange RJ, Harwig SSL, Lehrer RI. Primary structures of six antimicrobial peptides of rabbit peritoneal neutrophils. J Biol Chem 1985; 260:4579.

43. Pereira HA, Erdem I, Pohl J, Spitznagel JL. Synthetic bactericidal peptide based on CAP37:a 37 kDa human neutrophil granule-associated cationic antimicrobial protein chemotactic for macrophages. Proc Natl Acad Sci USA 1993; 90:4733.

44. Granger DL, Hibbs JB Jr, Perfect JR, Durack DT. Metabolic fate of L-arginine in relation to microbiostatic capability of murine macrophages. J Clin Invest 1990; 85:264.
45. Hibbs JB Jr, Taintor RR, Vavrin Z. Macrophage cytotoxicity: role of L-arginine deiminase activity and imino nitrogen oxidation to nitrate. Science 1987; 235:473.
46. Stueher D, Nathan CF. Nitric oxide: a macrophage product responsible for cytostasis and respiratory inhibition in tumor target cells. J Exp Med 1989; 169:1543.
47. Hibbs JB Jr, Taintor RR, Vavrin Z, Rachlin EM. Nitric oxide: a cytotoxic activated effector molecule. Biochem Biophys Res Commun 1988; 156:87.
48. Drapier JC, Hibbs JB Jr. Differentiation of murine macrophages to express nonspecific cytotoxicity for tumor cells results in L-arginine-dependent inhibition of mitochondrial iron-sulfur enzymes in the macrophage effector cells. J Immunol 1988; 140:2829.
49. Amber IJ, Hibbs JB Jr, Taintor RR, Vavrin Z. The L-arginine dependent effector mechanism is induced in murine adenocarcinoma cells by culture supernatant from cytotoxic activated macrophages. J Leuk Biol 1988; 43:187.
50. Palmer RMJ, Ferrige AG, Moncada S. Nitric oxide release accounts for biological activity of EDRF. Nature 1987; 327:524.
51. Ignarro LJ, Buga GM, Wood KW, Byrns RE, Chaudhuri G. EDRF produced and released from artery and vein is nitric oxide. Proc Natl Acad Sci USA 1987; 84:9265.
52. Kilbourn RG, Gross SS, Jubran A, et al. N^G-methyl-L-arginine inhibits TNF-induced hypotension: implications for the involvement of nitric oxide. Proc Natl Acad Sci USA 1990; 87:3629–3632.
53. McCartney AC. Endotoxemia in septic shock: clinical and post mortem correlations. Intensive Care Med 1983; 9:117.
54. Vaara M. Agents that increase the permeability of the outer membrane. Microbiol Rev 1992; 56:395.
55. Tossi A, Scocchi M, Skerlauaj B, Gennaro R. Identification and characterization of primary antibacterial domain in CAP18, a LPS-building protein from rabbit leukocytes. FEBS Lett 1994; 339:108–112.
56. Del Sal G, Storici P, Schnerider C, Romeo D, Zanetti. M. cDNA cloning of the neutrophil bactericidal peptide indolicidin. Biochem Biophys Res Commun 1992; 187:467.
57. Lehrer RI, Lichtenstein AK, Ganz T. Defensins: antimicrobial and cytotoxic peptide of mammalian cells. Annu Rev Immunol 1993; 11:105.
58. Brade L, Brade H, Fischer W. A 28 kDa protein of normal mouse serum binds lipopolysaccharide of gram-negative and lipoteichoic acids of gram-positive bacteria. Microb Pathogen 1990; 355.

6

Therapeutic Potential of a Recombinant Endotoxin-Neutralizing Protein from *Limulus polyphemus*

Richard A. Saladino and Gary R. Fleisher
Harvard Medical School and Children's Hospital
Boston, Massachusetts

George R. Siber
Dana-Farber Cancer Institute, Harvard Medical School
and Massachusetts Public Health Biologic Laboratories
Boston, Massachusetts

Claudette Thompson
Dana-Farber Cancer Institute, Harvard Medical School
Boston, Massachusetts

Thomas J. Novitsky
Associates of Cape Cod, Inc.
Woods Hole, Massachusetts

I. INTRODUCTION

Neutralizing or enhancing the clearance of endotoxin in vivo for treatment of gram-negative bacterial sepsis has been an important focus of research during the last decade. The polymyxin compounds (1), polyclonal (2) or monoclonal antibodies to the lipid A moiety of endotoxin (3,4), and bactericidal/permeability-increasing protein (5,6) have been evaluated as potential adjunctive strategies to current antimicrobial and supportive therapy for sepsis.

This chapter summarizes our studies of an endotoxin-neutralizing protein for treatment of high-mortality models of endotoxin shock and *Escherichia coli* sepsis in small animals. We have evaluated the native endotoxin-neutralizing protein isolated from the horseshoe crab, *Limulus polyphemus*, termed anti-LPS factor (LALF), and the recombinant form of this factor expressed in yeast, termed endotoxin-neutralizing protein (ENP).

II. BACKGROUND

Native endotoxin-neutralizing proteins isolated from the hemolymph of horseshoe crabs, *Tachypleus tridentatus* (7) and *Limulus polyphemus* (8), have been termed anti-LPS factors (LALF). These proteins have molecular weights of approximately 12 kDa and are thought to function as a part of the crab's primitive host defense mechanism against endotoxin exposure. As well, these endotoxin-neutralizing proteins may function as part of a feedback regulation of the clotting of amebocytes that occurs in the presence of endotoxin (9,10). *Limulus* anti-LPS factors may also have native antimicrobial capacity, as purified LALF directly inhibits the growth of rough gram-negative bacteria (9).

Purified *Limulus* anti-LPS factor binds the lipid A portion of endotoxin and inhibits the biologic activities of LPS in vitro, including gelation of *Limulus* amebocyte lysate (9–12) and activation of cultured murine splenocytes (11), human endothelial cells (13), and peripheral blood monocytes (J. Parsonnet and G. Siber, unpublished observations). Our initial investigations indicated that LALF mixed with LPS in vitro reduced mortality in rats (10) and mice (11), and reduced fever in rabbits and fever, neutropenia, and pulmonary hypertension in sheep (11), compared to animals challenged with LPS alone.

III. INVESTIGATIONS

A. Endotoxin-Neutralizing Protein from *Limulus polyphemus*

Native *Limulus* anti-LPS factor (LALF) was purified from the amebocyte membranes of *L. polyphemus* as described previously (10). A recombinant version of this factor, termed endotoxin-neutralizing protein (ENP), was expressed in *Saccharomyces cerevisiae*. Recombinant ENP differs from LALF by having four additional N-terminal amino acids (Glu-Ala-Glu-Ala).

The activities of LALF and ENP in neutralizing *E. coli* O111b4 LPS-induced gelation of *Limulus* amebocyte lysate (LAL) are shown in Fig. 1, and are similar. Using titration curves as shown in Fig. 1, we evaluated the ability of ENP at a concentration of 1 µg/mL to neutralize a variety of gram-negative endotoxins (Table 1). The concentration of LPS which induces 50 % of the maximal increase in 405-nm optical density (OD) is defined as the *Limulus* response 50% (LR^{50}) (14).

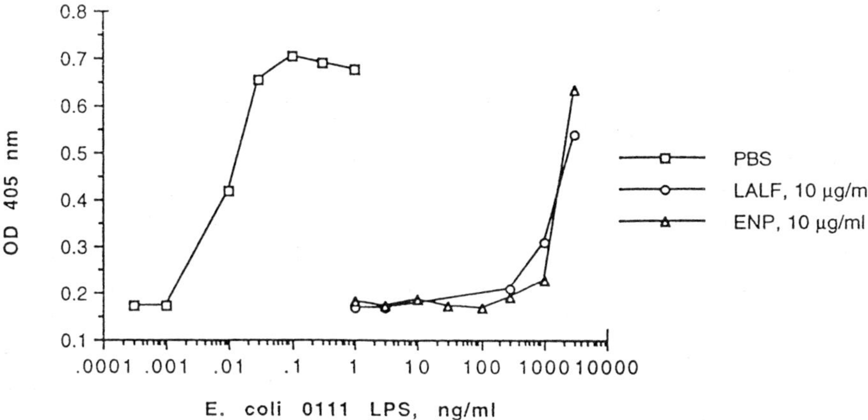

Figure 1 Effect of LALF and ENP on *E. coli* O111b4-induced gelation of LAL measured by increased OD at 405 nm. The LPS and LALF/ENP were preincubated for 1 h at 37°C prior to the addition of LAL.

Table 1 Inhibition of LAL Activity of Various Endotoxins by ENP at 1 µg/mL LPS

	LR_{50} response (pg/mL)	Fold inhibition by ENP
Salmonella minnesota		
WT	20	60 ×
Ra	1.5	170
Rb	<1.5	>100
Rc	7	20
Rd	7	20
Re	7	20
Salmonella typhimurium	7	70
Shigella flexneri	7	100
E. coli O113	3	200
E. coli J5	5	>300
Klebsiella pneumoniae	7	40
Pseudomonas aeruginosa	8	10
Proteus mirabilis	7	25
Yersinia enterocolitica	10	10
Bordetella pertussis	3	2.5
Vibrio cholerae Inaba	9	0
Serratia marcescens	9	2.5

B. Pharmacology of ENP (15)

New Zealand White rabbits were used as the investigational animal model for ENP serum half-life determination, measurement of the physiological response to infusion of ENP, and immune response to ENP challenge.

ENP and LALF were measured by an ELISA method utilizing lipid A coated to plastic microtiter plates to capture ENP/LALF and rabbit anti-ENP serum followed by alkaline phosphatase-labeled goat anti-rabbit IgG. ENP was detected quantitatively in phosphate-buffered saline or normal rabbit serum in this assay. LPS inhibited the assay, suggesting that ENP-LPS complexes are not measured.

Rabbits administered intravenous ENP 1.2, 2.5, 5.0, and 10 mg/kg showed progressive increases in peak serum concentrations of ENP, measured 5 min after infusion, from 0.86 to 17.2 μg/mL. The peak concentrations and half-life in rabbits given LALF at 1.2 mg/kg did not differ significantly from those given ENP at the same dose. The mean serum half-life was 45 min and was not influenced by dose.

Physiological monitoring of rabbits during a 6-h period after ENP and LALF administration showed no changes from normal baseline mean arterial pressure, temperature, arterial pH, or serum bicarbonate.

In order to evaluate the immune response to ENP administration, 8 rabbits were administered a dose of ENP (5 mg/kg). IgG antibody response measured 3 weeks after the initial infusion ranged from 0.29 to 1.89 μg/mL (mean: 0.69). A second infusion of ENP (5 mg/kg) in 4 of the rabbits produced no detectable effects on physiological monitoring over 6 h. A booster antibody response was noted in 2 of 4 rabbits (mean: 6.01 μg/mL; range: 0.01 to 16.0 μg/mL).

C. LALF and ENP for Treatment of Endotoxin Shock in Rabbits

LALF and ENP were initially evaluated as treatment for endotoxic shock in New Zealand White rabbits. In this intravenous challenge model, the LD_{90} of *N. meningitidis* group B M986 LOS in rabbits was 10 μg/kg (16). When the LOS was premixed in vitro with LALF 1.2 mg/kg, mean arterial pressure, arterial pH, serum bicarbonate, and survival were significantly higher than in controls. Prophylaxis of rabbits with LALF 1.2 mg/kg administered intravenously just prior to LOS challenge also significantly improved physiological measurements and survival. Even when therapy was delayed until 30 min after LOS challenge, LALF significantly improved physiological measurements and survival (12) (Fig. 2a).

Recombinant ENP was evaluated in a similar model of *E. coli* endotoxin shock in which the LD_{80} of *E. coli* O111b4LPS in rabbits was 100 μg/kg, 10-fold higher than for meningococcal LOS. Increasing prophylactic doses of ENP (1.2 to 5.0 mg/kg prior to intravenous challenge) resulted in progressively and

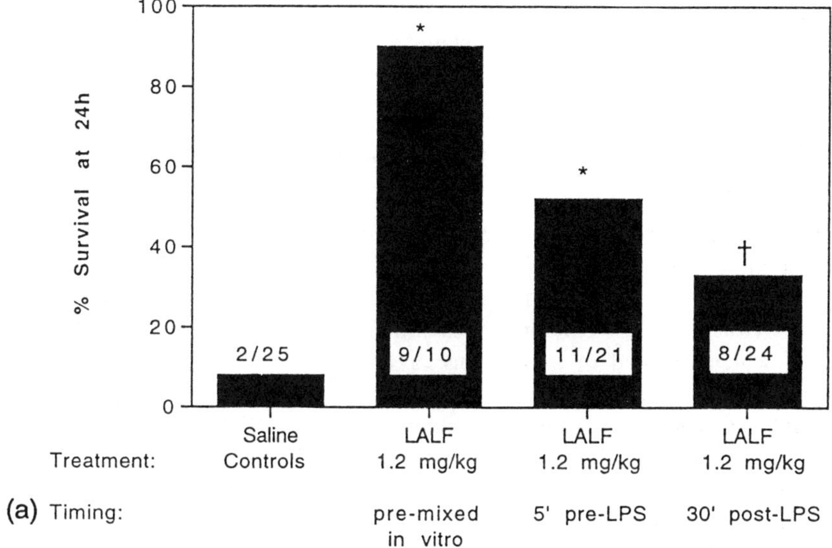

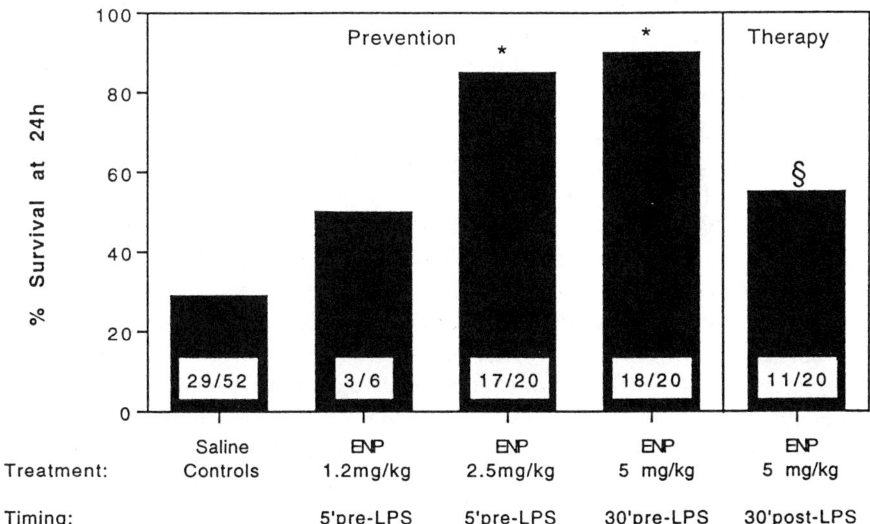

Figure 2 (a) Effect of LALF on mortality of rabbits 24 h after meningococcal LOS challenge (10 µg/kg) (10). *$p < 0.01$ versus saline control. †$p = 0.028$ versus saline control. (b) Effect of ENP on survival of rabbits 24 h after *E. coli* O111b4 LPS challenge (100 µg/kg) (16). *$p < 0.001$ versus saline control. §$p = 0.055$ versus saline control.

significantly improved survival (17). Treatment with ENP at 5.0 mg/kg improved survival of animals even when administered 30 min after LPS challenge, although not significantly so (Fig. 2b).

D. ENP for Treatment of *E. coli* sepsis in Rabbits and Rats

Our next objective was to evaluate the protective effects of ENP in the more complex milieu of bacterial sepsis. A model of peritoneal sepsis with *E. coli* O18ac K1 administered with a porcine mucin adjuvant was developed. New Zealand White rabbits were challenged intraperitoneally with 2.5×10^8 CFU *E. coli*, which resulted in reliable bacteremia (4×10^4 CFU/mL) 1 h after challenge and produced 80–90% mortality at 24 h despite gentamicin therapy (2.5 mg/kg) at 1 h (18). Paired rabbits received saline or ENP (5 mg/kg) concurrently with gentamicin 1 h after intraperitoneal challenge with *E. coli*. ENP-treated animals had similar mean bacterial densities in blood and peritoneal fluid as saline controls. Peak geometric mean serum endotoxin concentrations (262 in ENP-treated rabbits versus 1054 pg/mL in controls, $p = 0.013$) and tumor necrosis factor concentrations (2540 in ENP-treated rabbits versus 6438 pg/mL in controls, $p = 0.046$) measured 2 h after challenge were significantly lower in ENP-treated animals compared to controls. In this model, gentamicin failed to clear bacteremia in 11 of 24 pairs of rabbits. ENP treatment did not improve survival when all 24 rabbit pairs were analyzed (7 of 24 ENP -treated rabbits versus 4 of 24 controls, $p = 0.19$); however, analysis of the subgroup of 13 pairs who cleared bacteremia demonstrated improved survival in the ENP-treated group (5 of 13 ENP-treated rabbits versus 1 of 13 controls) (Fig. 3).

To establish the optimal dose of ENP for treatment of sepsis, we performed a dose-response trial in Wistar rats. We established a model of peritoneal sepsis utilizing *E. coli* O18ac K1 with sterile cecal contents as adjuvant encapsulated in gelatin capsules and implanted intraperitoneally, according to the method of Weinstein et al. (19). Rats challenged with 5×10^7 CFU *E. coli* were reliably bacteremic (2.4×10^4 CFU/mL); this resulted in 100% mortality at 24 h without treatment and 70–80% mortality with intramuscular gentamicin treatment (5 mg/kg) administered 1 h after *E. coli* challenge. Gentamicin transiently decreased blood bacterial density but did not clear bacteria from blood or peritoneal fluid. Nonetheless, administration of ENP at doses of 5, 25, or 50 mg/kg 1 h after challenge significantly improved survival in a dose-related fashion (Fig. 4).

In light of the results from our initial live bacterial sepsis study in rabbits and those of the ENP dose-response trial in rats, the model of *E. coli* peritoneal sepsis in rabbits was modified to include optimal antibiotic treatment while maintaining a high mortality. Rabbits challenged with 7×10^9 CFU *E. coli* were consistently bacteremic 1 h after challenge (3.6×10^5 CFU/mL). Treatment

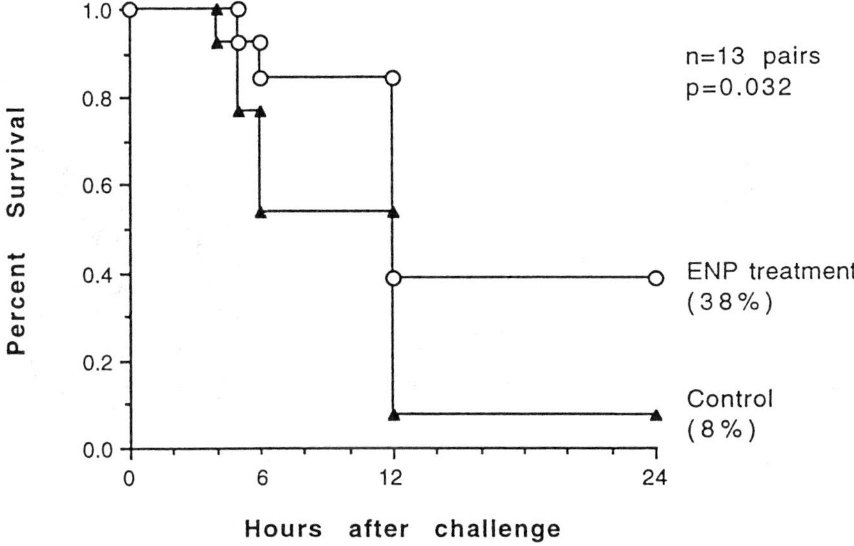

Figure 3 Effect of ENP (5 mg/kg) on survival of rabbits 24 h after challenge with intraperitoneal *E. coli* O18ac K1. Treatment was given 1 h after challenge.

with intravenous gentamicin (2.5 mg/kg) and ceftriaxone (100 mg/kg) 1 h after challenge (immediately after the blood for culture was obtained) reliably eliminated bacteremia, but continued to have nearly 60% mortality (20). Paired rabbits received saline or the high dose of ENP (50 mg/kg) concurrently with antibiotic therapy. Between-groups analysis did not demonstrate a significant difference in peak serum endotoxin concentrations measured 2 h after challenge, likely due to the mean endotoxin concentration 1 h after challenge in the ENP-treated group, which was 1.5-fold higher than controls. However, within-groups analysis demonstrated that from 1 to 2 h after *E. coli* challenge, serum endotoxin concentrations increased only 1.2-fold in ENP-treated rabbits (2040 to 2380 pg/mL, p = ns), versus 2.5-fold in controls (1310 to 3290 pg/mL, p = 0.024). Although serum TNF concentrations were not significantly different between groups, ENP-treatment significantly improved survival (18 of 25 ENP-treated rabbits versus 11 of 25 controls) ($p < 0.05$). (Fig. 5).

The model of *E. coli* peritoneal sepsis in rats was again used to evaluate early versus late treatment with ENP. The model was modified by giving animals lead acetate to increase their sensitivity to endotoxin (21) and by maximizing antibiotic treatment at 1 h by the addition of ceftriaxone (100 mg/kg) to gentamicin (5 mg/kg). The challenge dose of *E. coli* O18ac of 2.5 to 5×10^7 CFU resulted in a mean bacteremia 1 h after challenge of 5×10^2 CFU/mL, nearly 50-fold lower

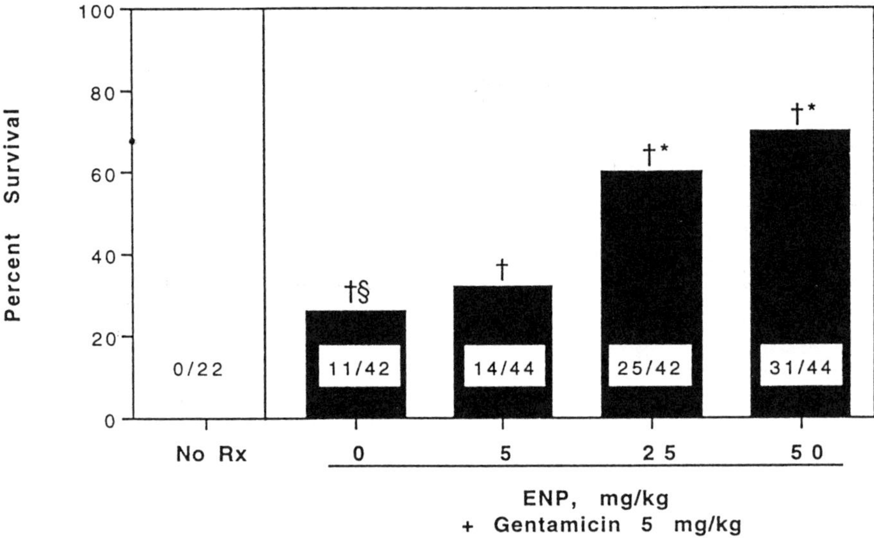

Figure 4 Effect of increasing doses of ENP on survival in rats after challenge with intraperitoneal *E. coli* O18ac K1. ENP was administered 1 h after challenge. $\S p<0.05$ versus no gentamicin by Fisher exact test. $*p<0.01$ versus 0 ENP + gentamicin by Fisher exact test. $^{\dagger}p<0.001$ by trend analysis of indicated groups for dose-response effect by Cox-Armitage test.

than in nonsensitized rats. Despite this, mortality for sensitized control rats treated with ceftriaxone and gentamicin alone was 96%. In order to determine the efficacy of ENP administered at various times after antibiotic treatment for sepsis, rats received either saline 1 h after *E. coli* challenge, or high-dose ENP (50 mg/kg) 1, 2, or 3 h after challenge (22). ENP administration resulted in significantly improved survival in rats treated at both 1 and 2 h postchallenge (Fig. 6). Survival was slightly improved with treatment at 3 h postchallenge, but not significantly so ($p = 0.32$)

Finally, the efficacy of ENP (50 mg/kg) for treatment of gram-negative sepsis was compared to that of the HA-1A human IgM monoclonal antibody to lipid A (Centoxin, Centocor, Leiden, Holland) (5 mg/kg). The rat model of *E. coli* O18ac K1 peritoneal sepsis was modified only slightly from previous. The challenge dose of *E. coli* was reduced to 5×10^6 CFU, 10-fold lower than in the nonsensitized rats, and the mean blood bacterial density 1 h after challenge was 3.6×10^3 CFU/mL, about sevenfold lower than in nonsensitized rats. Animals reliably cleared bacteremia 1 h after treatment but continued to have 80–90% mortality at 24 h.

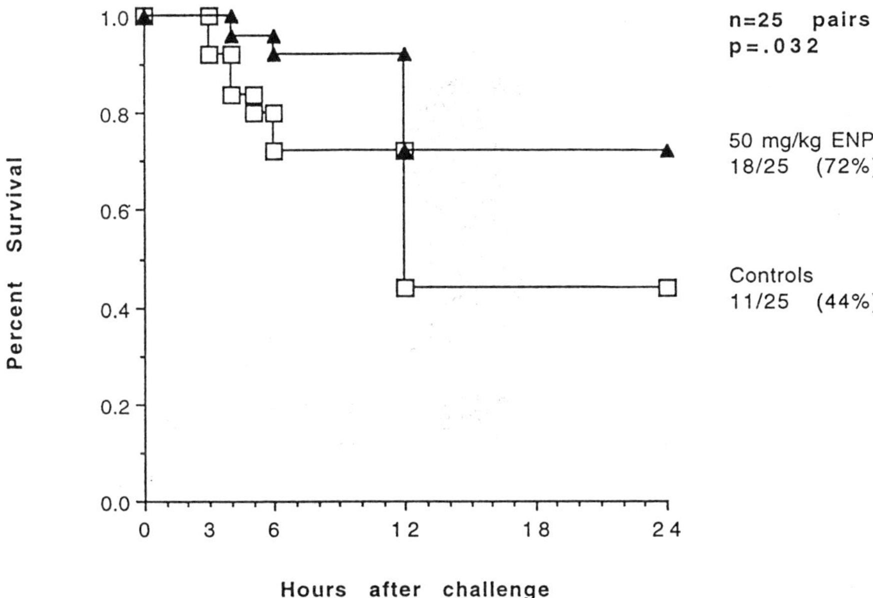

Figure 5 Effect of high-dose ENP (50 mg/kg) treatment (1 h after intraperitoneal challenge) in gentamicin- and ceftriaxone-treated *E. coli* O18ac K1 sepsis in rabbits.

Rats were treated with ENP, the monoclonal antibody, or saline concomitantly with antibiotics 1 h after intraperitoneal challenge. ENP therapy resulted in a significant improvement in 24-h survival to 85% versus 14% in controls ($p<0.001$, Fig. 7), whereas HA-1A had no detectable benefit for survival (19%) (23).

IV. DISCUSSION

The broad-spectrum antiendotoxin capacity of LALF and ENP, as shown by our in-vitro data, was applied to both the meningococcal LOS and *E. coli* LPS intravenous endotoxin challenge models in rabbits. Improvements in physiological changes and survival were noted even when LALF or ENP treatment was initiated 30 min after intravenous endotoxin challenge.

Given those encouraging results, recombinant ENP was used as therapy in animal models that more closely resembled human gram-negative sepsis. *E. coli* O18ac K1, a human pathogen, was administered intraperitoneally at a dose which reliably produced high-grade bacteremia 1 h after challenge. Notably, gentamicin treatment alone did not consistently eliminate bacteria from the blood and peritoneum in rabbits or rats.

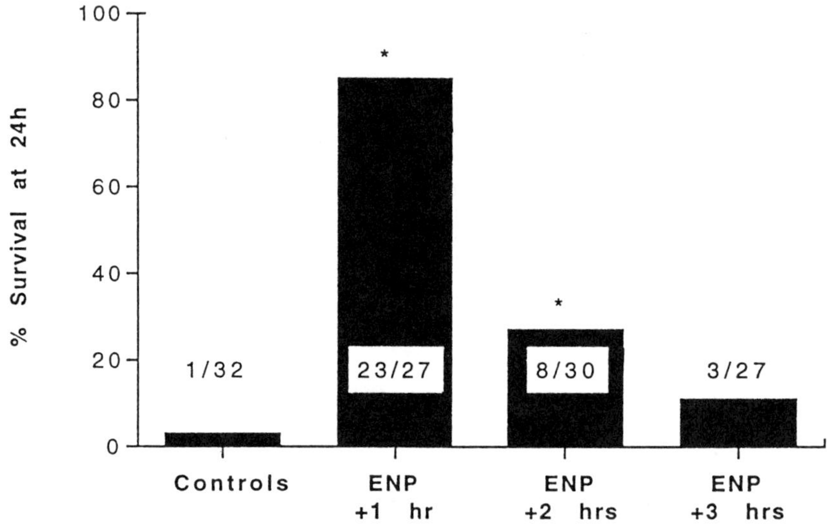

Figure 6 Early versus late ENP treatment in *E. coli* O18ac sepsis in rats. *$p<0.01$ versus saline control.

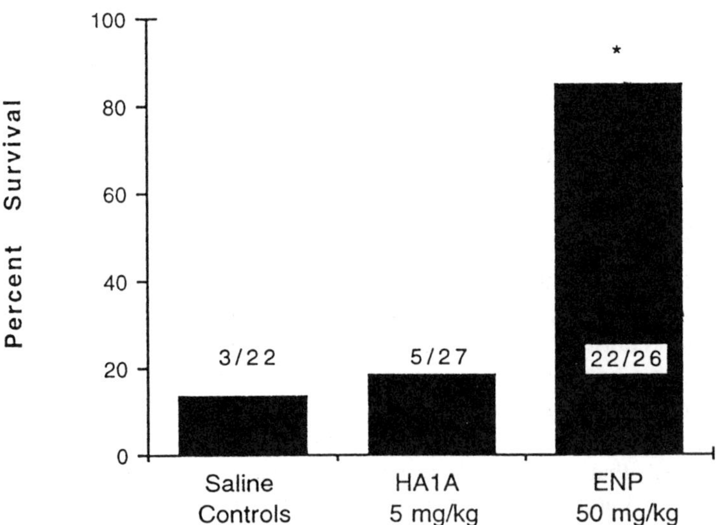

Figure 7 Effect of ENP and HA-1A on mortality of lead acetate-sensitized rats 24 h after i.p. challenge with *E. coli* O18ac K1. Treatments were given 1 h after challenge. All animals received gentamicin and ceftriaxone. *$p<0.001$ versus saline control.

In the rabbit model of gentamicin-treated *E. coli* peritonitis and sepsis, ENP treatment (5 mg/kg) significantly reduced serum endotoxin and tumor necrosis factor concentrations, and improved survival in the subgroup that cleared bacteremia. Furthermore, the rat model of gentamicin-treated *E. coli* sepsis demonstrated ENP dose-related improved survival. In this model, ENP treatment reduced serum tumor necrosis factor concentrations significantly, but for reasons that are not clear, did not reduce serum endotoxin concentrations, as measured by LAL [23]. Large variations in endotoxin concentrations could have precluded the detection of twofold or greater differences between groups. Despite the lack of apparent effect on endotoxin concentrations, we speculate that ENP neutralized the biological effects of endotoxin sufficiently to permit increased survival.

Our next goal was to optimize ENP treatment and antimicrobial killing. We added ceftriaxone to gentamicin treatment in the rabbit model of sepsis to provide optimal antibiotic treatment. As noted, endotoxin concentrations measured 2 h postchallenge and 1 h after ENP 50 mg/kg were not significantly different between groups, likely a consequence of the relatively lower initial endotoxin concentrations in the control animals. Between-groups analysis demonstrated that ENP prevented a significant rise in endotoxin concentrations after antibiotic treatment, and we speculate that ENP therefore blocked the lethal effects of endotoxin. The high-dose regimen of ENP in this model significantly improved survival, demonstrating the efficacy of ENP in an optimally treated high-mortality animal model of sepsis.

Finally, we evaluated delayed treatment with ENP in our rat model of *E. coli* sepsis. This model was modified to sensitize the rats to the effects of endotoxin by the addition of intravenous lead acetate, such that 80–90% mortality was achieved despite a 10-fold lower challenge of intraperitoneal *E. coli* prior to gentamicin and ceftriaxone treatment. ENP treatment, even when delayed 2 h after intraperitoneal *E. coli* challenge in rats, resulted in significantly improved survival compared to control animals.

In addition, we sought to compare the efficacy of ENP to HA-1A human monoclonal antibody in this lead-sensitized rat model of sepsis. As reported, whereas ENP had a dramatic therapeutic effect (improving survival from 14% to 85%), HA-1A had no such benefit. It has been postulated that HA-1A does not directly neutralize the biological activities of endotoxin as ENP does, but rather fixes complement and enhances its clearance. As well, CR-1 receptors on red blood cells may be important for clearance of endotoxin, although these receptors are present on human but not rat red cells. Hence, HA-1A may lack protective mechanisms in the rat model. Direct neutralization of endotoxin without requirement of other host defense mechanisms may be an important advantage for ENP over certain monoclonal antibodies to endotoxin.

We have noted the induction of an immune response to the *Limulus* protein, and this is a potential clinical limitation. It is unlikely, though, that a single treatment with ENP would cause immunologically mediated side effects, given its short serum half-life (45 min). The booster response that we noted, though, may demonstrate that repeated administration should be avoided.

In summary, our investigations regarding the endotoxin-neutralizing capacity of LALF and recombinant endotoxin-neutralizing protein demonstrate amelioration of the physiological effects of endotoxin shock and significant survival benefit for treatment of both endotoxin shock and *E. coli* septic shock in rats and rabbits. Although not all of our animal studies are directly comparable, overall survival was significantly improved in ENP-treated groups compared to controls (Table 2). Hence, in-vitro data demonstrating that ENP binds and neutralizes the biological activity of various gram-negative lipopolysaccharides in the LAL assay and on mammalian target cells (7–13), is corroborated by our in-vivo data. Taken together, all of these data support further investigation of the use of a recombinant endotoxin-neutralizing protein from *Limulus* for treatment of gram-negative sepsis.

Table 2   Summary Data

Model	ENP dose (mg/kg)	Survival Treated	Survival Control	Totals Treated	Totals Control
Endotoxin challenge:					
N. meningitidis		28/55	2/25		
LOS challenge i.v.					
—rabbit	1.2–5.0				
E. coli		46/60	15/52		
LPS challenge i.v.					
—rabbit	2.5–5.0				
				74/115	17/77[a]
Live bacterial challenge:					
E. coli	5.0	7/24	4/24		
peritonitis/sepsis					
—rabbit					
—rat	5.0, 25, 50	70/130	11/42		
—rabbit	50	18/25	11/25		
—rat	50 (1 h vs. 2 h)	31/57	1/32		
—rat	50	22/26	3/22		
				148/262	30/145[a]
Summary total:				222/377	47/222[a]

[a] $p < 0.001$.

REFERENCES

1. Baldwin G, Alpert G, Caputo GL, et al. Effect of polymyxin B on experimental shock from meningococcal and *Escharichia coli* endotoxins. J Infect Dis 1991; 164:542–549.

2. Ziegler EJ, McCutchan JA, Fierer J, et al. Treatment of gram negative bacteremia and shock with human antiserum to a mutant *E. coli*. N Engl J Med 1982; 307:1225–1230.

3. Ziegler EJ, Fisher CJ Jr., Sprung CL, et al. Treatment of gram-negative bacteremia and septic shock with HA-1A human monoclonal antibody against endotoxin. N Engl J Med 1991; 324:429–436.

4. Greenman RL, Schein RMH, Martin MA, et al. A controlled trial of E5 murine monoclonal IgM antibody to endotoxin in the treatment of gram-negative sepsis. JAMA 1991; 266:1097–1102.

5. Marra MN, Thornton MB, Snable JL, Wilde CG, Scott RW. Endotoxin-binding and neutralizing properties of recombinant bactericidal/permeability-increasing protein and monoclonal antibodies HA-1A and E5. Crit Care Med 1994; 22:559–565.

6. Fisher CJ Jr, Marra MN, Palardy JE, Marchbanks CR, Scott RW, Opal SM. Human neutrophil bactericidal/permeability-increasing protein reduces mortality rate from endotoxin challenge: a placebo-controlled study. Crit Care Med 1994; 22:553–558.

7. Aketagawa J, Miyata T, Ohtsubo S, et al. Primary structure of *Limulus* anticoagulant anti-lipspolysaccharide factor. J Biol Chem 1986; 261:7357–7365.

8. Muta T, Miyata T, Tokunaga F, Nakamura T, Iwanaga S. Primary structure of anti-lipopolysaccharide factor from American horseshoe crab, *Limulus polyphemus*. J Biochem 1987; 101:1321–1330.

9. Morita T, Ohtsubo, Nakamura T, Tanaka S, Iwanaga S, Ohashi K, Niwa M. Isolation and biological activities of *Limulus* anticoagulant (anti-LPS factor) which interacts with lipopolysaccharide (LPS). J Biochem 1985; 97:1611–1620.

10. Wainwright NR, Miller RJ, Paus E, et al. Endotoxin binding and neutralizing activity by a protein from *Limulus polyphemus*. In: Nowotny A, Spitzer JJ, Ziegler EJ, eds. Cellular and Molecular Aspects of Endotoxin Reactions. Amsterdam: Elsevier Science 1990:315–325.

11. Warren HS, Glennon ML, Wainwright N, et al. Binding and neutralization of endotoxin by *Limulus* atnilipopolysaccharide factor. Infect Immun 1992; 60:2506–2513.

12. Alpert G, Baldwin G, Thompson C, et al. *Limulus* antilipopolysaccharide factor protects rabbits from meningococcal endotoxin shock. J Infect Dis 1992; 165:494–500.

13. Desch CE, O'Hara P, Harlan JM. Antilipopolysaccharide factor from horseshoe crab, *Tachypleus tridentatus*, inhibits lipopolysaccharide activation of cultured human endothelial cells. Infect Immun 1989; 57:1612–1614.

14. Novitsky TJ, Roslansky PF, Siber GR, Warren HS. Turbidimetric method for quantifying serum inhibition of *Limulus* amoebocyte lysate. J Clin Microbiol 1985; 20:211–216.

15. Saladino R, Garcia C, Thompson C, Hammer B, Siber G, Fleisher G. Assessment

of intravenous endotoxin neutralizing protein in a rabbit model. Pediatr Res 1991; N182:33A.

16. Caputo GL, Baldwin G, Alpert G, et al. Effect of meningococcal endotoxin in a rabbit model of shock. Circ Shock 1992; 36:104–112.

17. Garcia C, Saladino R, Thompson C, et al. Effect of a recombinant endotoxin-neutralizing protein on endotoxin shock in rabbits. Crit Care Med 1994; 22:1211–1218.

18. Saladino R, Garcia C, Thompson C, et al. Efficacy of a recombinant endotoxin neutralizing protein in rabbits with *E. coli* sepsis. Circ Shock 1994; 42:104–110.

19. Weinstein WM, Onderdonk AB, Bartlett JG, Gorbach SL. Experimental intraabdominal abscesses in rats; development of an experimental model. Infect Immun 1974; 10:1250–1255.

20. Saladino R, Stack A, Thompson C, et al. High-dose recombinant endotoxin neutralizing protein improves survival from *E. coli* sepsis in rabbits (Abstr). Pediatr Res 1994; 35:N332,58A.

21. Selye H, Tuchweber B, Bertok L. Effect of lead acetate on the susceptibility of rats to bacterial endotoxins. Bacteriology 1966; 91:884–890.

22. Weiner D, Kuppermann N, Saladino R, et al. Comparison of early vs late treatment with recombinant endotoxin neutralizing protein (ENP) in a rat model of *E. coli* sepsis (abstr). Pediatr Res 1994; N1185,200A.

23. Nelson DS, Kuppermann N, Fleisher GR, et al. Recombinant endotoxin neutralizing protein improves survival from *E. coli* sepsis in a rat model. Crit Care Med 1995, 23:92–98.

7

Diphosphoryl Lipid A from *Rhodobacter sphaeroides*
A Novel Lipopolysaccharide Antagonist

Nilofer Qureshi and Jaroslav Hofman
University of Wisconsin
Madison, Wisconsin

Kuni Takayama
William S. Middleton Memorial Veterans Hospital
Madison, Wisconsin

Stefanie N. Vogel
Uniformed Services University of the Health Sciences
Bethesda, Maryland

David C. Morrison
University of Kansas Medical Center
Kansas City, Kansas

I. INTRODUCTION

Lipopolysaccharide (LPS) is an amphipathic glycolipid found on the outer surface of the outer membrane of gram-negative bacteria (1,2). The isolated LPS has been shown to have a wide range of immunological and pathophysiological effects (3,4). The LPS of the Enterobacteriaceae consists of three structural regions: the O-antigen (highly variable), the core consisting primarily of heptose and 2-keto-3-deoxyoctonate (Kdo) (relatively conserved region), and the lipid A (lipophilic region). The structures of the lipid A moiety of LPS from *Escherichia coli* and the *Salmonella* strains have been established (5,6). The lipid A consists of the glucosamine disaccharide with a $\beta(1\rightarrow6)$ linkage, phosphate groups are attached to the sugar at the 1- and 4'-positions, and the 3-hydroxytetradecanoate group is attached to the 2-, 3-, 2′-, and 3′-positions. The myristate and laurate groups are attached to the 3-hydroxytetradecanoic acids in acyloxyacyl linkages as shown in Fig. 1A. The hexaacyl diphosphoryl lipid A is the most toxic lipid A (5).

LPS is recognized to play a fundamental role in the pathophysiology of gram-negative septic shock (3,4). The sepsis syndrome is defined as hypothermia or fever, tachycardia, tachypnea, inadequate organ perfusion, elevated plasma lactate, low blood glucose, and a decrease in blood pressure (7). This syndrome often leads to multiorgan failure, adult respiratory distress syndrome, and death. Much of the sequellae associated with endotoxin shock occur from involvement of cytokine cascades initiated by LPS, and result in uncontrolled amplification of the inflammatory response (8–10). Early recognition of the signs and symptoms of circulatory compromise in patients with presumed sepsis and early treatment are crucial for reducing the mortality due to septic shock. Attempts to treat patients who are already in septic shock have met with relatively little success. This has prompted researchers to develop innovative approaches, which will ultimately lead to effective drugs for septic shock.

Theoretically, intervention in septic shock could be achieved by blocking LPS-binding sites on cells with nontoxic lipid A or LPS. Several groups are interested in developing nontoxic structural analogs of lipid A which may be used as LPS antagonists. In this review we focus on the purification and structural determination of the pentaacyl diphosphoryl lipid A (Rs-DPLA) derived from the LPS of *Rhodobacter sphaeroides*, its biological properties, and its usage as a potent LPS antagonist both at the cellular level and in animal models.

II. STRUCTURE AND BIOLOGICAL ACTIVITIES OF LPS ANTAGONISTS

Three effective disaccharide antagonists of LPS have been extensively described in the literature, precursor lipid IV_A, partially deacylated LPS, and Rs-DPLA (11,12). Both lipid IV_A and deacylated LPS are antagonists in human cells only, whereas Rs-DPLA is effective in both human and murine cells (12).

Lipid X, a glucosamine monosaccharide lipid A precursor, was first tried as an LPS antagonist, and the conclusion from these studies was that it is a weak antagonist (Table 1) (12). Subsequently, a large number of synthetic monosaccharide lipid X analogs have been prepared and tested for antagonist activity. SDZ 880.431 (3-aza lipid X-phosphate) is threefold more potent than lipid X at blocking LPS-induced procoagulant activity in cultures of human peripheral blood mononuclear cells (13,14).

Munford et al. have deacylated LPS using an acyloxyacyl hydrolase, which specifically releases the normal fatty acids from the lipid A moiety. This partially deacylated LPS was used to inhibit the LPS-induced adherence of human umbili-

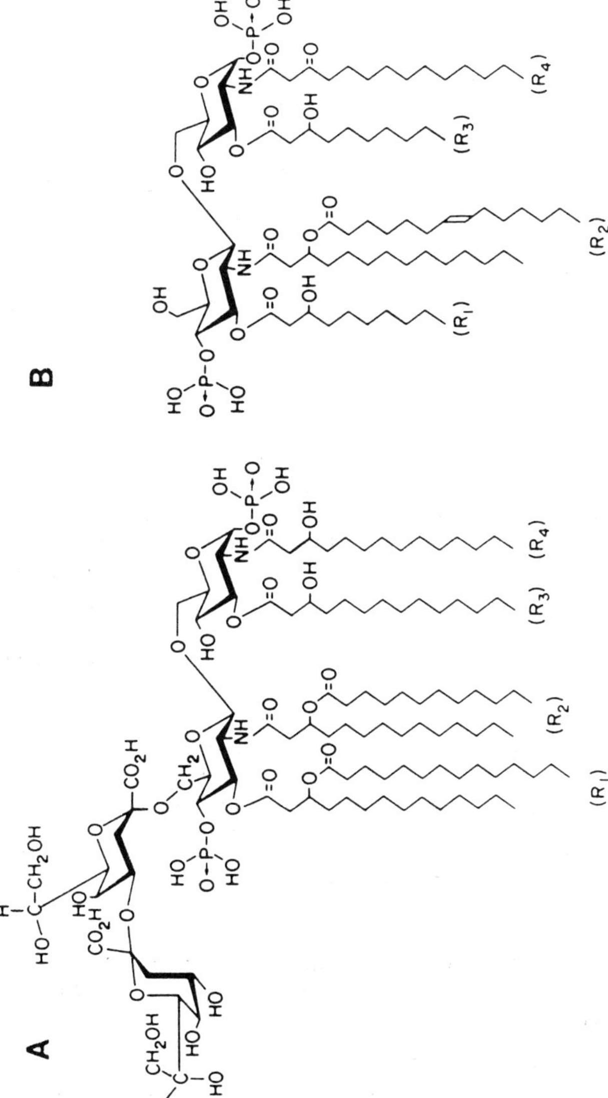

Figure 1 Structures of (A) Re-LPS isolated from *E. coli* (the diphosphoryl lipid A lacks the two Kdo's) and (B) Rs-DPLA prepared from the LPS of *R. sphaeroides*. R_1, R_2, R_3, and R_4 denotes the fatty acyl groups at the 3'-, 2'-, 3-, and 2-positions of the glucosamine disaccharide backbone, respectively. Structure B is the predominant form of two major components of Rs-DPLA. The other form lacks the unsaturation in the fatty acyl group of R_2.

Table 1 LPS Antagonists

Antagonist	Cell type used	LPS action inhibited
Lipid X (weak antagonist)	70Z/3 cells	k Light-chain expression
	Neutrophils	Priming
Precursor IV_A (works only with human cells)	Human mononuclear cells	TNF-α, IL-1β, IL-6, and PGE$_2$ induction
	Neutrophils	Activation
Deacylated LPS (similar to IV_A)	Monocytes	TNF-α, IL-1β, and IL-6 induction
	Neutrophils	Activation
	Endothelial cells	Adherence of PMN
Rs-DPLA (potent antagonist)	Murine RAW 264.7	TNF-α induction and AA release
	THP-1 human cell	TNF-α induction
	Human mononuclear cells	IL-β and IL-6 induction
	Murine peritoneal macrophage	IL-1β induction, in-vitro tolerance, IL-1β, IP-10, TNFR-2, D3, D8, and TNF-α gene expression
	Alveolar macrophage	Priming of macrophage, neopterin synthesis
	Human macrophage	PGE2 release
	Murine 70Z/3 cell line	Synthesis of surface immunoglobulin and k mRNA
	Human PMN	CD11/CD18 expression

Abbreviations: IL-6, interleukin-6; PGE$_2$, prostaglandin E$_2$; AA, arachidonic acid; TNFR-2, type 2 TNF receptor; k, kappa; and PMN, polymorphonuclear cells.

cal vein endothelial cells to polymorphonuclear leukocytes, and expression of plasminogen activator inhibitor-1, prostacyclin, and prostaglandin PGE2 by human umbilical vein endothelial cells (15–17).

Later, diglucosamine disaccharide precursor lipid IV_A (Table 1) Rs-DPLA (11, 12), and later LPS from *Rhodobacter capsulatus* were used to inhibit toxic LPS-induced interleukin-1 (IL-1β), interleukin-6 (IL-6), and tumor necrosis factor (TNF-α) synthesis in human monocytes (18–20). Recently, phosphonooxyethyl analogs of lipid IV_A and other lipid A have also been synthesized and tested for antagonist activity (21). These derivatives will be discussed in another chapter. Both deacylated LPS and IV_A are agonists in murine cell types (12). In contrast, Rs-DPLA is unique in that it has been shown to be the first potent LPS-antagonist in both human and murine cells (Table 1) (11,22,23).

III. PURIFICATION AND STRUCTURE OF Rs-DPLA

A. Early Studies

Early studies were carried out by Strittmatter et al., who reported the isolation and chemical analysis of the LPS and lipid A from *R. sphaeroides* (24). The LPS from this source was 10,000-fold less toxic in galactosamine (GalN)-sensitized mice and 160-fold less pyrogenic in rabbits than *Salmonella abortus equi* LPS. The unfractionated free lipid A was characterized by *Salimath* et al. (25). The sugar backbone is similar to that of the *Salmonella* lipid A. The ester-linked fatty acids were identified as 2-hydroxydecanoic acids (OHC_{10}), and the amide-linked fatty acids were Δ^7- tetradecenoyloxytetradecanoic (Δ^7 C14OC14) and 3-oxotetradecanoic acids. Later, Qureshi et al. purified the *R. sphaeroides* pentaacyl lipid A, completed the structural analysis of this lipid A, and studied its properties as an LPS antagonist (22,26,27).

In the study of the antagonist activity of Rs-DPLA, the highly purified and well-characterized deep rough chemotype hexaacyl LPS (Re-LPS) from *E. coli* was used. It served as the model toxic LPS (agonist) (28) (Fig. 1A). The nontoxic pentaacyl Rs-DPLA (Fig. 1B) (26,27) is unique, because the DPLA derived from the LPS of either *E. coli* or *Salmonella* strains is highly toxic. The monophosphoryl lipid A (MPLA) derived from this source has attenuated toxicity and biological activity due to absence of the reducing-end phosphate (5). This strongly suggests that the lack of toxicity in Rs-DPLA can be attributed directly to the number and nature of the fatty acyl groups present in the lipid A moiety (27).

B. Growth of Bacteria and Preparation of LPS

R. sphaeroides ATCC 17023 is grown photoheterotrophically in the ATCC medium 550 at 26°C for 12 days. The cell paste is extracted with solvents to remove the pigment. The pigment-depleted cells are used to extract the LPS (1%) as described previously (26).

C. Preparation and Purification of Rs-DPLA

Rs-DPLA is prepared by performing mild acid hydrolysis of LPS at 100°C, pH 2.5. The Rs-DPLA is recovered and purified using a DEAE cellulose column, which separates the MPLA, the polar pentaacyl Rs-DPLA (which probably contains a polar head group), the pentaacyl Rs-DPLA, and the tetraacyl Rs-DPLA. The fractions are analyzed by analytical TLC and pooled as described previously (27). The pentaacyl Rs-DPLA and Rs-MPLA are then methylated and fractionated by reverse-phase HPLC. Purified peak fractions are analyzed by plasma desorption mass spectrometry, laser desorption mass spectrometry, and proton-nuclear magnetic resonance spectroscopy. Rs-DPLA preparation consists predominantly of two isomers that differ from each other by 2 mass units. The molecular weights of these methylated lipid A's were established as 1555 and 1557 (27). The structure of one of the major pentaacyl Rs-DPLA is presented in Fig. 1B. Laser desorption mass spectrometry revealed the molecular weights of the corresponding Rs-MPLA as 1447, and 1449, respectively. These lipid A species differ only by the presence or absence of unsaturation and a keto group in the fatty acids (26). The isolated and purified Rs-DPLA is stable for over a year when frozen at $-20°C$.

A lipid A similar to Rs-DPLA has now been organically synthesized. The antagonist properties are similar to those described for Rs-DPLA. It has been claimed that Rs-DPLA "decomposes" in deuterated chloroform/methanol, yet chloroform/methanol has been used in all the purification steps without any problems (27). It is also not clear why Christ et al. tried neutralization of Rs-DPLA (free acid form) with a strong base like NaOH, when dissolving it in saline converts it to the sodium salt (29). They seem to be studying biological activities of breakdown products (29).

IV. IN-VITRO EFFECTS OF RS-DPLA

A. Effect of Rs-DPLA on Cytokines

TNF-α has been established as one of the most important mediators of septic shock (9,30,31). This conclusion is based on the following: (a) large amounts of TNF-α are present in rabbit and human serum after endotoxin administration; (b) administration of recombinant TNF-α in quantities such as those produced endogenously in response to endotoxin causes the appearance of symptoms of shock and death; (c) neutralizing this cytokine with anti-TNF-α antibody in a septic shock animal model confers significant increase in survival.

Other mediators of septic shock have also been identified. IL-1β is an important mediator of inflammatory response that is controlled in part by the neuroendocrine system (32,33). It probably plays a major role in septic shock. Interleukin-8 (IL-8) has neutrophil-activating and chemoattractant properties and as such is clearly involved in the sequellae of septic shock. TNF-α appears to increase the induction of IL-8 (34). Interleukin-10 (IL-10) is able to reduce the release of TNF-α and to prevent lethality in experimental endotoxemia (35). It antagonizes the production of interferon-γ (IFN-γ) (36). Pretreatment with cyclosporin A causes a marked enhancement of IL-10 in mice when exposed to endotoxin (37). Both transforming growth factor (TGF)-β and IL-10 inhibit LPS-induced macrophage production of TNF-α and IL-1β by posttranscriptional mechanisms (38). Anti-IL-6 monoclonal antibody (MAb) pretreatment of mice subsequently challenged intraperitoneally with a lethal dose of *E. coli* or intravenously with lethal doses of TNF protected mice from death caused by these treatments (39). However, a recent report by Libert et al. (40) suggests that IL-

6 has limited involvement in the pathogenesis of lethal septic shock in murine models.

Pentaacyl Rs-DPLA has been shown to be an LPS antagonist in murine cell systems. Rs-DPLA does not induce TNF-α in the RAW 264.7 macrophage cell line, and it blocks the induction of TNF-α by Re-LPS from *E. coli* in a dose-dependent manner. The Re-LPS/Rs-DPLA mass ratios of 1:10 and 1:100 (when 1 ng of Re-LPS/ml was used) gave 55% and 95% inhibition, respectively, of the induction of TNF (22). Rs-DPLA is also unable to induce IL-1β release by murine peritoneal macrophages. Rs-DPLA at a dose of 1 μg/mL at Re-LPS Rs-DPLA mass ratios of 1:10 and 1:100 inhibited induction of IL-1β release by 60% and >90%, respectively (23). These experiments suggested the possibility that Rs-DPLA is probably competing for the LPS-binding sites on cells.

The antagonistic effect of Rs-DPLA was also investigated in human cell types. Rs-DPLA is an antagonist of LPS-induced effects in the human promonomyelocytic cell line THP-1 and human monocytic cells (41). Complete inhibition of LPS activity is achieved at a 10- to 100-fold excess of Rs-DPLA or lipid IV$_A$ as judged by measuring the release of TNF-α, IL- 1β, and IL-6. Stimulation of monocytes by whole gram-negative bacteria is also antagonized in a dose-dependent manner. Although Rs-DPLA appears to inhibit LPS effects when tested with macrophages from humans and mice, lipid IV$_A$ acts as an LPS antagonist only with human-derived cells and is a potent agonist in murine cells.

B. Effect of Rs-DPLA on Other Mediators of Septic Shock

Other mediators of septic shock include oxygen metabolites, nitric oxide, prostaglandins, platelet-activating factor, tissue factor, and factors of the complement system. The importance of these mediators has been reviewed by Vogel (42), de Boer et al. (43), and Vadas and Pruzanski (44). IFN-γ and TNF-α can synergize for the induction of microbicidal activities. These cytokines can stimulate macrophages, neutrophils, or endothelial cells to release reactive oxygen and nitrogen intermediates essential for the destruction of pathogens (45). Incubation of macrophages with IFN-γ triggers production of both reactive oxygen (H_2O_2) and nitric oxide anion (NO_2-) products, while addition of TNF-α alone elicits only enhanced reactive oxygen intermediates (46,47). Nitric oxide (NO) has been widely studied for its role as a direct mediator of TNF-induced hypotension and shock (48).

Rs-DPLA also blocks the Re-LPS-induced "priming" for phorbol myristate acetate-stimulated superoxide anion release and neopterin synthesis in human alveolar macrophages (49). Similarly, LPS-stimulated PGE2 production in THP-1 cells can be inhibited by Rs-DPLA (41). Rs-DPLA does not induce NO production in macrophages (50).

C. Effect of Rs-DPLA on LPS-Binding Sites on the Cell Surface

It is generally assumed that the first step in the activation of responding cells by LPS (leading to the induction of cytokines) is the binding of this ligand to specific membrane receptors (51,52). The relationships between LPS-binding sites in the cell membranes and signaling pathways are not yet clearly defined. Several LPS-binding proteins have been identified on macrophages such as CD14, 73-kDa protein, CD11/18 adhesins, 38-kDa protein, 40/45-kDa protein, and scavenger receptor (acetyl LDL receptor).

1. Binding to the 73-kDa Protein

Lei and Morrison have shown that the 73-kDa LPS-binding protein is present in mouse lymphoreticular cells and peripheral blood mononuclear cells (53). They present other evidence that the 73-kDa protein is a physiological receptor for LPS (53). Mab5D3 with specificity for this 73-kDa protein has been generated and characterized. In-vitro studies have shown that Mab5D3 functions as an agonist for LPS and activates macrophages to become cytotoxic for tumor cells. Mab5D3 fails to trigger C3H/HeJ (Lps^d) macrophages. It also protects mice against the lethal effects of the LPS (54).

Rs-DPLA competes with Re-LPS for the putative physiological receptors on cells. Perhaps the strongest evidence to date for this is the recent observation that Rs-DPLA can displace the binding of radioiodinated-LPS to the murine 73-kDa protein (55). Rs-DPLA selectively inhibits binding of ^{125}I-ASD-LPS to the 73-kDa protein on mouse lymphocytes and macrophages (55).

2. Binding to CD14

CD14 is a cell-surface, 55-kDa phosphatidylinositol-linked protein on macrophages, monocytes, and neutrophils (56,57). Other LPS-responding cell types, i.e., lymphocytes, endothelial cells, and fibroblasts, are devoid of CD14. LPS can also complex with soluble CD14 in the bloodstream and be carried to cells that are devoid of CD14 (58). CD14 is the receptor protein that recognizes and binds complexes formed between LPS and circulating LPS-binding protein (LBP) and septins. Presently it is thought that CD14 may serve to ''focus'' the LPS-LBP complex to a true ''signaling'' receptor, which triggers the activation of the cells. Co-precipitation of the GPI-anchored cell surface molecules, including CD14 with protein kinase activity, suggests that CD14 signaling might occur through protein tyrosine phosphorylation (59).

Identifying receptors and signaling pathways for LPS is an important and emerging field of research. LPS binds to LBP and septins to form complexes which then bind to CD14 present on the surface of monocytes (60–62). Antibodies to CD14 block both binding and stimulation of monocytes to LPS. Kitchens et al. showed that both LPS and deacylated LPS (dLPS) bound to the human monocyte cell line THP-1 (exposed to vitamin D_3), with similar avidity in the presence of LBP. LPS stimulated these cells, whereas dLPS was an antagonist. However, dLPS did not block LPS binding via CD14 receptor. These results suggest that the dLPS is competing with LPS for the binding sites on a receptor that is distal to CD14 (63).

Recently, Kirikae et al. have shown that Rs-DPLA does not induce TNF-α or IL-6 release by the murine macrophagelike cell line J774.1. Rs-DPLA inhibits the induction of these two cytokines by the Re-LPS from *Salmonella minnesota* R595. Maximal inhibition occurs when the Re-LPS/Rs-DPLA mass ratio is 1:10. The binding study showed that the Rs-DPLA strongly inhibits the binding of ^{125}I-ASD-Re-LPS to the cells and this binding inhibition is about 16-fold greater than that by the unlabeled Re-LPS on a mass basis. These results provide further evidence that the Rs-DPLA is competing with Re-LPS for the physiological receptors on the J774.1 cells, possibly via a CD14 mechanism (64).

3. Binding to CD11b/CD18

Rs-DPLA blocks the LPS-induced upregulation of the expression of CD11b/CD18 in human neutrophils (PMN) (65). CD11b/CD18 is important for PMN margination. By using flow cytometry, LPS-induced expression of the β2 integrin CD11b/CD18 has been characterized. After exposure to *S. minnesota* R595 Re-LPS, expression of neutrophil CD11b/CD18 is rapidly upregulated, beginning within 5 min and achieving a peak fluorescence (typically two- to threefold over baseline) by 30 min. The increase in CD11b/CD18 expression is similar in kinetics and magnitude to that produced by f-Met-Leu-Phe (FMLP), phorbol myristic acid, and human rTNF-α. The upregulation of CD11b/CD18 by LPS is not interrupted by protein synthesis inhibitors. However, both Rs-DPLA and lipid IV_A were able to block the stimulatory effect of LPS. Monoclonal antibody against CD14 also specifically inhibits LPS-induced PMN CD11b/CD18 expression, in both the presence and absence of serum. These findings support the hypothesis that LPS stimulates neutrophils by interacting with specific cellular receptors.

4. LPS-Induced Early Gene Expression and Protein Tyrosine Phosphorylation

One of the earliest biochemical sequella of LPS binding to macrophages is the activation of kinase cascades, which are thought to be essential for gene expression. Within minutes of LPS stimulation of macrophages, tyrosine phosphorylation of 41-, 42-, and 45-kDa proteins is detectable. The 42- and 45-kDa proteins have been identified as "mitogen-activated protein kinase," isoforms of the *erk* family of kinases (66,67). Inhibition of TNF secretion and induction of invitro tolerance induced by LPS or MPLA of *Salmonella* LPS are blocked most efficiently with Rs-DPLA, and somewhat less efficiently by pentaacyl Rs-MPLA

(68), suggesting that the phosphoryl group at the one-position contributes significantly to the interaction of this analog with the putative LPS-signaling receptor. Rs-DPLA also blocks expression of a panel of six LPS-inducible "early" genes and protein-tyrosine phosphorylation in a competitive fashion when Rs-DPLA is present at a concentration of 1 μg/mL in murine macrophages (69).

5. Activation of NF-*k*B Transcription Factor and Induction of *k* in 7OZ/3 Pre-B Cell Line

LPS induction of *k* light-chain expression in B cells is dependent on the action of two transcription factors, NF-*k*B and Oct-2 (70,71). NF-*k*B is a transcription factor involved in the LPS-inducible expression of immunoglobulin *k* light chains in B lymphocytes (72). However, it is now recognized that NF-*k*B plays a central role in the activation of a large number of promoters that control the expression of genes involved in inflammatory responses. Prior to stimulation, NF-*k*B consists of a heterodimer composed of one 50-kDa DNA-binding subunit and one 65-kDa subunit of unknown function complexed with a protein inhibitor (I*k*B) which prevents its binding to DNA. Binding of NF-*k*B to the *k*B site stimulates synthesis of k mRNA. When 7OZ/3 cells are treated with LPS, one p50/65 subunit of the NF-*k*B heterodimer is released from the inhibitor. The inhibitor-free heterodimer then translocates to the nucleus, where it binds to the *k* intron enhancer at the *k*B site. Nuclear NF-*k*B DNA-binding activity can be measured with electrophoretic mobility shift assays. LPS induced a dramatic increase in NF-*k*B binding activity in 7OZ/3 cell nuclei after 15 min, which was sustained through 24 h. In contrast to NF-*k*B, the Oct-2 gene is activated transcriptionally by LPS. Newly synthesized Oct-2 binds to an octamer site just 5' to the *k* gene's TATA box. Since these cells produce μ mRNA constitutively, the initiation of *k* mRNA synthesis leads to the synthesis of surface immunoglobulin.

Rs-DPLA effectively blocked the Re-LPS-induced activation of murine 7OZ/3 pre-B-cell line (73). LPS activates mIgM expression by increasing the rate of *k* transcription. Rs-DPLA failed to induce mIgM expression in these cells, and Rs-DPLA can competitively inhibit the Re-LPS-induced activation of mIgM expression and *k* message synthesis. Rs-DPLA, however, can transiently activate as much NF-*k*B as LPS in 7OZ/3 cells after 1 h of exposure. This effect is not sustained after 24 h as observed with LPS. Both LPS and Rs-DPLA activate a p50/65 NF-kB heterodimer, but Rs-DPLA causes no increase in either Oct-2 or *k* message even after prolonged treatment. The difference between LPS and Rs-DPLA activation in this regard lies in the duration of NF-*k*B induction. The LPS receptor may have the capacity to discriminate molecules of very similar structure, especially with respect to the fatty acyl groups, and to send different signals accordingly, in this case leading to either transient or continuous activation of NF-*k*B. This suggests that Rs-DPLA is not entirely inert, yet does not elicit a signal sufficient to induce *k* transcription (74).

V. IN-VIVO EFFECTS OF Rs-DPLA

A. Effect of Rs-DPLA on Cytokine Production and LPS-Induced Lethality in Galactosamine-Sensitized Mice

Rs-DPLA also blocks the induction of TNF-α in animals due to LPS. Treatment of mice with Rs-DPLA blocks the rapid and transient rise of TNF-α caused by Re-LPS. Similar results were obtained with guinea pigs. Recently, Zuckerman and Qureshi (75) have shown that administration of a 100-fold excess of Rs-DPLA, 1 h prior to Re-LPS administration, inhibits the characteristic peak in serum TNF-α levels induced by LPS in both normal and GalN-sensitized mice. No changes in blood glucose or colony-stimulating factor levels were observed in mice treated with Rs-DPLA alone (Vogel and Qureshi, unpublished results).

There is normally an increase in IL-1β and TNF-α mRNA levels in Re-LPS stimulated mice. Rs-DPLA by itself does not result in a significant increase above constitutive splenic TNF-α or IL-1β mRNA levels. However, mice pretreated with Rs-DPLA prior to Re-LPS had a 90% reduction in the amount of serum TNF-α, and 70% and 34% reductions in the amounts of TNF-α and IL-1β mRNAs, respectively. Moreover, a decrease in the expression of these two genes is observed in Rs-DPLA-pretreated animals (75).

Rs-DPLA pretreatment protects GalN-sensitized mice from a lethal Re-LPS challenge. Rs-DPLA (1 mg) protected GalN-sensitized mice against an LD_{50} of Re-LPS (10 μg) and GalN (10 mg), with 100% survival in the Rs-DPLA-treated group (75).

B. Possible Role of Corticosterone and IFN-γ in Mice

Rs-DPLA pretreatment does not significantly increase the survival of adrenalectomized (Adrex) mice to a lethal challenge of Re-LPS. This experiment suggests that the protective effect of Rs-DPLA may be mediated largely through corticosterone induction (75).

Preliminary experiments on the time course of induction of corticosterone and adrenocorticotrophic hormone (ACTH) in mice by Rs-DPLA and Re-LPS showed the following: With Rs-DPLA (2 mg), an initial rise in corticosterone levels to 1000 ng/mL is observed immediately after injection, which is sustained for 2 h, and levels drop to basal values after 3–4 h. ACTH levels, however, rise moderately to 90 pg/mL within 15–30 min after injection of Rs-DPLA and return to basal values by 1–2 h.

With Re-LPS (10-100 μg), the corticosterone levels increase after 5 min, and rise to about 1300 ng/ml by 3 h. This rise is sustained, and even after 24 h, corticosterone levels are still above basal values. ACTH levels increase to 100 pg/ml at 5–30 min and then go down; ACTH starts rising again at 90–180 min to a peak value of 230 pg/mL (180 min), and by 24 h it approaches basal values. These results showed that Rs-DPLA produces a transient increase in corticosterone levels which lasts about 3–4 h, whereas Re-LPS produces a more sustained and prolonged rise in corticosterone levels. Both ACTH and corticosterone peaked at 3 h after injection. This suggests that the ACTH levels may be affected by several cytokines and inflammatory mediators. The first peak in ACTH is probably not due to IL-1β, since IL-1β is induced 2 h after LPS treatment and corticosterone levels rise 5 min after injection (76).

IFN-γ has been shown to be a mediator of lethal endotoxin-induced Shwartzman-like shock reaction in mice (77). The cellular sources of this cytokine are primarily T lymphocytes and NK cells (78), although recent studies have demonstrated the presence of IFN-γ-specific mRNA and highly cell-associated IFN-γ in LPS-stimulated macrophages (79). Treatment of mice with anti-IFN-γ-MAb up to 2 h after endotoxin injection significantly reduces mortality from endotoxin shock but causes only a slight decrease in serum TNF (80,81). A combination of anti-IFN-γ-Mab and antibody to the IFN-γ receptor administered together provides a substantially greater level of protection (82). IFN-γ has been shown to down-regulate CD14 expression and LPS following IFN-γ pretreatment potentiates this effect (83). This cytokine overcomes glucocorticoid suppression of TNF biosynthesis by murine macrophages (84). It may also act to increase macrophage sensitivity to feedback inhibition by glucocorticoids by increasing the number and/or affinity of available glucocorticoid receptor expressions (85). In contrast to IFN-γ, IFN-α has been reported to prevent endotoxin-induced mortality in mice (86).

The mechanisms by which IFN-γ contributes to LPS-induced toxicity are not known. IFN-γ has been demonstrated to synergize with TNF to induce Shwartzman-like histopathology and death, up-regulate expression of TNF receptors, augment binding of LPS to specific macrophage populations, increase the production of other LPS-induced cytokines (such as IL-1), as well as attenuate IL-1β gene expression in LPS-treated monocytes and macrophages. The effect of IFN-γ on cells has been reviewed recently (87). Recent studies with IFN-γ knockout mice show that these mice are highly resistant to septic shock, thus providing strong evidence for the involvement of IFN-γ in septic shock (88,89).

C.   Rs-DPLA and LPS-Induced Tolerance

Rs-DPLA induces a state of refractoriness to LPS in mice. Mice pretreated with either Rs-DPLA (1 mg) or ReLPS (10 μg), 20 h prior to a lethal challenge with Re-LPS, are endotoxin tolerant, and these mice show no increase in TNF-α upon challenge. However, Rs-DPLA does not induce TNF, and cannot induce tolerance in Adrex mice, so these results indicate that the Rs-DPLA pretreatment results in an endotoxin-tolerant state in normal mice, presumably by a corticosterone-dependent process (75).

The in-vivo protective effects of Rs-DPLA presumably involve a combination of receptor antagonism and corticosteroid elevation. Inhibiting either of these effects of Rs-DPLA as with adrenalectomy compromises the in-vivo protective effects of Rs-DPLA (75).

VI. CONCLUSIONS

The unique biological properties of Rs-DPLA are as follows.

1. Rs-DPLA is an effective antagonist in both human and murine cells types.
2. As an antagonist of toxic LPS, it (a) blocks the binding of toxic LPS to the putative physiological membrane surface signaling receptor; (b) blocks the expression of early and late gene products (mRNA) to TNF-α, IL-1β, TNFR-2, IP-10, D-3, and D-8 in macrophages by toxic LPS; (c) blocks the LPS-induced protein tyrosine phosphorylation in macrophages; (d) blocks the activation of 70Z/3 pre-B cells and yet allows the activation of NF-kB by toxic LPS at early time points; and (e) blocks the induction of TNF-α and IL-1β by toxic LPS at the in-vitro (macrophages) and in-vivo (mice) levels.
3. It induces both ACTH and corticosterone in mice.
4. It protects normal and GalN-sensitized mice against the lethal effects of toxic LPS.

These findings are important because they show that (a) pentaacyl Rs-DPLA can serve as a model ''nontoxic'' lipid A and as an LPS antagonist for structure-to-function and receptor-to-ligand studies; (b) as an LPS antagonist and inducer of corticosteroids, Rs-DPLA is potentially a useful drug for the prevention of gram-negative septic shock.

Based on our present knowledge, a simplified scheme to explain how LPS activates the immune and the neuroendocrine systems is presented in Fig. 2. LPS is shed from the surface of gram-negative bacteria and activates macrophages/monocytes to produce cytokines such as TNF-α, IL-1β, IL-6, and IL-8. LPS also induces the formation of arachidonic acid metabolites such as leukotrienes, prostaglandins, and thromboxanes. Other inflammatory mediators such as superoxide anion, hydrogen peroxide, and nitric oxide are also released. T cells and NK cells are also activated to induce IFN-γ, which further activates macrophages. TNF-α and IL-1β produced by the macrophages and other chemotactic factors such as FMLP stimulate the neutrophils to produce lysosomal enzymes, oxygen anion, and hydrogen peroxide. This is part of the inflammatory response due to LPS.

LPS also activates the production of ACTH and corticosteroids as a part of the antiinflammatory response. The mechanisms through which LPS stimulates the hypothalamic-pituitary-adrenal (HPA) axis and the exact site or sites of action are unclear (75). Production and release of corticosteroids by the adrenal glands

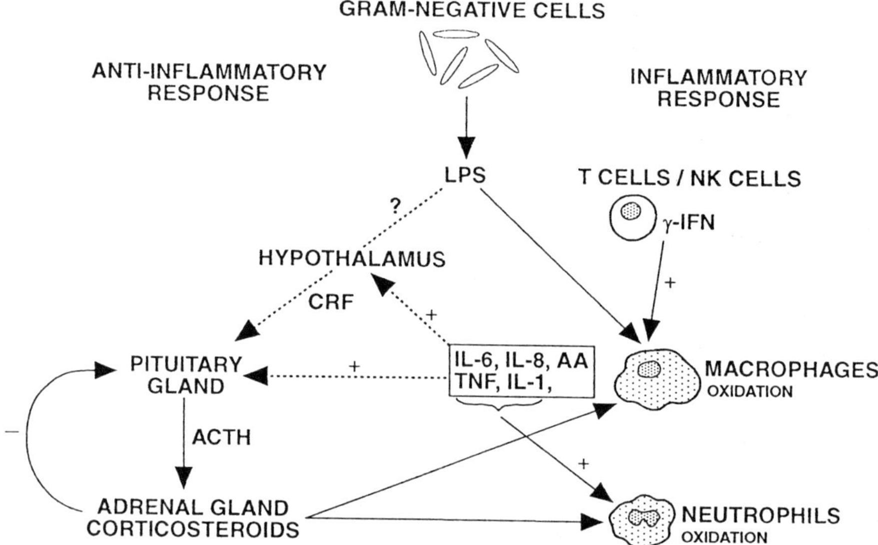

Figure 2 A scheme showing how LPS from gram-negative bacteria can induce both inflammatory and antiinflammatory responses by the immune cells. This is shown to be modulated by the neuroendocrine system.

is primarily under control of ACTH released from the anterior pituitary gland. In turn, the release of ACTH is regulated by corticotropin-releasing factor (CRF) and vasopressin, both of which are produced in the paraventricular nucleus (PVN, hypothalamic neurons) (90). Some investigators have suggested that the hypothalamus mediates stimulation of the HPA axis by LPS, while others have suggested that LPS can stimulate corticosterone secretion even after removal of the medial hypothalamus. LPS could have a direct effect on the pituitary gland or could act through an extrapituitary, nonparaventricular pathway to activate the HPA axis (91).

Recently, IL-1β, TNF-α and IL-6, produced mainly by activated macrophages and monocytes during stimulation with LPS, have been implicated in the activation of the HPA axis. Evidence for the stimulation of one or more of the components of the HPA axis by cytokines is considerable. TNF-α has a direct action on the pituitary to stimulate ACTH production. However, IL-1β activates the release of ACTH by a hypothalamic mechanism, with the release of CRF and possibly vasopressin, which then stimulates the release of corticosteroids (92). The cytokines may act on the pituitary gland to stimulate the release of ACTH directly. However, the role of LPS in the activation of the HPA axis is controversial, and more work is needed (93). Other inflammatory mediators such as

IFN-γ, histamine released from mast cells, serotonin, and leukotrienes also induce corticosteroids. This regulatory loop may have an essential role in preventing a vigorous ongoing acute-phase response. We have recently reviewed this topic (75).

Toxic LPS induces both inflammatory and antiinflammatory responses (a fact that is either ignored or not appreciated). This is in contrast to Rs-DPLA, which at high doses can only induce antiinflammatory responses in vivo. The important point to be made here is that Rs-DPLA can activate the HPA axis *without* the prior induction of TNF-α, IL-1β, and IL-6. The corticosteroids and ACTH are induced within 15–30 min after the administration of Rs-DPLA or Re-LPS in mice. Rs-DPLA (up to 4 mg) does not induce TNF-α in vivo. Corticosteroids produced then reduce the splenic mRNA for TNF-α and IL-1β in macrophages and the activity of the neutrophils. A equilibrium is established between the inflammatory and the antiinflammatory responses. Any defect in the biosynthesis of corticosteroids or the expression of glucocorticoid receptors would increase the inflammatory response and potentially lead to septic shock in this model. The macrophage-neuroendocrine axis is clearly important in the development of septic shock. A concept has emerged that endogenous glucocorticoids can modulate the endotoxic effects of LPS by inhibiting the synthesis of inflammatory cytokines (75).

ACKNOWLEDGMENTS

This review and related work were supported in part by the Medical Research Service of the Department of Veterans Affairs and by National Institutes of Health grants GM-36054 and GM-50870. We thank Cindi Birch for excellent editorial assistance.

REFERENCES

1. Muhlradt L, Golecki JR. Asymmetrical distribution and artificial reorientation of lipopolysaccharide in the outer membrane bilayer of *Salmonella typhimurium*. Eur J Biochem 1975; 51:343–352.
2. Funahara LY, Nikaido H. Asymmetrical localization of lipopolysaccharides on the outer membrane of *Salmonella typhimurium*. J Bacteriol 1980; 141:1463–1465.
3. Morrison DC, Ulevitch RJ. The effects of bacterial endotoxins on host mediation systems. Am J Pathol 1978; 93:527–617.
4. Beutler B, Cerami A. Cachectin: more than a tumor necrosis factor. N Engl J Med 1987; 316:379–385.
5. Qureshi N, Takayama K. Structure and function of lipid A. In: Iglewski BH, Clark VL, eds. The Bacteria, Vol. XI, Molecular Basis of Bacterial Pathogenesis. New York: Academic Press, 1990: 319–338.
6. Takayama K, Qureshi N. Chemical structure of lipid A. In: Morrison DC, Ryan

JL, eds. Bacterial Endotoxic Lipopolysaccharides, Vol. 1, Molecular Biochemistry and Cellular Biology, Boca Raton, FL: CRC Press, 1992: 43–65.

7. Bone RC, Fisher CJ, Clemmer TP, Slotman GJ, Metz CA, Balk RA. Sepsis syndrome: a valid clinical entity. Crit Care Med 1989; 17:389–393.

8. Beutler B, Greenwald JD, Hulmes JD, et al. Identity of tumor necrosis factor and the macrophage-secreted factor. Nature (London) 1985; 316:552–554.

9. Beutler B, Cerami A. The common mediator of shock, cachexia and tumor necrosis. Adv Immunol 1988; 42:213–231.

10. Dinarello CA. Interleukin-1: amino acid sequences, multiple biological activities and comparison with tumor necrosis factor (cachectin). Year Immunol 1986; 2:68–89.

11. Qureshi N, Takayama K, Hofman J, Zuckerman SH. Diphosphoryl lipid A obtained from nontoxic lipopolysaccharide (LPS) of *Rhodobacter sphaeroides* is an LPS antagonist and an inducer of corticosteroids. In: Bacterial Endotoxins: Recognition and Effector Mechanisms. eds. Stutz PL, eds. Levin J, Alving CR, Munford RS, Elsevier, 1993: 361–371.

12. Lynn WA, Golenbock DT. Lipopolysaccharide antagonists. Immunol Today 1992; 13:271–276.

13. Stuetz PL, Aschauer H, Hildebrandt J, et al. Chemical synthesis of endotoxin analogues and some structure activity relationships. In: Nowotny A, Spitzer JJ, Ziegler EJ, eds. Endotoxin Series, Vol. 1, Cellular and Molecular Aspects of Endotoxin Reactions. Belle Mead, NJ: Excerpta Medica, 1991:129–144.

14. Perera PY, Manthey CL, Stuetz PL, Vogel SN. Induction of early gene expression in murine macrophages by toxic and non-toxic synthetic lipid A analogues. Infect Immun 1993; 61:2015–2023.

15. Erwin AL, Munford RS. Deacylation of structurally diverse lipopolysaccharides by human acyloxyacyl hydrolase. J Biol Chem 1990; 265:16444–16449.

16. Pohlman TH, Stanness KA, Beatty PG, Ochs HD, Harlan JD. An endothelial cell surface factor (s) induced in vitro by lipopolysaccharide, interleukin 1, and tumor necrosis factor-alpha increases neutrophil adherence by a Cdw18-dependent mechanism. J Immunol 1986; 136:4548–4554.

17. Riedo FX, Munford RS, Campbell WB, Reisch JS, Chien KR, Gerard RD. Deacylated lipopolysaccharide inhibits plasminogen activator inhibitor-1, prostacyclin, and prostaglandin E2 induction by lipolysaccharide but not by tumor necrosis factor-alpha. J Immunol 1990; 144:3506–3512.

18. Loppnow H, Brade H, Durrbaum I, et al. Interleukin 1 induction capacity of defined lipolysaccharide partial structures. J Immunol 1989; 142:3229–3238.

19. Loppnow H, Libby P, Freundenberg M, Krauss JH, Weckesser J, Mayer H. Cytokine induction by lipopolysaccharide (LPS) corresponds to lethal toxicity and is inhibited by nontoxic *Rhodobacter capsulatus* LPS. Infect Immun 1990; 58:3743–750.

20. Feist W, Ulmer AJ, Wang MH, et al. Modulation of lipolysaccharide-induced production of tumor necrosis factor, interleukin 1, and interleukin 6 by synthetic precursor la of lipid A. FEMS Microbiol Immunol 1992; 89:73–90.

21. Heine H, Brade H, Kusumoto S, et al. Inhibition of LPS binding on human

monocytes by phosphonooxyethyl analogs of lipid A. J Endotoxin Res 1994; 1:14–20.

22. Takayama K, Qureshi N, Beutler B, Kirkland TN. Diphosphoryl lipid A obtained from *Rhodopseudomonas sphaeroides* ATCC 17023 blocks induction of cachectin in macrophage by lipopolysaccharide. Infect Immun 1989; 57:1336–1338.

23. Qureshi N, Takayama K, Kurtz R. Diphosphoryl lipid A obtained from the nontoxic lipopolysaccharide of *Rhodopseudomonas sphaeroides* is an endotoxin antagonist in mice. Infect Immun 1991; 59:441–444.

24. Strittmatter W, Weckesser J, Salimath PV, Galanos C. Nontoxic lipoplysaccharide from *Rhodopseudomonas sphaeroides* ATCC 17023. J. Bacteriol 1983; 155:153–158.

25. Salimath PV, Weckesser J, Strittmatter W, Mayer H. Structural studies on the non-toxic lipid A from *Rhodopseudomonas sphaeroides*. Eur J Biochem 1983; 136:195–200.

26. Qureshi N, Honovich JP, Hara H, Cotter RJ, Takayama K. Location of fatty acids in lipid A obtained from lipopolysaccharides of *Rhodopseudomonas sphaeroides* ATCC 17023. J Biol Chem 1988; 263:5502–5504.

27. Qureshi N, Takayama K, Meyer KC, et al. Chemical reduction of 3-oxo and unsaturated groups in fatty acids of diphosphoryl lipid A from the lipopolysaccharide of *Rhodopseudomonas sphaeroides*. Comparison of biological properties before and after reduction. J Biol Chem 1991; 266:6532–6538.

28. Qureshi N, Takayama K, Mascagni P, Honovich J, Wong R, Cotter RJ. Complete structural determination of lipopolysaccharides obtained from deep rough mutant of *Escherichia coli*. Purification by high performance liquid chromatography and direct analysis by plasma desorption mass spectrometry. J Biol Chem 1988; 263:11971–11976.

29. Christ WJ, McGuinness PD, Asano O, et al. Total synthesis of the proposed structure of *Rhodobacter sphaeroides* lipid A resulting in the synthesis of new potent lipopoly-saccharide antagonists. J Am Chem Soc 1994; 116:3637–3638.

30. Tracey KJ. The acute and pathophysiologic effects of TNF: mediation of septic shock and wasting (cachexia). In: Beutler B, ed. Tumor Necrosis Factors: The Molecules and Their Emerging Role in Medicine. New York: Raven Press, 1992:255–269.

31. Poll TDV, Sauerwein HP. Tumour necrosis factor-α: its role in the metabolic response to sepsis. Clin Sci 1993; 84:247–256.

32. Dinarello CA. Biology of interleukin 1. FASEB J 1988; 2:108–115.

33. Lumpkin MD. The regulation of ACTH secretion by IL-1. Science 1987; 238:452–454.

34. Van Deventer SJH, Hart H, van der Poll T, Hack CE, Arden LA. Endotoxin and tumor necrosis factor-α-induced interleukin-8 release in humans. J Infect Dis 1993; 167:461–464.

35. Gerard C, Bruyns C, Merchant A, et al. Interleukin 10 reduces the release of tumor necrosis factor and prevents lethality in experimental endotoxemia. J Exp Med 1993; 177:547–550.

36. Chomarat P, Rissoan M-C, Banchereau J, Miossec P. Interferon-γ inhibits interleu-
     kin 10 production by monocytes. J Exp Med 1993; 177:523–527.
37. Durez P, Abramowicz L, Gerard C, et al. In vivo induction of interleukin 10 by
     anti-CD3 monoclonal antibody or bacterial lipopolysaccharide: differential modula-
     tion by cyclosporin A. J Exp Med 1993; 177:551–555.
38. Bogdan C, Paik J, Vodovitz Y, Nathan C. Contrasting mechanisms for suppression
     of macrophage cytokine release by transforming growth factor-β and interleukin-
     10. J Biol Chem 1992; 267:23301–23308.
39. Fletcher Starnes HFV Jr, Pearce MK, Tewari A, Yim JH, Zou J-C, Abrams JS.
     Anti-IL-6 monoclonal antibodies protect against lethal *Escherichia coli* infection in
     mice. J Immunol 1990; 145:4185–4191.
40. Libert C, Vink A, Coulie P, et al. Limited involvement of interleukin-6 in the
     pathogenesis of lethal septic shock as revealed by the effect of monoclonal antibodies
     against interleukin-6 or its receptor in various murine models. Eur J Immunol 1992;
     22:2625–2630.
41. Golenbock DT, Hampton RY, Qureshi N, Takayama K, Raetz CRH. Lipid A-like
     molecules that antagonize the effects of endotoxins on human monocytes. J Biol
     Chem 1991; 266:19490–19498.
42. Vogel SN. The Lps gene: insights into the genetic and molecular basis of LPS
     responsiveness and macrophage differentiation. In: Beutler B, ed. Tumor Necrosis
     Factors: The Molecules and Their Emerging Role in Medicine. New York: Raven
     Press, 1992: 485–513.
43. De Boer JP, Wolbink G-J, Thijs LG, Baars JW, Wagstaff J, Hack CE. Interplay
     of complement and cytokines in the pathogenesis of septic shock. Immunopharma-
     cology 1992; 24:135–148.
44. Vadas P, Pruzanski W. Induction of group II phospholipase A2 expression and
     pathogenesis of the sepsis syndrome. Circulatory Shock 1993; 39:160–167.
45. Sheehan KCF, Schreiber RD. The synergy and antagonism of interferon-γ and
     TNF. In: Beutler B, ed. Tumor Necrosis Factors: The molecules and their emerging
     role in medicine. New York: Raven Press, 1992: 145–178
46. Ding A, Nathan CF, Stuehr DJ. Release of reactive nitrogen intermediates from
     mouse peritoneal macrophages: comparison of activating cytokines and evidence
     for independent production. J Immunol 1988; 141:2407–2412.
47. Ding A, Nathan CF, Graycar J, Derynck R, Stuehr DJ, Srimal S. Macrophage
     deactivating factor and transforming growth factors-beta 1, -beta 2 and -beta 3
     inhibit induction of macrophage nitrogen oxide synthesis by IFN-gamma. J Immunol
     1990; 145:940–944.
48. Kilbourne RG, Gross SS, Jubran A., et al. N^g- methyl-L-arginine inhibits tumor
     necrosis factor-induced hypotension: implications for the involvement of nitric ox-
     ide. Proc Natl Acad Sci USA 1990; 87:3629–3633.
49. Meyer KC, Qureshi N, Powers C, Takayama K. Priming of human alveolar macro-
     phages for superoxide anion release. Lipopolysaccharides from *Rhodobacter sphaer-
     oides* antagonize priming effects of endotoxic lipopolysaccharide. Submitted.
50. Kirikae F, Kirikae T, Qureshi N, Takayama K, Morrison DC, Nakano M. *Rhodo-
     bacter sphaeroides* diphosphoryl lipid A inhibits tumor necrosis factor-alpha and

nitric oxide production induced by taxol, a lipopolysaccharide agonist, via a LPS receptor(s) on murine macrophages. Infect Immun 1995; 63: 486–497.

51. Morrison DC, Ryan JL. Endotoxin and disease mechanisms. Ann Rev Med 1987; 38:417–432.

52. Wright SD. Multiple receptors for endotoxin. Curr Opinion Immunol 1988; 3:83–90.

53. Lei M, Stimpson SA, Morrison DC. Specific endotoxic lipopolysaccharide-binding receptors on murine splenocytes III. Binding specificity and characterization. J Immunol 1991; 147:1925–1932.

54. Morrison DC, Silverstein R, Bright SW, Chen TY, Flebbe LM, Lei MG. Monoclonal antibody to mouse lipolysaccharide receptor protects mice against the lethal effects of endotoxin. J Infect Dis 1990; 162:1063–1068.

55. Lei M-G, Qureshi N, Morrison DC. *Rhodopseudomonas sphaeroides* lipid A competes with LPS for binding to the 73 kDa receptor but not to a 38 kDa LPS binding protein on lymphoreticular cells. Immunol Lett 1993; 36:245–250.

56. Schumann RR, Leong SR, Flaggs GW, et al. Structure and function of lipopolysaccharide-binding protein. Science 1990; 249:1429–1431.

57. Wright SD, Ramos RA, Tobias PS, Ulevitch RJ, Mathison JC. CD14, a receptor for complexes of lipopolysaccharides (LPS) and LPS binding protein. Science 1990; 249:1431–1433.

58. Frey EA, Miller DS, Jahr TG, et al. Soluble CD14 participates in the response of cells to lipopolysaccharide. J Exp Med. 1992; 176:1665–1671.

59. Stefanova I, Corcoran ML, Horak EM, Wahl LM, Bolen JB, Horak ID. Lipopolysaccharide induces activation of CD14-associated protein tyrosine kinase p53/56^{lyn}. J Biol Chem 1993; 268:20725–20728.

60. Wright SD, Ramos RA, Patel M, Miller DS. Septin: a factor in plasma that opsonizes lipopolysaccharide bearing particles for recognition by CD14 on phagocytes. J Exp Med 1992; 176:719–727.

61. Schumann RR. Function of lipopolysaccharide (LPS) -binding protein (LBP) and CD14, the receptor for LPS/LBP complexes: a short review. Res Immunol 1992; 143:11–15.

62. Ulevitch R. Recognition of bacterial endotoxin in biological systems. Lab Invest 1991; 65:121–122.

63. Kitchens RL, Ulevitch RJ, Munford RS. Lipopolysaccharide (LPS) partial structures inhibit responses to LPS in a human macrophage cell line without inhibiting LPS uptake by a CD14-mediated pathway. J Exp Med 1992; 176:485–494.

64. Kirikae T, Schade FU, Kirikae F, Qureshi N, Takayama K, Rietschel ET. Diphosphoryl lipid derived from the lipopolysaccharide (LPS) of *Rhodobacter sphaeroides* is a potent competitive LPS inhibitor in murine macrophage-like J774.1. FEMS Immunol Med Microbiol, 1994; 9: 237–243.

65. Lynn WA, Raetz CRH, Qureshi N, Golenbock DT. LPS induced stimulation of CD11b/CD18 expression on neutrophils. Evidence of specific receptor-based response and inhibition by lipid A-based antagonists. J Immunol 1991; 147:3072–3079.

66. Weinstein SL, Gold MR, DeFranco AL. Bacterial lipopolysaccharide stimulate

tyrosine phosphorylation in macrophages. Proc Natl Acad Sci USA 1991; 88:4148–4152.

67. Weinstein SL, Sanghera JS, DeFranco AL, Pelech SL. LPS induces tyrosine phosphorylation and activation of MAP kinases in macrophages. J Cell Biochem Suppl 16C:169 (abstr), 1992.

68. Henricson BE, Perera PY, Qureshi N, Takayama K, Vogel SN. *Rhodopseudomonas sphaeroides* lipid A derivative block in vitro induction of tumor necrosis factor and endotoxin tolerance by smooth lipopolysaccharide and monophosphoryl lipid A. Infect Immun 1992; 60:4285–4290.

69. Manthey CL, Perera PY, Qureshi N, Stutz PL, Hamilton TA, Vogel SN. Inhibition of lipopolysaccharide-induced macrophage gene expression by *Rhodobacter sphaeroides* lipid A and SDZ 880.431. Infect Immun 1993; 61:3518–3526.

70. Sen R, Baltimore D. Multiple nuclear factors interact with the immunoglobulin enhancer sequences. Cell 1986; 46:705–716.

71. Rooney JW, Emery DW, Sibley CH. 1.3E2, a variant of the B lymphoma 70Z/3 defective in activation of NF-kB and OTF-2. Immunogenetics 1990; 31:73–78.

72. Zabel U, Bauerle P. Purified IkB can rapidly dissociate the complex of the NF-kB transcription factor with its cognate DNA. Cell 1990; 61:255–265.

73. Kirkland TN, Qureshi N, Takayama K. Diphosphoryl lipid A derived from lipopolysaccharide (LPS) of *Rhodopseudomonas sphaeroides* inhibits activation of 70Z/3 cells by LPS. Infect Immun 1991; 59:131–136.

74. Lawrence O, Rachie N, Qureshi N, Bomsztyk K, Sibley CH. Diphosphoryl lipid A from *Rhodobacter sphaeroides* transiently activates NF-*k*B but inhibits lipolysaccharide (LPS) induction of kappa immunoglobin and Oct-2 in the B cell lymphoma 70Z/3. Infect Immun 1995; 63: 1040–1046

75. Zuckerman SH and Qureshi N. In vivo inhibition of LPS induced lethality and TNF synthesis by *Rhodobacter sphaeroides* diphosphoryl lipid A is dependent on corticosterone induction. Infect Immun 1992; 60:2581–2587.

76. Hofman J, Qureshi N, Takayama K, Kalin N, Vogel SN, Morrison DC. LPS-antagonizing effects of diphosphoryl-lipid A from *Rhodobacter sphaeroides* (Rs-DPLA). In: Bacterial Endotoxins: Basic Science to Anti-sepsis Strategies. New York. Wiley-Liss, 1994, 95–106.

77. Heremans H, Van Damme J, Dillen C, Dijkmans L, Billiau A. Interferon-γ, a mediator of lethal lipopolysaccharide-induced Shwartzman-like shock reactions in mice. J Exp Med 1990; 171:1853–1869.

78. Vogel SN. Lipopolysaccharide-induced interferon. In: Ryan JL and Morrison DC, eds. Bacterial Endotoxic Lipopolysaccharides, Vol. 2, Boca Raton, Fl: CRC Press, 1992: 165–195.

79. Fultz MJ, Barber SA, Dieffenbach CW, Vogel SN. Induction of interferon-γ in macrophages by lipopolysaccharide. Immunol 1993; 5:1383–1392.

80. Heinzel FP. The role of IFN-γ in the pathology of experimental endotoxemia. J Immunol 1990; 145:2920–2924.

81. Silva AT, Cohen J. Role of interferon-γ in experimental endotoxemia. J Infect Dis 1992; 166:331–335.

82. Bucklins, Russells, and Morrison DC. Augmentation of anti-cytokine immunotherapy by combining neutralizing monoclonal antibodies to interferon-γ and the interferon-γ receptor: protection in endotoxin shock. J Endotoxin Res, 1994; 1:45–51.

83. Payne JB, Nichols FC, Peluso JF. The effects of interferon-γ and bacterial lipopolysaccharide on CD14 expression in human monocytes. J Infect Dis 1992; 166:331–335.

84. Leudke CE, Cerami A. Interferon-γ overcomes glucocorticoid suppression of cachectin/tumor necrosis factor biosynthesis of murine macrophages. J Clin Invest 1990; 86:1234–1240.

85. Salkowski CA, Vogel SN. Lipopolysaccharide increases glucocorticoid receptor expression in murine macrophages. A possible mechanism for glucocorticoid-mediated suppression of endotoxicity. J Immunol 1992; 149:4041–4047.

86. Tzung S-P, Mahl TC, Lance P, Andersen V, Cohen SA. Interferon-α prevents endotoxin-induced mortality in mice. Eur J Immunol 1992; 22:3097–3101.

87. Vogel SN. Lipopolysaccharide-induced interferon. In: Ryan JL, Morrison DC, ed. Bacterial Endotoxic Lipopolysaccharides, Vol. II. Boca Raton, FL: CRC Press, 1993: 165–195.

88. Barinaga M. Interfering with interferon. Science 1993; 259:1693–1694.

89. Car BD, Eng VM, Schnyder B, et al. Interferon γ receptor deficient mice are resistant to endotoxic shock. J Exp Med 1994; 179:1437–1444.

90. Bateman A, Singh A, Kral T, and Solomon S. The immune-hypothalamic-pituitary-adrenal axis. Endocrine Rev 1989; 10:92–112.

91. Elenkov IJ, Kovacs K, Kiss J, Bertok L, Vizi ES. Lipopolysaccharide is able to bypass corticotrophin releasing factor in affecting plasma ACTH and corticosterone levels: evidence from rats with lesions of the paraventricular nucleus. J Endocrinol 1992; 133:231–236.

92. Dunn AJ. The role of interleukin-1 and tumor necrosis factor-α in the neurochemical and neuroendocrine responses to endotoxin. Brain Res Bull 1992; 29:807–812.

8

Inhibition of Endotoxin-Induced Monocyte and T-Lymphocyte Activation by Lipopolysaccharide Partial Structures

Artur J. Ulmer, Taila Mattern, Holger Heine, Birgit Weidemann, Helmut Brade, Ernst Th. Rietschel, and Hans-Dieter Flad
Forschungsinstitut Borstel
Borstel, Germany

Shoichi Kusumoto
Osaka University
Osaka, Japan

I. INTRODUCTION

Endotoxin, a constituent of the outer leaflet of gram-negative bacteria, plays a prominent role during infection. It is released from multiplying and, in higher amounts, from dying bacteria, e.g., during treatment with antibiotics. Endotoxin induces in an infected host a variety of systemic pathophysiological effects, including fever, hypotension, disseminated intravascular coagulation, multiorgan failure, miscarriages, and/or endotoxic shock, which in most severe situations may cause death (1).

Today it is well established that toxic effects of endotoxin are not due to direct action of endotoxin, but are elicited by secondary mediators. Interleukin 1 (IL-1), interleukin 6 (IL-6), and tumor necrosis factor (TNF) are such hormonelike proteins that are released by a variety of cells [fibroblasts, endothelial cells, epithelial cells, Langerhans cells, macrophages, keratinocytes, and/or astrocytes (2–4)] after exposure to endotoxin.

Endotoxin is an amphiphilic structure consisting of a hydrophilic polysaccharide and a covalently bound hydrophobic lipid component, termed lipid A. Hence, it is chemically a "lipopolysaccharide" (LPS). The major conspicuous function of LPS in the manifestation of gram-negative infections has been greatly stimulated by its structure elucidation, by the determination of its biologically active moiety, and by the development of antagonistic partial structures.

Figure 1 shows the chemical structure of two of the most important synthetic compounds, compound 506 and compound 406. Compound 506 is a synthetic hexaacyl lipid A consisting of a bisphosphorylated β 1,6-linked D-glucosamine disaccharide carrying six acyl residues and structurally corresponding to free lipid A prepared from LPS of the *Escherichia coli* Re-mutant strain F515 (5–8). Compound 406 is a synthetic tetraacyl lipid A precursor Ia (also termed lipid IV_a or LA-14-PP), which was synthesized as described elsewhere (9,10). Beside these two compounds, a variety of other lipid A analogs have been synthesized, which differ in their phosphorylation and acylation pattern. A list of the most essential compounds tested in our laboratory is given elsewhere (11).

II. LPS, LIPID A, STRUCTURE–ACTIVITY RELATIONSHIP

Based on the finding that the monokines IL-1, IL-6, and/or TNF are involved in the reactions during septicemia, our approaches to study the structure–activity

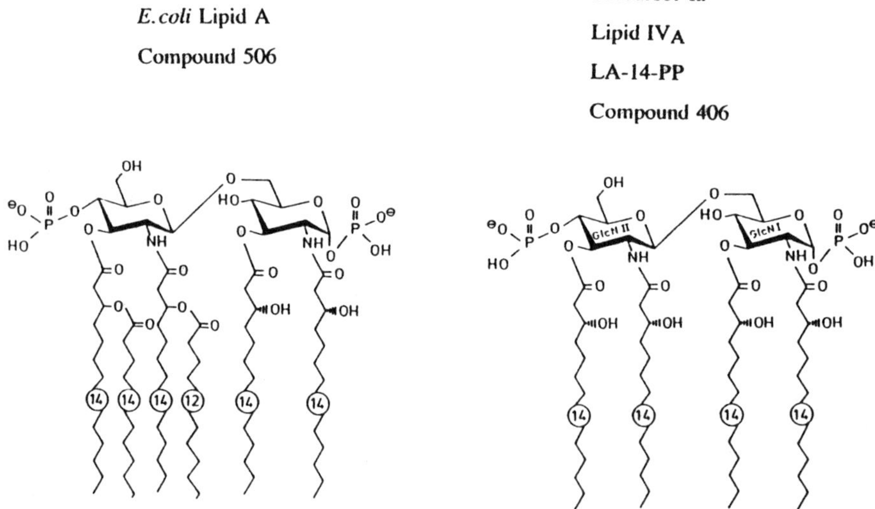

Figure 1 Chemical structure of synthetic *E. coli*-type lipid A (compound 506) and synthetic lipid A precursor Ia (compound 406).

relationship of LPS, lipid A, and their defined partial structures focused on the induction of monokine production in vitro. We used human peripheral blood mononuclear cells (MNC) or monocytes as effector cells. LPS, lipid A, or lipid A partial structures were either of bacterial or of synthetic origin.

We were able to demonstrate a structure-dependent hierarchy of LPS and defined LPS partial structures in their capacity to induce IL-1, IL-6, and TNF (12–14). Figure 2 shows the results of an experiment with compound 506 and compound 406 with respect to IL-1 production. Determination of TNF and IL-6 revealed similar results. These in vitro experiments enabled us to confirm in-vivo experiments showing that lipid A is the principle expressing all the activities of LPS. However, lipid A is not as active as LPS in inducing monokines. First, the minimal concentration of lipid A necessary for the stimulation of monokine production by human MNC is about 10-fold higher than the minimal bioactive concentration of LPS. Second, the amount of monokines (IL-1, IL-6, or TNF) produced after stimulation with lipid A is lower than after stimulation with LPS. In contrast to compound 506, the tetraacylated lipid A precursor Ia (compound 406) is a lipid A partial structure with no agonistic biological activity on human monocytes (Fig. 2). This indicates that the induction of monokines in human monocytes requires a lipid A structure with more than four fatty acid residues. The acyl residues at the lipid A backbone are significant for the biological activity not only of lipid A but also of LPS. This has been demonstrated previously by Loppnow et al. (15), reporting that LPS from *Rhodobacter capsulatus* LPS shows only minor monokine-inducing activities. LPS from *R. capsulatus* is composed of a lipid A backbone containing only two amide-linked 3-oxo-myristic acids and two ester-linked 3-OH-10:0 fatty acids. Therefore, we conclude that results regarding the biological activity of lipid A are also of relevance for the evaluation of the biological activity of LPS having different lipid A backbones.

Besides the acylation pattern, the phosphorylation of lipid A is also of significance for the biological activity of these compounds. When comparing different phosphorylated *E. coli*-type lipid A structures, the results indicate that biphosphorylated lipid A structures are more active than monophosphorylated structures (12,13).

It should be noted that not only the lipophilic part of LPS but also the hydrophilic oligosaccharides derived from the core region of LPS are of great relevance for the biological activity of LPS. However, data on the monokine-inducing activity of the oligosaccharides alone are so far conflicting (16–18).

In past years, knowledge has been accumulated on the effects of LPS on murine B-lymphocytes (19) and on murine or human monocytes/ macrophages (reviewed in Refs. 5 and 7). Less known are the effects of LPS on T lymphocytes. Whereas in-vitro proliferative responses of murine T cells to LPS have been reported (20,21), a proliferation of human T cells has not been observed (22–24).

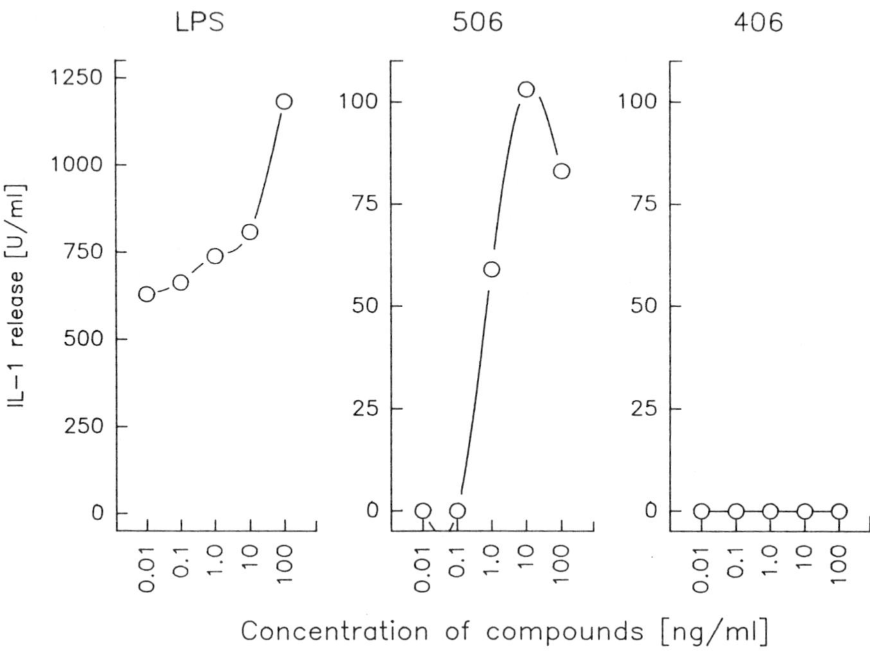

Figure 2 Induction of IL-1 by LPS, compound 506, and compound 406 in human MNC. MNC (4×10^6/mL) were stimulated with LPS, synthetic compound 506, or synthetic compound 406 at concentrations ranging from 0.01 ng/mL to 100 ng/mL. After an incubation period of 12 h, the supernatants were harvested and tested for IL-1 production in a bioassay. Each value represents the mean of triplicate cultures.

Recently we found that human T lymphocytes can be stimulated by LPS (25). Dose-response experiments revealed induction of T-cell proliferation at 10 pg/mL of LPS with a maximum at 100–10,000 ng/mL. By testing synthetic compounds we could show that the bioactive region of LPS for the activation of T cells also is lipid A: *E. coli*-type lipid A (compound 506) induces T-cell proliferation, whereas the tetraacylated partial structure of lipid A (precursor Ia, compound 406) is not active (see Fig. 3). This proliferation is accompanied by the expression of mRNA for the TH_1 lymphokines IFN-γ and IL-2, but not for the TH_2 lymphokines IL-4, IL-5, or IL-10. $CD4^+$ as well as $CD8^+$ T cells belong to the responder population. Limiting dilution analyses revealed that the frequency of responding cells is about 1/800 cells. Activation of human T lymphocytes by LPS needs accessory functions provided by viable monocytes during direct cell-to-cell contact. Viable monocytes cannot be replaced by B lymphocytes, fixed monocytes, or monokine cocktails (IL-1, IL -6, and/or TNF). Monocytes, preincubated with

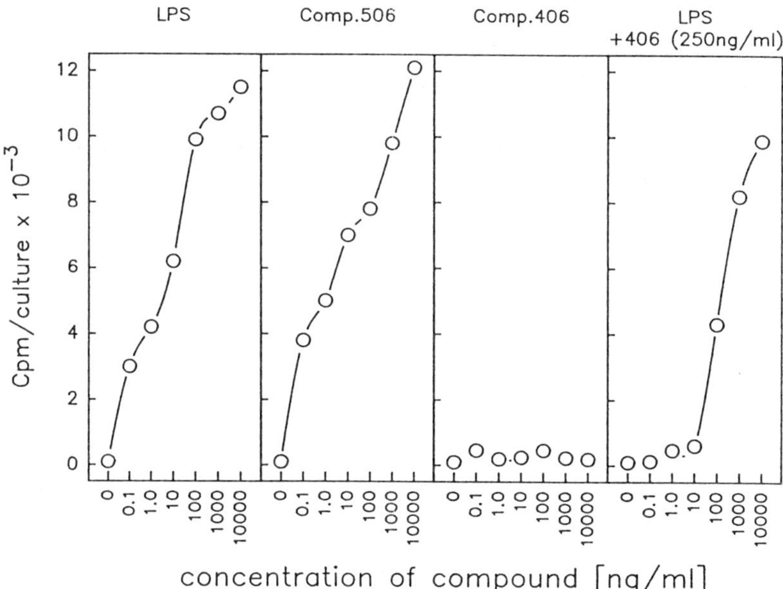

Figure 3 Dose response curves of purified LPS from *S. friedenau*, compound 506, compound 406, and a combination of LPS and compound 406. Human MNC (1 × 10^6/mL) were stimulated with the indicated amounts of LPS or LPS partial structures. After 7 days of culture, the thymidine incorporation was determined. Each value represents the mean of triplicate cultures.

LPS, are able to activate T lymphocytes, which leads to the assumption that a kind of presentation of LPS by monocytes is involved in the activation mechanism. This hypothesis could be confirmed by the finding that purified T lymphocytes did not bind FITC-LPS even in the presence of soluble CD14. Furthermore, CD14 was not detectable on T cells. Our results indicate that human T cells respond to LPS exposure by proliferation and lymphokine production in a monocyte-dependent manner. This finding may be of clinical relevance because of the known contribution of T-cell-derived cytokines in septic shock.

III. ANTAGONISTIC ACTION OF LIPID A ANALOGS

After we had analyzed the effect of LPS and its partial structures alone on their monokine-inducing capacity and on T-cell activation, it was obvious to investigate the combined interaction of these components in the hope that nonactive partial structures might compete endotoxin-mediated reactions. Such antagonistic compounds may be valuable therapeutic agents in endotoxin-mediated

                                                          Ulmer et al.

diseases such as septic shock. This antagonistic action should differ from the so-called endotoxin-induced LPS resistance or LPS tolerance, which is a refractory state of cells (in vitro) or animals (in vivo) rather than a competitive inhibitory effect (26–28). Up to now a variety of different lipid A analogs has been tested regarding their antagonistic effect on LPS-induced reactions in vitro and in vivo.

Less antagonistic action has been reported for lipid X, the monosaccharide lipid A precursor in different animal or cellular models (14,29–31). More efficient antagonists of the endotoxic effects of LPS were found within disaccharide lipid A analogs. Of special interest was the action of lipid A precursor Ia (compound 406) on endotoxin-induced IL-1, IL-6, and TNF production by human monocytes. We and others (14,17,29,32,33) found that the synthetic compound 406 is able to effectively inhibit LPS-induced monokine production (Fig. 4) as

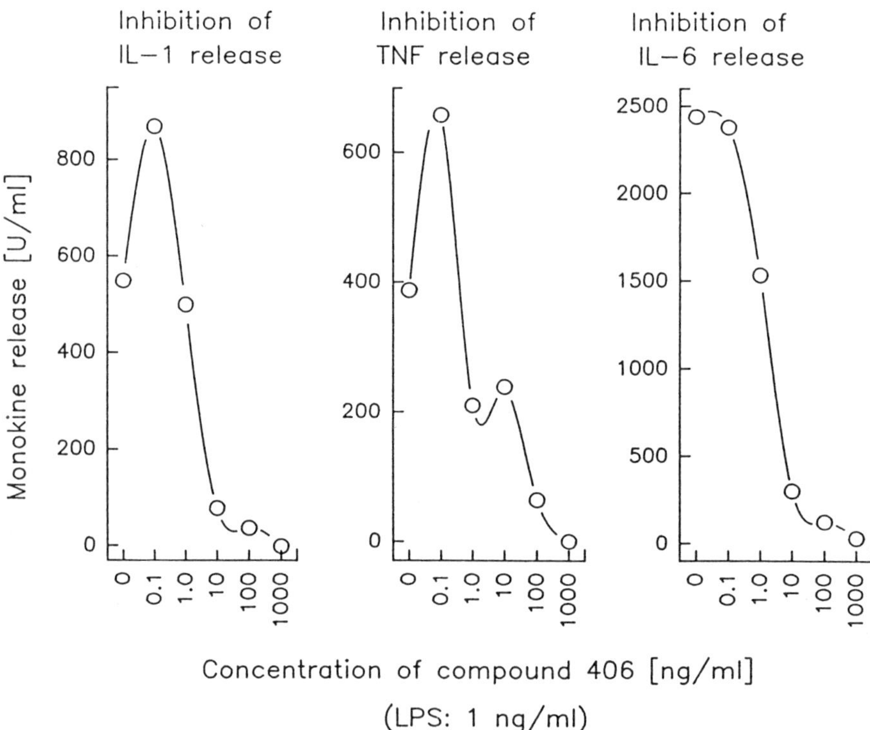

Figure 4 Inhibition of LPS-induced IL-1, TNF, and IL-6 production by compound 406. MNC (4 × 10^6/mL) were preincubated in the presence of compound 406 at concentrations as indicated. After 1 h, LPS was added at a concentration of 1 ng/mL. The release of IL-1, TNF, and IL-6 in the culture supernatant was determined after 12 h of incubation. Each value represents the mean of triplicate cultures.

well as T-cell proliferation (Fig. 3, and Ref. 25). Compound 406 exerted its inhibitory effect on monocyte activation not only by inhibition of the release of monokines, but at an earlier stage of monokine production. The LPS-induced specific mRNA production for monokines (IL-1 and TNF) was found to be blocked by compound 406, as shown by Northern blot analysis (33). Similar results were obtained by Kovach et al. (34) using lipid IV_a isolated from *S. typhimurium*, and by Takayama et al. (35), who investigated the inhibitory effect of pentaacyl diphosphoryl lipid A isolated from *Rhodopseudomonas sphaeroides* ATCC 17023. Furthermore, the non-active LPS of *Rhodobacter capsulatus*, having only five acyl residues bound to the lipid A backbone, also shows inhibitory activity when investigated regarding LPS (e.g., from *Pseudomonas diminuta*)-induced monokine production in a specific manner (15).

Investigation of the structure–activity relationship of the inhibitory effects of lipid A analogs proved that compound 406 and its phosphonooxyethyl analog PE-4 are the most potent inhibitory compounds tested (36). Compounds with a higher number of acid residues become agonists (37,38). A lipid A composed of a reduced number of acid residues (e.g., compound 606) has less inhibitory activity than compound 406 (37,40). Furthermore, the phosphorylation of these compounds is of important significance (37). These findings indicate that the structure–activity requirement for the antagonistic activity of lipid A analogs follows the same rule as the structure requirements for the agonistic activity.

All previous investigations on the specificity of the antagonistic action of compound 406 have shown that compound 406 exerted its inhibitory activity in a specific way and only on LPS induction. Monokine production induced by phorbolester, *S. epidermidis*, *Bacillus Calmette-Guérin*, *Staphylococcus aureus* COWAN I, or by a lipopeptide (N-palmitoyl-(S)-[2,3- bis(palmitoyloxy)-(2RS)-propyl]-(R)-cysteinylseryl-lysyl-lysyl-lysyl-lysine) was absolutely not affected (14,17,33). This has led to the assumption that a competitive mechanism for the inhibition by 406 on LPS-induced monokine production is effective. However, more recently (39) we reported that compound 406 not only antagonizes monokine induction by LPS but also by soluble peptidoglycan (sPG) in human monocytes (Fig. 5). In addition, monokine production induced by sPG was also blocked by anti-CD14 monoclonal antibodies. These findings may indicate that CD14 is involved in common activation steps during the induction of human monocytes by LPS or sPG. However, since biochemical analyses of the interaction of sPG and CD14 (e.g., binding experiments) have not been performed so far, this hypothesis still needs to be verified.

The above results show that low acylated lipid A analogs, such as compound 406, are potent antagonists of LPS-induced activities in human systems in vitro. In this manner they may be able to prevent the LPS-mediated production of shock-inducing monokines in vivo and represent a new approach in managing systemic endotoxemia. It should be mentioned, however, that compound 406

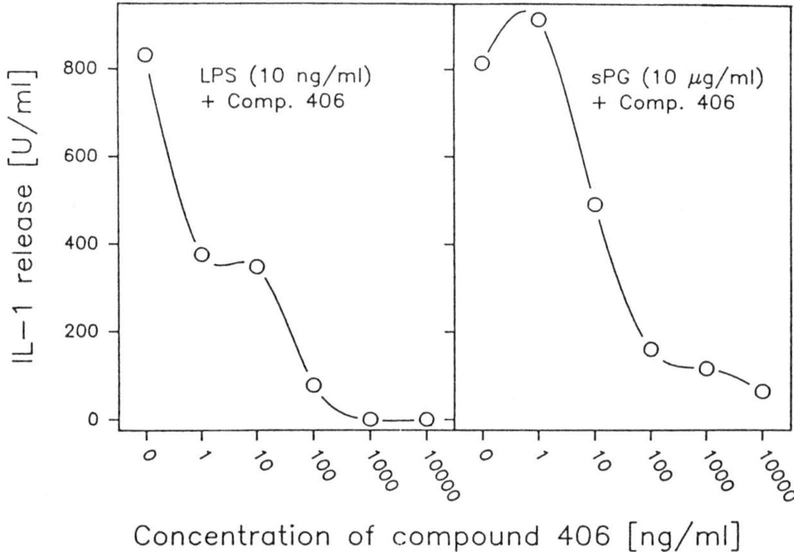

Figure 5 Inhibition of LPS- and sPG-induced Il-1 release by compound 406. MNC (4 × 10⁶/mL) were preincubated in the presence of compound 406 at increasing concentrations as indicated for 1 h. After 8 h of stimulation with LPS (1 ng/mL) or sPG (10 μg/mL), the supernatants were harvested, and IL-1 activity was determined in a bioassay. Each value represents the mean of triplicate cultures.

exerts endotoxic activities in mice and other animal models. Therefore, this compound cannot be pretested for its antagonistic action on endotoxemia or septic shock in an animal model. More recently, a new lipid A analog has been described which effectively antagonizes the action of LPS. E5531 is a synthetic analog of the nontoxic lipid A from *Rhodobacter capsulatus* which inhibits at nanomolar concentrations the TNF production induced by LPS in human monocytes as well as LPS-responsive murine cells (40). It showed a therapeutical effect in mice, reducing the lethality to *E. coli* under antibiotic treatment nearly completely. These results give hope that antagonistic lipid A partial structures will be useful drugs for therapeutic intervention in endotoxin-mediated septic shock.

IV. BINDING OF LPS, LIPID A, OR LIPID A ANALOGS TO MONOCYTES/MACROPHAGES

Interaction of LPS with a target cell (e.g., monocytes /macrophages) of an infected host is a prerequisite for the induction of its biological effects. The first event which can be observed is the binding to the surface membrane. Different structures for binding of LPS have been described so far: CD18 recognizes *E. coli* via LPS and is present on all leukocytes (41). It is noncovalently linked to either CD11a (LFA-1), CD11b (iC3b receptor), or CD11c (42). However, this LPS-recognizing antigen does not seem to be involved in the activation of cytokine secretion in monocytes/ macrophages by LPS (43). Another LPS-binding protein on monocytes/macrophages is a 40-kDa protein detected by Kirikae et al. (44). However, there is no evidence that this protein may serve as a functional receptor for LPS. There is no question that CD14 is the prominent LPS-binding structure on monocytes/macrophages. It has been shown that interaction of LPS with CD14 is necessary for the specific binding and activation of human monocytes or murine macrophages (38,45,46). The binding of LPS to CD14 has been a special feature, as reviewed recently by Tobias and Ulevitch (47). In the absence of serum factor(s), this binding seems to be rather low, but can be mediated by an LPS-binding protein (LBP) or septins (45,48,49). LBP forms a complex together with LPS and enhances binding to CD14 manyfold. LBP seems to be responsible for the fact that only minute amounts of LPS are necessary to stimulate monocytes/macrophages. CD14 is only phosphoinsositol-anchored into the membrane and, in this way, may be unable to activate transmembrane signals (50). However, anti-CD14 monoclonal antibodies alone, like other phosphoinositol-anchored membrane proteins, are able to induce intracellular signals such as Ca^{2+} flux, protein tyrosine phosphorylation, and NF-κ B activation (51,52). Nevertheless, an additional, undefined membrane structure may be involved in the activation of the cells. Indeed, there is growing evidence for more than one specific LPS-binding site on monocytes/macrophages which may recognize different substructures of LPS or lipid A, respectively (53–56). One of the best candidates for such a receptor is a recently discovered 80-kDa LPS-binding protein found on human monocytes and endothelial cells (57). This protein binds LPS and lipid A only in the presence of soluble CD14 and LBP.

The knowledge of the LPS receptors/binding structures leads to the question of whether the different biological activity of lipid A partial structures is the result of a different binding strength and whether the antagonistic lipid A partial structures simply block the binding of LPS to cells. Therefore, structure–activity relationships were performed using human monocytes or the murine macrophagelike cell line J774.1 (37,38). Since different radiolabeled lipid A partial structures were not available, the experiments were designed as inhibition experiments to measure the inhibition of binding of ^{125}I-LPS by unlabeled structures. If one assumes that inhibition of ^{125}I-LPS by lipid A partial structures is of competitive nature, there should be a correlation between inhibition of binding and affinity to a given binding structure (or receptor). These studies show that inhibition of binding of ^{125}I-LPS by lipid A analogs is again a function of the acylation pattern *and* the degree of phosphorylation (37). For example, the tetraacylated compound 406 shows more inhibitory activity than compound 606, which has only two fatty acids (37,38). The *E. coli*-type lipid A compound 506 is a stronger competitor than compound LA-22-PP, which is a hexaacylated lipid A of the *Chromobacterium violaceum* type with, in contrast to compound 506, a symetrical distribution of fatty acids. In addition, the nature of the acyl residues is also of importance for the binding of lipid A analogs. Compound LA-23-PP, which contains four residues of nonhydroxylated decanoic acid (10:0), as well as compound LA-24-PP, which carries two moles of nonhydroxylated decanoic acid in addition to two hydroxylated acyl residues, have a pronounced reduced binding capacity compared to compound 406 (37,38).

The influence of the phosphorylation pattern was demonstrated by experiments which show that compound 404 (lacking the 1-phosphate group) as well as compound 405 (lacking the 4′- phosphate group) are less inhibitory to the binding of ^{125}I-LPS than compound 406 (37). In addition, the anomeric configuration of GlcN I was found to be of great biological relevance, as the α-anomer expressed high, the β-anomer low binding capacity (58).

Our results raised the question for the mode of action of the inhibition by "cold" compounds. Using a Lineweaver-Burk- plot we could show (58) that unlabeled LPS as well as PE-4 (the phosphonooxyethyl analog of compound 406) inhibited the binding of FITC-LPS in a competitive manner (Fig. 6). This indicates that the binding of LPS as well as the inhibition of binding of LPS by the investigated compounds is a specific phenomenon. However, it should be mentioned that in THP-1 cells inhibition of LPS-induced NF-κB-binding activity and IL-1 release is blocked by compound 406 under conditions in which the binding of LPS was not affected (59). This indicates that at least in THP-1 cells compound 406 may inhibit activation of cells by LPS also in a noncompetitive manner.

T lymphocytes are able to become activated under treatment with LPS in the presence of monocytes (25). However, we were unable to detect any specific binding of LPS to isolated T cells. Only unspecific unsaturable binding was observed, even in the presence of soluble CD14 (unpublished observations). Therefore, the stimulation of T cells by LPS seems not to be due to a direct specific binding of LPS to these cells. However, it has to be investigated whether monocytes present LPS motifs to a low number of specific T cells. Following this line, compound 406 may antagonize LPS-induced T-cell activation by preventing accessory cell (e.g., monocytes) activation rather than by a direct effect of compound 406 on T lymphocytes.

The data show that the structure–activity relationship for biological activity as well as for binding capacity depends on the acylation and phosphorylation pattern. Interestingly, the optimal structure for biological activity and for optimal binding affinity differ markedly. Whereas the optimal activity is represented in both cases by a bisphosphorylated hydrophilic βGlcN(1–6)αGlcN disaccharide backbone, the optimal hydrophobic structure for a biologically active lipid A is

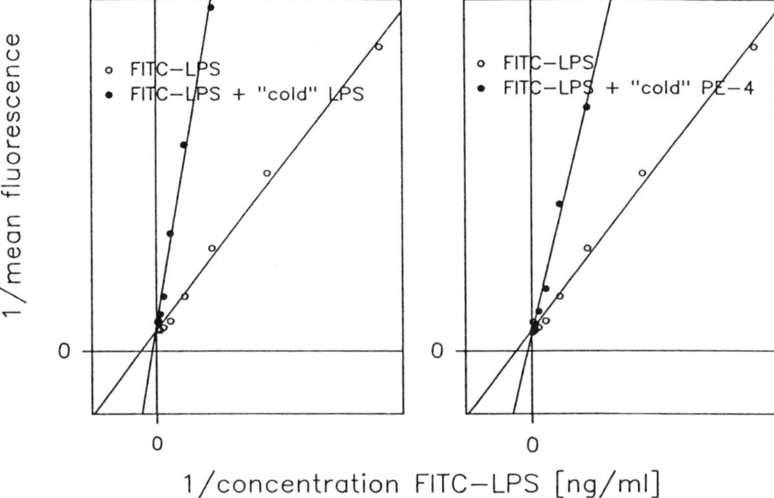

Figure 6 Lineweaver-Burk plot of binding inhibition of FITC-LPS by unlabeled LPS or PE-4. Human MNCs were labeled with FITC-LPS (0.01–20 μg/mL) in the presence of PE-4 (1 μg/mL) or unlabeled LPS (1 μg/mL). The fluorescence of labeled monocytes was determined by flow cytometry in an Epics Profile II. The results were presented in a Lineweaver-Burk plot. The regression coefficients were > 0.99, respectively.

expressed by the bisphosphorylated compound 506, having six acyl residues, the maximal binding affinity is displayed by the bisphosphorylated lipid A possessing four acyl residues (compound 406). These results prove that an optimal binding is not sufficient for optimal biological activity.

Taken together, our results provide strong evidence for the concept that inhibition of LPS–cell interaction by compound 406 and other lipid A partial structures is based on a competitive inhibition of specific LPS binding to a protein on the responder cell. In this way these compounds may be able to prevent the fatal endotoxin-induced reactions of an infected host. Therefore, synthetic lipid A analogs, compound 406, PE-4, and E5531, may be good candidates for the development of new immunomodulators which may be used to prevent gram-negative septic shock and related disorders.

ACKNOWLEDGMENTS

We thank Mrs. I. Goroncy and Mrs. C. Schneider and for excellent technical, and Mrs. R. Hinz for secretarial assistance. This study was supported in part by Deutsche Forschungsgemeinschaft [SFB 367, Projects B1 (H.B.), B2 (E.Th.R.), and C5 (A.J.U.)], a grant from the Fonds der Chemischen Industrie, Frankfurt/ Main, Germany (H.-D.F., E.Th.R.), and by BMBF [grant no. 01KI9471 (A.J.U.)].

REFERENCES

1. Young LS, Stevens P, Kaijser B. Gram-negative pathogens in septicaemicy infections. Scand J infect Dis (suppl) 1982; 31:78–94.
2. Schindler R, Dinarello CA. Interleukin 1. In: Habenicht A, ed. Growth Factors, Differentiation Factors, and Cytokines. Berlin: Springer Verlag, 1990:85–102.
3. Van Snick J, Nordan RP. Interleukin 6. In: Habenicht A, ed. Growth Factors, Differentiation Factors, and Cytokines. Berlin: Springer Verlag, 1990:163–176.
4. Bendtzen K. Interleukin 1, interleukin 6 and tumor necrosis factor in infection, inflammation and immunity. Immunol Lett 1988; 19:183–192.
5. Rietschel ET, Brade H. Bacterial endotoxins. Sci Am 1992; 267:2–54.
6. Galanos C, Lüeritz O, Rietschel Et, et al. Synthetic and natural *Escherichia coli* free lipid A express identical endotoxic activities. Eur J Biochem 1985; 148:1–5.
7. Rietschel ET, Kirikae T, Schade FU, et al. Bacterial endotoxins: molecular relationships of structure to activity and function. FASEB 1994; 8:217–225.
8. Imoto M, Yoshimura H, Shimamoto T, Sakaguchi N, Kusumoto S, Shiba T. Total synthesis of *Escherichia coli* lipid A. The endotoxically active principle of cell-surface lipopolysaccharide. Bull Chem Soc Jpn 1987; 60:2205–2214.
9. Imoto M, Yoshimura H, Sakaguchi N, Kusumoto S, Shiba T. Total synthesis of *Escherichia coli* lipid A. Tetrahedron Lett 1985; 26:1545–1548.
10. Imoto M, Yoshimura H, Yamamoto M, Shimamoto T, Kusumoto S, Shiba T. Chemical synthesis of phosphorylated tetraacyl disaccharide corresponding to a precursor of lipid A. Tetrahedron Lett 1984; 25:2667–2670.
11. Ulmer AJ, Heine H, Feist W, et al, Biological activity of lipid A partial structures. In: Levin J, Sturk, A, v.d.Poll T, v.Deventer SJH, eds. Bacterial Endotoxins: Basic Science to Anti-Sepsis Strategies. New York: Wiley, 1994: 71–83.
12. Loppnow H, Brade L, Brade H, et al. Induction of human interleukin 1 by bacterial and synthetic lipid A. Eur J Immunol 1986; 16:1263–1267.
13. Feist W, Ulmer AJ, Musehold J, Brade H, Kusumoto S, Flad H-D. Induction of Tumor necrosis factor-alpha release by lipopolysaccharide and defined lipopolysaccharide partial structures. Immunobiol 1989; 179:293–307.
14. Wang M-H, Flad H-D, Feist W, et al. Inhibition of endotoxin-induced interleukin 6 production by synthetic lipid A partial structures in human peripheral blood mononuclear cells. Infect Immun 1991; 59:4655–4664.
15. Loppnow H, Libby P, Freudenberg M, Kraus JH, Weckesser J, Mayer H. Cytokine induction by lipopolysaccharide (LPS) corresponds to the lethal toxicity and is inhibited by nontoxic *Rhodobacter capsulatus* LPS. Infect Immun 1990; 58:3743–3750.
16. Lebbar S, Cavaillon J-M, Caroff M, et al. Molecular requirement for interleukin 1 induction by lipopolysaccharide-stimulated human monocytes: involvement of the heptosyl-2-keto 3-deoxyoctulosonate region. Eur J Immunol 1986; 16:87–91.

17. Loppnow H, Brade H, Duerrbaum I, et al. IL-1 induction-capacity of defined lipopolysaccharide and partial structures. J Immunol 1989; 142–3229–3238.

18. Lasfargues A, Ledur A, Charon D, Szabo L, Chaby R. Induction by lipopolysaccharide of intracellular and extracellular interleukin 1 production: analysis with synthetic models. J Immunol 1987; 139:429–436.

19. Peavy D, Adler W, Smith R. The mitogenic effects of endotoxin and staphylococcal enterotoxin B on mouse spleen cells and human peripheral lymphocytes. J Immunol 1970; 105:1453–1458.

20. Milner ECB, Rudbach JA, von Eschen KB. Cellular responses to bacterial lipopolysaccharide: T cells recognize LPS determinants. Scand J Immunol 1983; 18:21–28.

21. Vogel SN, Hilfiker ML, Caulfield MJ. Endotoxin-induced T lymphocyte proliferation. J Immunol 1983; 130:1774–1779.

22. Greaves M, Janossy G, Doenhoff M. Selective triggering of human T and B lymphocytes in vitro by polyclonal mitogens. J Exp Med 1974; 140:1–18.

23. Miller RA, Gartner S, Kaplan HS. Stimulation of mitogenic responses in human peripheral blood lymphocytes by lipopolysaccharide: serum and T helper cell requirements. J Immunol 1978; 121:2160–2164.

24. Schmidtke J, Najarian J. Synergistic effects on DNA synthesis of phytohemagglutinin or concanavalin A and lipopolysaccharide in human peripheral blood lymphocytes. J Immunol 1975; 114:742–746.

25. Mattern T, Thanhäuser A, Reiling N, et al. Endotoxin and lipid A stimulate proliferation of human T cells in the presence of autologous monocytes. J Immunol 1994; 153:2996–3004.

26. Beeson PB. Tolerance to bacterial pyrogens. J Exp Med 1947; 86:29–38.

27. Freudenberg MA, Galanos C. Induction of tolerance to lipopolysaccharide (LPS)-D-galactoseamine lethality by pretreatment with LPS is mediated by macrophages. Infect Immun 1988; 56:1352–1357.

28. Mathison JC, Virca GD, Wolfson E, Tobias PS, Glaser K, Ulevitch RJ. Adaption to bacterial lipopolysaccharide controls lipopolysaccharide-induced tumor necrosis factor production in rabbit macrophages. J Clin Invest 1990; 85:1108–1118.

29. Wang M-H, Flad H-D, Feist W, et al. Inhibition of endotoxin or lipid A-induced tumor necrosis factor production by synthetic lipid A partial structures in human peripheral blood mononuclear cells. Lymphokine Cytokine Res 1992; 11:23–31.

30. Golenbock DT, Will JA, Raetz CRH, Proctor RA. Lipid X ameliorates pulmonary hypertension and protects sheep from death due to endotoxin. Infect Immun 1987; 55:2471–2476.

31. Lam C, Hildebrandt J, Schütze E, et al. Immunostimulatory, but not antiendotoxin, activity of lipid X is due to small amounts of contaminating N, O-acylated disaccharide- 1-phosphate: in vitro and in vivo reevaluation of the biological activity of synthetic lipid X. Infect Immun 1991; 59:2351–2358.

32. Wang M-H, Feist W, Herzbeck H, et al, Suppressive effect of lipid A partial structures on lipopolysaccharide or lipid A-induced release of interleukin 1 by human monocytes. FEMS Microbiol Immunol 1990; 64:179–186.

33. Feist W, Ulmer AJ, Wang M-H, et al. Modulation of lipopolysaccharide-induced production of tumor necrosis factor, interleukin 1, and interleukin 6 by synthetic precursor Ia of lipid A. FEMS Microbiol Immunol 1992; 89:73–90.

34. Kovach NL, Yee E, Munford RS, Raetz CRH, Harlan JM. Lipid IVa inhibits synthesis and release of tumor necrosis factor induced by lipopolysaccharide in human whole blood ex vivo. J Exp Med 1990; 172:77–84.

35. Takayama K, Quereshi N, Beutler B, Kirkland TN. Diphosphoryl lipid A from *Rhodopseudomonas sphaeroides* ATCC 17023 blocks induction of cachectin in macrophages by lipopolysaccharide. Infect Immun 1989; 57:1336–1338.

36. Ulmer AJ, Heine H, Feist W, et al. Biological effects of synthetic phosphonooxyethyl analogues of lipid A and lipid A partial structures. Infect Immun 1992; 60:3309–3314.

37. Kirikae T, Schade UF, Zähringer U, et al. The significance of the hydrophilic backbone and the hydrophobic fatty acid regions of lipid A for macrophage binding and cytokine induction. FEMS Immunol Microbiol 1994; 8:13–26.

38. Ulmer AJ, Feist W, Heine H, et al. Modulation of endotoxin-induced monokine release in human monocytes by lipid A partial structures inhibiting the binding of ^{125}I-LPS. Infect Immun 1992; 60:5145–5152.

39. Weidemann B, Brade H, Rietschel ET, et al. Soluble peptidoglycan-induced monokine production can be blocked by anti CD14 and by lipid A partial structures. Infect Immun 1994; 62:4709–4715.

40. Christ WJ, Asano O, Robidoux ALC, et al. E5531, a pure endotoxin antagonist of high potency. Science 1995; 268:80–83.

41. Wright SD, Jong MTC. Adhesion-promoting receptors on human macrophages recognize *E. coli* by binding to lipopolysaccharide. J Exp Med 1986; 164:1876–1888.

42. Detmers PA, Wright SD. Adhesion-promoting receptors on leukocytes. Curr Opin Immunol 1988; 1:10–15.

43. Wright SD, Detmers PA, Aida Y, et al. CD18-deficient cells respond to lipopolysaccharide *in vitro*. J Immunol 1990; 144:2566–2571.

44. Kirikae T, Kirikae F, Schade UF, et al. Detection of lipopolysaccharide-binding proteins on membrane of murine lymphocyte and macrophage-like cell lines. FEMS Microbiol Immunol 1991; 76:327–336.

45. Wright SD, Ramos RA, Tobias PS, Ulevitch RJ, Mathison JC. CD14, a receptor for complexes of lipopolysaccaride (LPS) and LPS binding protein. Science 1990; 249:1431–1433.

46. Schütt C, Ringel B, Nausch M, et al. Human monocyte activation induced by an anti-CD14 monoclonal antibody. Immunol Lett 1988; 19:321–328.

47. Tobias PS, Ulevitch RJ. Lipopolysaccharide binding protein and CD14 in LPS dependent macrophage activation. Immunobiology 1993; 187:227–232.

48. Schuman RR, Leong SR, Flaggs GW, et al. Structure and function of lipopolysacchiride binding protein. Science 1990; 249:1429–1431.

49. Wright SD, Ramos RA, Tatel M, Miller DS. Septin: a factor in plasma that opsonizes lipopolysaccharide-bearing particels for recognition by CD14 on phagocytes. J Exp Med 1992; 176:719–727.

50. Haziot A, Chen S, Ferrero E, Low MG, Silber R, Goyert SM. The monocyte differentiation antigen, CD14, is anchored to the cell membrane by a phosphatidylinositol linkage. J Immunol 1988; 141:547–552.

51. Lund-Johansen F, Olweus J, Symington FW, et al. Activation of human monocytes and granulocytes by monoclonal antibodies to glycosylphosphatidylinositol-anchored antigens. Eur J Immunol 1993; 23:2782–2791.

52. Lee JD, Kravchenko V, Kirkland TN, et al. Glycosyl-phosphatidylinositol-anchored or integral membrane forms of CD14 mediate identical cellular responses to endotoxin. Proc Natl Acad Sci USA 1993; 90:9930–9934.

53. Golenbock DT, Hampton RY, Raetz CRH, Wright SD. Human phagocytes have multiple lipid A-binding sites. Infect Immun 1990; 58:4069–4075.

54. Haeffner-Cavaillon N, Cavaillon J-M. Involvement of the LPS receptor in the induction of interleukin-1 in human monocytes stimulated with endotoxins. Ann Inst Pasteur Immunol 1987; 138:473–477.

55. Tahri-Jouti M-A, Mondange M, Le Dur A, et al. Specific binding of lipopolysaccharides to mouse macrophages. II. Involvement of distinct lipid A substructures. Mol Immunol 1990; 27:763–770.

56. Morrison DC. The case for specific lipopolysaccharide receptors expressed on mammalian cells. Microbial Pathogenesis 1989; 7:389–398.

57. Schletter J, Brade H, Brade L, et al. Binding of lipopolysaccharide (LPS) to an 80 kD membrane protein of human cells is mediated by soluble CD14 and LPS-binding protein. Infect. Immun. (in press).

58. Heine H, Brade H, Kusumoto S, et al. Inhibition of LPS-binding on human monocytes by phosphonooxyethyl analogs of lipid A. J Endotox Res 1994: 1:14–20.

59. Kitchens RL, Ulevitch RJ, Munford RS. Lipopolysaccharide (LPS) partial structures inhibit response to LPS in a human macrophage cell line without inhibiting LPS uptake by a CD14-mediated pathway. J Exp Med 1992; 176:485–492.

9

Induction of Endotoxin Tolerance in Humans with Monophosphoryl Lipid A

Kenneth B. Von Eschen
Ribi ImmunoChem Research, Inc.
Hamilton, Montana

I. INTRODUCTION

Endotoxin, a lipopolysaccharide component of gram-negative bacterial cell walls, is believed to play a key role in serious adverse systemic reactions associated with bacteremia and sepsis (1–4). This is demonstrated by experimentally reproducing many of the physiological changes that occur in septic shock after injecting purified endotoxin into the circulation (2,3,5–7). Circulating endotoxin interacts with plasma proteins and cellular components of blood and tissues, stimulating production and release of pro-inflammatory cytokines such as interleukin-1 (IL-1), interleukin-6 (IL-6), and tumor necrosis factor-alpha (TNF-α); components of complement; platelet-activating factor; kinins; and other mediators which can have a devastating effect on the cardiovascular system and other organs (4,6,8–11). Once activated, this cascade of endogenous mediators contributes greatly to the morbidity and mortality associated with septic shock.

In humans, four different approaches have been used alone or in combination in an attempt to treat patients with septic shock. These approaches included antibiotics (12,13), glucocorticoids (14,15), monoclonal antibodies directed against the lipid A moiety of endotoxin (16–21), and inhibitors of pro-inflammatory cytokines (22–26). In general, these therapeutic approaches were directed at interfering with the endotoxin source or endotoxin itself (antibiotics and anti-lipid A monoclonals) or at modulating the host response once it was already activated (glucocorticoids and cytokine inhibitors). Unfortunately, these approaches have not proven to be efficacious in the treatment of septic shock.

We choose to pursue a novel approach to the clinical management of septic shock. This approach involves *prevention* of shock by prophylactic treatment to induce a state of endotoxin tolerance in patients at high risk of developing sepsis and septic shock. Endotoxin tolerance refers to a state of hyporesponsiveness to the pathophysiological effects of endotoxin. Such tolerance is observed in both animals and humans following repeated intravenous injections of endotoxin (7,27–38). As evidenced by results of several animal studies, endotoxin tolerance is associated with reduced secretion of pro-inflammatory mediators upon reexposure to endotoxin (39). Therefore, it is reasonable to predict prophylactic induction of endotoxin tolerance in high-risk patients will down-modulate their subsequent response to endotoxin, attenuate the sepsis cascade of endogenous mediators, and, as a result, prevent or ameliorate septic shock in these patients.

Tolerance resulting from repeated injections of endotoxin is nonspecific and results in hyporesponsiveness to endotoxins from a broad spectrum of gram-negative bacteria (29–31). However, practical application of this treatment in patients at high risk for sepsis is limited by the severe toxicity of the endotoxin products used (3,5,6,7,11,27). To overcome this limitation, we have focused on the development of Monophosphoryl Lipid A (MLA; manufactured by Ribi ImmunoChem Research, Inc., Hamilton, MT, under the trade name MPL-immunostimulant). MLA, a structure created by selective hydrolysis of the lipid A moiety of endotoxin, is markedly less toxic than purified endotoxin but is still a potent immunostimulant (40). Pretreatment with MLA has been shown to induce endotoxin tolerance in several animal models (37,38,41–45) and to inhibit endotoxin priming of human neutrophils in vitro (46). MLA, therefore, may be a reasonable molecule to induce endotoxin tolerance in high-risk patients.

To evaluate the safety and biological activity of MLA in humans, we conducted a double-blind, randomized, vehicle-controlled, ascending-dose study in healthy male volunteers. Also, as "proof of concept," a second part of the study evaluated the ability of MLA pretreatment to induce a state of tolerance to a subsequent challenge dose of purified endotoxin in normal volunteers. Data from both parts of this clinical trial are presented in this chapter.

II. METHODS

This study was conducted at the Clinical Research Center, New Orleans, LA, and the protocol was approved by the Institutional Review Board of the Clinical Research Center. Written informed consent was obtained from all subjects in the study, and each subject was admitted as an inpatient at the Clinical Research Center.

A. Subject Selection

Forty-four healthy male volunteers ranging in age from 18 to 35 years (mean age 27 years) were recruited to participate in the study. All volunteers had normal physical examinations, electrocardiograms, and routine screening laboratory studies prior to enrollment. Subjects were not eligible for study enrollment if they were less than 18 or more than 35 years old; if they had a history of septic shock or significant disease or organ dysfunction; if they had a history of allergy to any components of the study materials; if they had participated in any investigational drug study in the previous month; if they had used any medication in the previous 7 days; if they had used glucocorticoids or other immunologically active drugs in the previous 3 months; if they had used nicotine-containing products in the previous month; or if they had a history of substance abuse in the previous year. All subjects had negative urine drug screens and negative tests for hepatitis B surface antigen and HIV antibodies. The subjects were admitted to the Clinical Research Center on the day prior to first study treatment and were discharged 24 h after final treatment with an investigational drug.

B. Administration of Study Treatments

The study was conducted as a double-blind, randomized, vehicle-controlled trial. In Part A of the study, eight groups of three volunteers each were randomized in a 2:1 ratio to receive a single intravenous infusion of MLA or the vehicle control. Physical and laboratory parameters were monitored after dosing to assess the safety and immunostimulant effects of MLA. Dosing progressed from 1.0 to 20 μg of MLA per kilogram of body weight in an ascending fashion, with determination of safety at each dose required prior to testing of the next highest dose. After evaluating responses to the 20 μg/kg dose, 5 additional subjects were tested at this dose in a 4:1 MLA:vehicle control ratio.

Part B of the study was conducted to evaluate the effects of MLA pretreatment on responses to purified endotoxin in normal volunteers. In this part, 12 new subjects were randomized equally to receive a single intravenous infusion of either 20 μg/kg of MLA or vehicle control. Twenty-four hours later, all subjects received infusion of a standard dose (20 endotoxin units per kilogram = 2 ng/kg) of U.S. reference *Escherichia coli* endotoxin (Lot Ec-5). This dose of Ec-5 endotoxin was previously demonstrated to be pyrogenic and to induce subjective side effects in normal male volunteers (3,11,47). As in study Part A, physical and laboratory parameters were monitored after dosing to evaluate the safety and immunostimulant effects of MLA. In addition, the effects of MLA pretreatment on the physical and biological responses to the Ec-5 purified endotoxin were evaluated.

C. MLA and Endotoxin

MLA is a modified form of lipid A prepared by sequential acid and alkaline hydrolyses of glycolipid from *Salmonella minnesota* Re595. The preparation and chemical structure of MLA were described previously by Myers et al. (48). In the present study, MLA was provided in 2.5-mL vials as a sterile solution of 100μg/mL of MLA in 9.5% ethanol and 40% propylene glycol in USP Water for Injection. The vehicle control consisted of the same formulation without the MLA and was provided in vials identical to the active drug. Immediately before use, MLA or vehicle control was diluted in 5% dextrose in water (D5W) to a total volume of 20 mL and administered intravenously by syringe pump over 3–10 min.

U.S. reference *E. coli* endotoxin (Lot Ec-5) was obtained for use in this study from the Center for Biologics Evaluation and Research, Food and Drug Administration, Bethesda, MD. The Clinical Research Center holds an IND approved by the U.S. FDA to use this endotoxin in human investigations. Endotoxin was supplied as a lyophilized powder which was reconstituted in 5 mL of USP Water for Injection and immediately vortex mixed for at least 30 min. Within 5 min of mixing, the endotoxin solution was administered intravenously as a single bolus injection at a dose of 20 endotoxin units per kilogram of body weight (2 ng/kg).

D. Measurements

Vital signs were monitored 1 h before and 5 min, 13 min, and 1, 1.5, 2, 3, 4, 8, 12, and 24 h after the start of MLA or vehicle control infusion (Part A) and after endotoxin infusion (Part B). Temperature was measured orally with a digital thermometer. Heart rate was determined by peripheral pulse count, and blood pressure was measured with a standard sphygmomanometer.

Blood samples were obtained from an indwelling venous catheter fitted with a heparin lock. In study Part A, routine serum chemistries were determined from samples taken 1 day before and 24 h, 3 days, and 6 days after the start of infusion with MLA or vehicle control. Samples for hematology studies in Part A were taken 1 day before and 2, 6, 12, 24 h, 3 days, and 6 days after the start of MLA or vehicle control infusion. In study Part B, samples for routine serum chemistries were taken 2 days before, 1 h before, and 24 h, 2 days, and 5 days after endotoxin infusion. Samples for hematology studies in Part B were taken 1 day before and 2, 6, 12, and 23 h after pretreatment with MLA or vehicle control; then 2, 6, 12, and 24 h, and 2 and 5 days after infusion of endotoxin.

Subjects were monitored continuously for spontaneous reporting of subjective side effects from 1 h before the first drug infusion until discharge from the

Clinical Research Center 24 h after the last infusion. The severity of each reported side effect was assessed as mild, moderate, severe, or life-threatening by the research staff at the bedside.

E. Special Laboratory Measurements

Blood samples for measuring epinephrine, norepinephrine, and cortisol were obtained 1 h before and 1, 2, 4, 6, 8, and 12 h after the start of MLA or vehicle control infusion in study Part A and 1 h before and 1, 2, 4, 6, 8, and 12 h after endotoxin infusion in Part B. Serum concentrations of catecholamines were determined by high-performance liquid chromatography (Division of Clinical Pharmacology, Medical School, Vanderbilt University, Nashville, TN) and cortisol by radioimmunoassay (SmithKline Beecham Laboratories, St. Louis, MO).

Cytokine concentrations were determined from blood samples obtained 1 h before and 13 min and 0.5, 1, 1.5, 2, 4, 6, and 24 h after the start of MLA or vehicle control infusion in study Part A. In Part B, samples for cytokines were obtained 1 h before and 13 min and 0.5, 1, 1.5, 2, 4, 6, and 24 h after endotoxin challenge. Serum concentrations of TNF-α, IL-1, IL-6, interleukin-8 (IL-8), and interleukin-1 receptor antagonist (IL-1RA) were determined by enzyme-linked immunosorbent assay (Quantine, R&D Systems, Minneapolis, MN).

Blood samples for measurement of C-reactive protein (CRP), alpha-1-antitrypsin, and neopterin were obtained 1 h before and 6 and 24 h after MLA or vehicle control administration in Part A and endotoxin administration in Part B. CRP and alpha-1-antitrypsin were measured by radial immunodiffusion (The Binding Site, Inc., San Diego, CA) using the endpoint-tabular method, with a calibrator standard on each plate. Neopterin concentrations were determined by radioimmunoassay (Specialty Laboratories, Inc., Santa Monica, CA). Cytokine, CRP and alpha-1-antitrypsin assays were performed in the laboratories of Dr. J. T. Ulrich, Ribi ImmounoChem Research, Inc., Hamilton, MT.

F. Data Analysis

Data from all subjects who received the 20-μg/kg MLA dose in study Part A were inspected, then combined for analysis. Vital-sign and laboratory parameter changes after MLA infusion were compared to changes after vehicle control infusion. For Part B, analysis of changes from baseline values and differences in vital signs and laboratory parameters after endotoxin challenge between MLA and vehicle-control pretreated subjects was performed. Wilcoxon's ranked-sum statistic was used to compare all quantitative data. Data are expressed as the group mean $\pm$ one standard error of the mean. A level of $p \leq 0.05$ indicated a statistically significant difference.

III. RESULTS

A. Effects of MLA on Normal Volunteers—Part A

The first part of this study was a dose-escalation trial of 1, 3, 5, 7, 10, 12.5, 15, and 20 µg MLA/kg administered i.v. to healthy volunteers. In general, consistent effects of MLA were not observed at doses lower than 20 µg/kg. Therefore, the effects of MLA at 20 µg/kg, the highest dose used in this study, will be reported.

1. Subjective Side Effects and Vital Signs

Subjective side effects after administration of 20 µg/kg of MLA were evaluated in 12 volunteers, 6 in Part A and 6 in Part B of the study (Table 1). Eight volunteers experienced systemic symptoms beginning 1–4 h after MLA administration, including headache (3 subjects), chills (6 subjects), and myalgias (1 subject). Pain at the infusion site was reported by 1 subject shortly after completion of MLA infusion. All symptoms were characterized as mild or moderate, most resolved within 3 h of onset, and none required treatment.

Changes in vital signs after the 20µg/kg MLA dose were evaluated in 6 volunteers in study Part A and compared with those of the 9 volunteers who received vehicle control. Four hours after infusion, oral temperatures were clearly

Table 1 Subjective Side Effects After Administration of MLA (20 µg/kg)

Subject number	Side effect	Severity	Onset after infusion (h)	Duration (h)	Treatment given
762	Chills	Mild	1.5	2.5	None
763	None				
801	Chills	Moderate	3.0	0.3	None
802	Chills	Moderate	2.4	1.5	None
	Myalgias	Mild	3.3	0.5	None
804	Chills	Mild	1.2	0.4	None
805	Chills	Mild	1.4	2.2	None
901	Headache	Mild	4.0	9.0	None
904	None				
905	None				
908	Chills	Mild	3.0	2.1	None
909	Headache	Mild	0.4	1.4	None
	Chills	Mild	1.4	1.2	None
912	Pain at infusion site[a]	Mild	0.1	0.6	None

[a]Pain at infusion site was not considered a systemic side effect.

elevated from baseline values in subjects who received MLA and were significantly higher than those of the vehicle control subjects (38.4 ± 0.28 versus $36.3 \pm 0.06°C$, $p = 0.004$) (Fig. 1a). Heart rates of subjects receiving MLA were similarly elevated at 4 h compared to controls (89.7 ± 6.3 versus 61.6 ± 2.0 beats/min, $p = 0.031$) (Fig. 1b). Temperatures and heart rates subsequently declined rapidly, returning to near baseline values by 12 h postinfusion. No significant changes in temperatures or heart rates were seen in subjects who received vehicle control. There were no significant changes in respiratory rates or blood pressures following either MLA or vehicle control infusion.

2. Hematology and Serum Chemistry

Changes in hematological and serum chemistry parameters were evaluated in the 6 volunteers who received 20μg/kg MLA in study Part A and compared with the pooled responses of the 9 volunteers who received vehicle control. Significant changes were seen only for total WBC count, percent segmented neutrophils, and percent lymphocytes (Figs. 1c, 1d, 1e). Six hours after infusion, total WBC counts were significantly elevated in the MLA-treated subjects compared with those of control subjects (9.6 ± 0.7 versus $5.5 \pm 0.4 \times 10^3/mm^3$, $p = 0.016$). The proportion of neutrophils in MLA-treated subjects was also significantly elevated at 6 h compared with controls ($89.2 \pm 0.8\%$ versus $57.3 \pm 4.4\%$, $p = 0.008$). A corresponding decrease in lymphocyte proportions was seen in MLA-treated subjects compared with controls ($7.3 \pm 0.6\%$ versus $36.0 \pm 4.0\%$ at 6 h, $p = 0.001$). WBC and differential counts returned to near baseline values by 12–24 h after infusion. There were no consistent changes in any other hematological, coagulation, or routine serum chemical parameters after either MLA or vehicle control infusion.

3. Cytokines

Changes in serum TNF-α, IL-6, IL-8, and IL-1RA were evaluated in the 6 volunteers who received 20μg/kg MLA in study Part A and compared with those of 9 volunteers who received vehicle control (Fig. 2). Two hours after MLA infusion, serum TNF-α concentrations were significantly elevated compared with those after vehicle control (91.7 ± 27.0 pg/mL versus 0 pg/mL, $p = 0.004$). The first significant increases in TNF-α occurred 1 h after infusion, and concentrations decreased rapidly after the peak at 2 h, returning to near baseline values at 6 h postinfusion. Only 2 of 9 control subjects had detectable TNF-α concentrations at any of the sampling times. Serum concentrations of IL-6 and IL-8 also increased in response to MLA administration. Two hours after MLA infusion, IL-6 concentrations were significantly elevated (192 ± 86 pg/mL as compared with 0 pg/mL after vehicle control, $p = 0.004$). Similarly, IL-8 concentrations were significantly elevated at 2 h after MLA infusion (474 ± 122 pg/mL as compared with 0 pg/mL after vehicle control, $p = 0.004$). Concentrations of

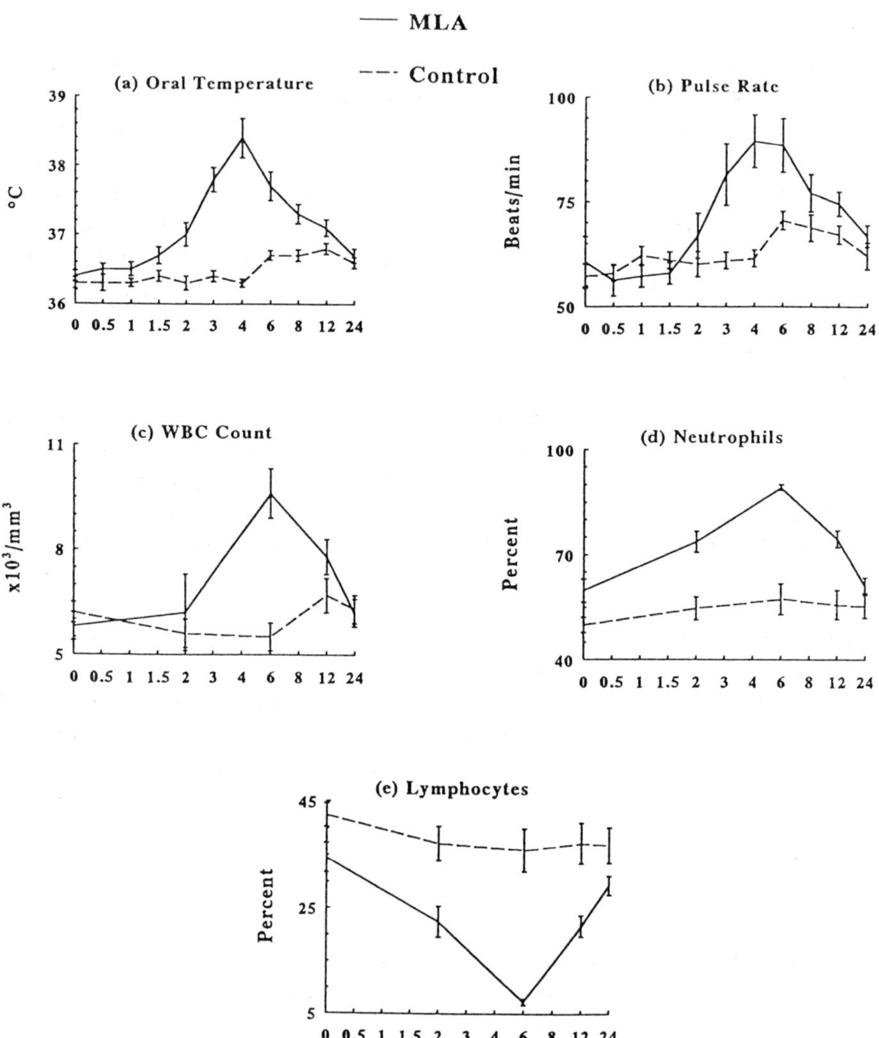

Figure 1 Changes in vital signs and hematological parameters in the 24 h after MLA (20 μg/kg) (solid lines) or vehicle control (dashed lines) was administered to healthy human volunteers (infusions began at time 0). Peak changes in all parameters of MLA-treated volunteers are significantly different from controls (see text). The mean value for each parameter is given, and the bars denote standard errors of the mean.

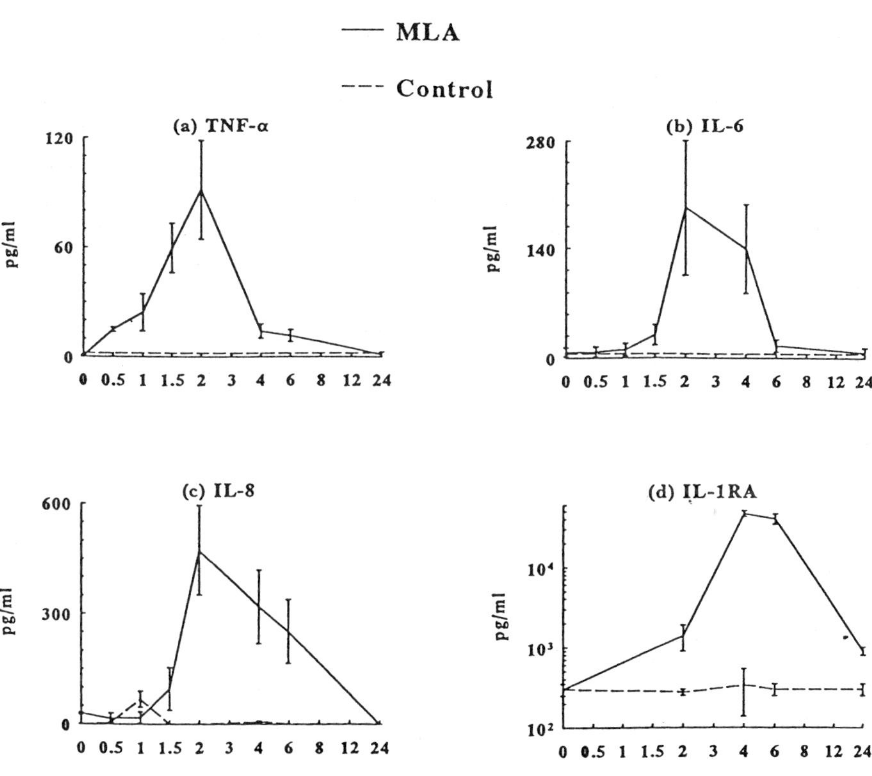

Figure 2 Changes in serum cytokine concentrations in the 24 h after MLA (20 μg/ kg) (solid lines) or vehicle control (dashed lines) was administered to healthy human volunteers (infusions began at time 0). Peak TNF-α, IL-6, IL-8, and IL-1RA levels were significantly elevated in the MLA-treated volunteers compared to controls (see text). The mean value for each cytokine is given, and the bars denote standard errors of the mean.

IL-6 and IL-8 then declined rapidly, returning to near baseline values at 6 and 24 h postinfusion, respectively. None of the volunteers who received the vehicle control had detectable levels of IL-6 or IL-8 at any of the sampling times. There were no detectable serum levels of IL-1 in any of the volunteers treated with MLA or vehicle control. However, IL-1RA levels increased significantly following MLA infusion and reached a maximum concentration of $4.67 \pm .41 \times 10^4$ pg/mL at 4 h postdosing. No increase in IL-1RA was observed following administration of vehicle control.

4. Changes in Acute-Phase Reactants and Neopterin

The effects of MLA administration on CRP, alpha-1-antitrypsin, and neopterin were evaluated in the 6 volunteers who received the 20μg/kg dose and compared with those of the 9 volunteers who received the vehicle control in study Part A. Twenty-four hours after MLA infusion, CRP concentrations were significantly elevated compared with those after vehicle control (52.9 ± 7.7 mg/L versus 6.8 ± 1.9 mg/L, $p = 0.0004$). Neopterin was also significantly elevated at 24 h after MLA infusion (7.7 ± 0.8 nmol/L as compared with 4.8 ± 0.6 nmol/L after vehicle control, $p = 0.0004$). Alpha-1-antitrypsin concentrations did not increase significantly after MLA infusion compared to those after vehicle control. No significant changes in concentrations of CRP, alpha-1-antitrypsin, or neopterin were seen in the volunteers who received vehicle control.

5. Changes in Catecholamines and Cortisol

Changes in catecholamine and cortisol concentrations after administration of 20μg/kg MLA were evaluated in the same subject groups in study Part A described above. Norepinephrine concentrations were significantly elevated 2 h after MLA infusion compared with those after vehicle control (462 ± 105 pg/mL versus 228 ± 76 pg/mL, $p = 0.012$). Cortisol concentrations increased in a similar fashion after MLA infusion (27.2 ± 1.4 μg/dL at 4 h postinfusion compared with 9.8 ± 1.9 μg/dL after vehicle control, $p = 0.0004$). Norepinephrine and cortisol levels returned to normal 8 h after MLA infusion. Epinephrine concentrations did not increase significantly after MLA infusion.

B. Effects of MLA Pretreatment on Response to Endotoxin—Part B

In Part B of the study, 12 volunteers were randomized equally to receive a single infusion of 20 μg/kg of MLA or vehicle control, followed 24 h later by challenge with a single infusion of 2 ng/kg of Ec-5 endotoxin. Changes in physical and laboratory parameters were evaluated, and the effects of MLA pretreatment on responses to endotoxin were compared with those of the subjects pretreated with vehicle control.

1. Subjective Side Effects and Vital Signs

All 6 subjects pretreated with vehicle control experienced one or more systemic side effects after challenge with endotoxin, compared with 3 of the 6 MLA-pretreated subjects. Seventeen side effects were reported by the vehicle control-pretreated subjects, compared to five in the MLA-pretreated subjects (Table 2). Side effects were mild or moderate in all cases. Onset ranged from 6 min to 3.5 h after endotoxin infusion, all resolved within 8 h, and none required treatment. The average duration of systemic side effects was similar in the two subject groups (3.1 h for MLA-pretreated subjects versus 2.7 h for controls). Pain at

Table 2 MLA Pretreatment Reduces Subjective Side Effects to
Ec-5 Endotoxin (2 ng/kg, i.v.)

Pretreatment	Patient number	Side effect	Severity	Onset after endotoxin (h)	Duration (h)	Treatment given
Vehicle control	902	Headache	Moderate	1.2	6.3	None
		Chills	Mild	1.5	1.5	None
	903	Headache	Moderate	1.3	3.3	None
		Chills	Mild	1.0	1.8	None
		Myalgia	Mild	1.3	6.5	None
	906	Headache	Mild	1.25	1.75	None
		Chills	Mild	1.25	2.25	None
	910	Chills	Mild	1.3	1.6	None
	911	Headache	Moderate	1.3	6.75	None
		Chills	Mild	1.2	4.0	None
		Myalgia	Moderate	1.2	4.0	None
		Nausea	Moderate	1.3	3.8	None
		Vomiting	Mild	3.5	0.2	None
		Diaphoresis	Mild	3.5	0.1	None
	919	Headache	Mild	1.3	1.5	None
		Chills	Mild	1.3	0.8	None
		Myalgia	Mild	1.3	0.2	None
MLA	901	Headache	Mild	3.0	8.0	None
		Pain at infusion site[a]	Mild	3.0	1.0	Topical
	904	None				
	905	None				
	908	Chills	Mild	1.3	1.6	None
	909	Headache	Moderate	1.2	2.9	None
		Chills	Moderate	1.2	0.5	None
		Nasal Congestion	Moderate	2.5	2.5	None
	912	None				

[a]Pain at infusion site was not considered a systemic side effect.

the infusion site, not considered a systemic side effect, was reported by one
MLA-pretreated subject shortly after endotoxin infusion and was treated topically
with warm compresses.

Oral temperatures in both control and MLA-pretreated groups increased modestly from baseline values after endotoxin infusion (Fig. 3a). There was no
significant difference in the peak temperatures in the vehicle control group and
the MLA pretreated group at 4 h postendotoxin. However, when the areas under

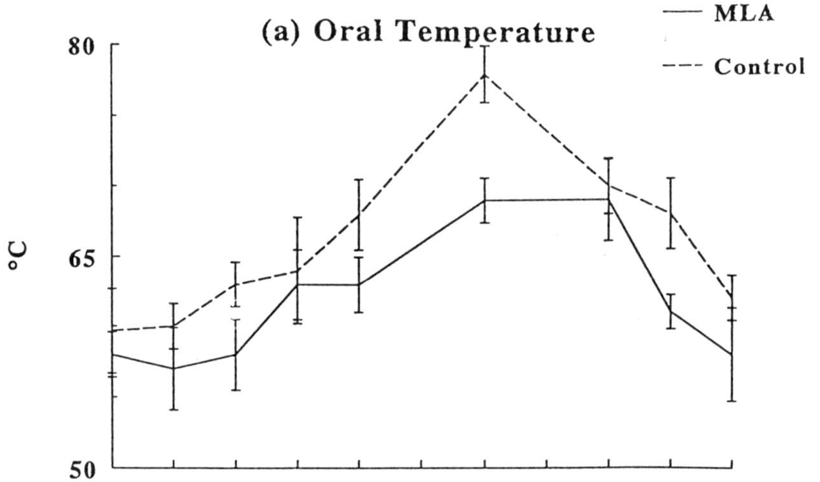

(a) Oral Temperature
MLA
Control
°C
80
65
50

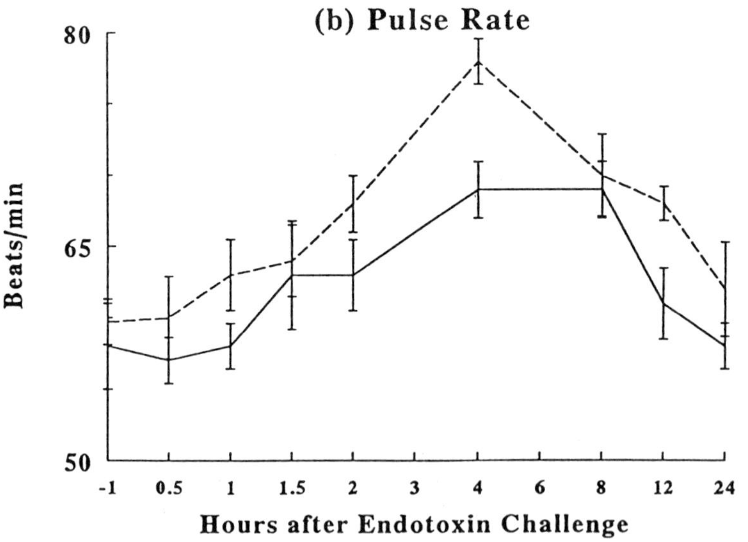

(b) Pulse Rate
Beats/min
80
65
50
-1 0.5 1 1.5 2 3 4 6 8 12 24
Hours after Endotoxin Challenge

the mean temperature curves (AUC) were measured, diminution of fever response to endotoxin by MLA pretreatment was suggested (15.0 ± 6.4 versus 7.2 ± 2.0, $p = <0.05$).

Heart rates also increased in both subject groups in response to endotoxin, reaching peak values at 4 h postinfusion (Fig. 3b). MLA pretreatment significantly reduced the peak heart rate response compared to vehicle control pretreatment (69.0 ± 5.3 versus 78.0 ± 4.0 beats/min, $p = 0.002$). No significant changes in respiratory rates or blood pressures from baseline values were seen in response to endotoxin infusion in either subject group.

2. Effect on Leukocyte Responses

Total WBC counts increased modestly after endotoxin challenge in both MLA- and vehicle control-pretreated subjects, reaching peak values at 6 h postinfusion. MLA pretreatment appeared to diminish the leukocyte response compared with control pretreatment, but the difference was not significant (8.1 ± 1.4 versus 10.7 ± 2.3 × 10^3/mm^3, $p = 0.18$). Mild diminutions in neutrophilic and lymphopenic responses to endotoxin were also seen in MLA-pretreated subjects compared to control subjects, but the differences were not statistically significant.

3. Effect on Cytokines

The effects of MLA pretreatment on changes in serum cytokine concentrations after endotoxin infusion are shown in Fig. 4. At 1.5 h after endotoxin infusion, serum TNF-α was 83.7 ± 76.2 pg/mL in MLA-pretreated subjects, compared with 244.3 ± 128.0 pg/mL in vehicle control-pretreated subjects ($p = 0.026$ for peak responses). Similar effects were seen on serum IL-6 and IL-8 concentrations at 2 h after endotoxin administration in MLA-pretreated subjects compared to controls. After endotoxin challenge, peak IL-6 concentrations were 100.0 ± 90.7 pg/mL in the MLA-pretreated group, compared to 267.8 ± 171.2 pg/mL in the vehicle control group ($p = 0.093$). Peak IL-8 concentrations were 136.0 ± 86.3 pg/mL in the MLA-pretreated group, compared to 632.2 ± 323.4 pg/mL in the vehicle control group ($p = 0.041$). Serum IL-1RA levels increased significantly in both the MLA- and vehicle control-pretreated subjects following endotoxin challenge; however, MLA pretreatment diminished peak IL-1RA re-

---

Figure 3 Effects of MLA (20 μg/kg) pretreatment on changes in oral temperature and pulse rate after endotoxin challenge (2 ng/kg). MLA (solid lines) or vehicle control (dashed lines) pretreatment began at time 0 and endotoxin infusion at 24 h. Increases in these parameters after endotoxin infusion were significantly reduced by pretreatment with MLA compared to vehicle control (see text). The mean value for each assessment is given, and the bars denote standard errors of the mean.

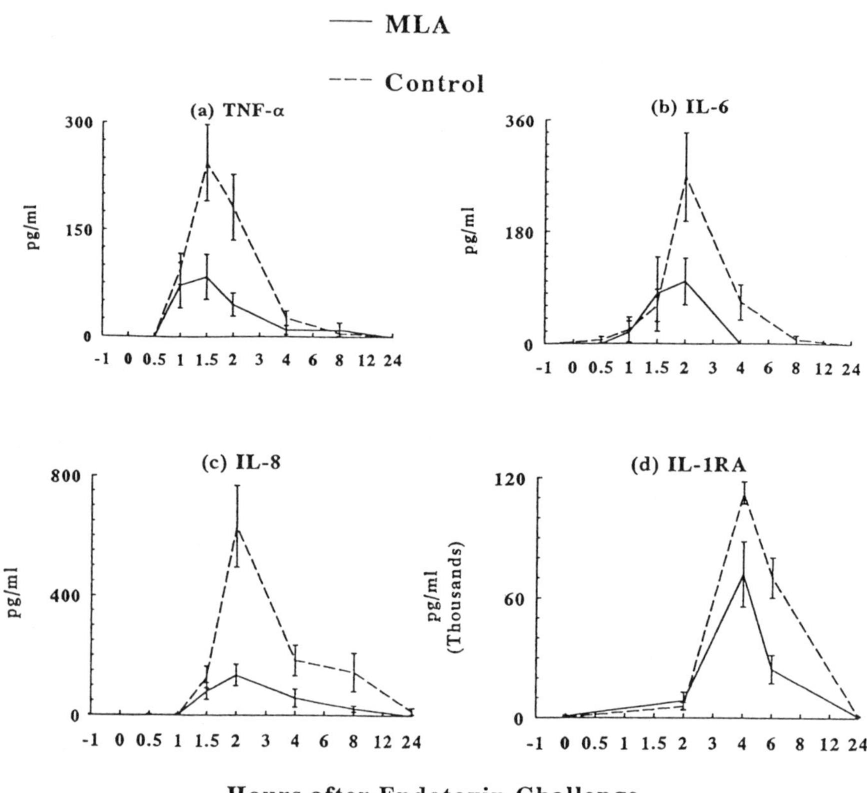

Figure 4 Effects of MLA (20 μg/kg) pretreatment on cytokine responses to an endotoxin challenge (2 ng/kg). MLA (solid lines) or vehicle control (dashed lines) pretreatment began at time 0 and endotoxin infusion at 24 h. Pretreatment with MLA significantly reduced these cytokine responses to endotoxin challenge (see text). The mean value for each assessment is given, and the bars denote standard errors of the mean.

sponses compared to pretreatment with vehicle control ($p = 0.025$ for peak responses). Cytokine concentrations in all subjects returned to baseline levels within 6–24 h after endotoxin challenge.

4. Effect on C-Reactive Protein and Neopterin

Serum CRP and neopterin concentrations in vehicle control-pretreated subjects increased significantly over the 24 h following endotoxin infusion. However, at the time of endotoxin challenge, CRP and neopterin concentrations in MLA-pretreated subjects were already significantly elevated from baseline values in response to MLA infusion. Therefore, no evaluation of the effects of MLA pretreatment on CRP and neopterin response to endotoxin infusion was attempted.

5. Effect on Catecholamines and Cortisol

Serum epinephrine and norepinephrine concentrations increased in both MLA- and vehicle control-pretreated subjects in response to endotoxin challenge. However, there were no significant differences in mean values between the two groups, indicating that MLA pretreatment had no measurable effect on the catecholamine response to endotoxin. Catecholamine concentrations returned rapidly to near baseline values by 4–6 h after endotoxin challenge.

Cortisol concentrations increased significantly from baseline values after endotoxin challenge in the vehicle control-pretreated subjects, reaching peak values at 2–4 h postinfusion. MLA pretreatment diminished the cortisol response to endotoxin, but the difference from control values did not reach significance (16.8 ± 6.3 versus 22.3 ± 2.4 μg/dL, MLA-pretreated subjects versus controls, p = 0.065). Cortisol concentrations returned to near baseline values by 6 h after endotoxin challenge.

IV. DISCUSSION

MLA is a modified form of lipid A, the principal toxic component of the endotoxin molecule (49). In the first part of this study, MLA infusion (20 μg/kg) produced side effects in some subjects similar to those usually associated with endotoxin, including headache, chills, myalgias, fever, and tachycardia. However, these side effects were generally well tolerated and required no treatment. Although less toxic, MLA retains many of the immunostimulatory properties of lipid A. This was demonstrated in the present study by increased circulating concentrations of cytokines, leukocytes, CRP, and neopterin in response to MLA (20 μg/kg) infusion. These increases were similar to those seen in previous studies after administration of much smaller doses (2 ng/kg) of endotoxin (3,5–7,11). Therefore, the systemic response to MLA, although of lesser magnitude, appeared similar to the response to endotoxin and included the following biological sequence of events: (a) macrophage priming and stimulation of neutrophil activity; (b) release of various cytokines such as TNF-α and interleukins; (c) secondary acute phase responses, e.g., increases in CRP; and (d) stress responses that enhanced host tolerance to toxic effects of cytokines and other mediators in the sepsis cascade (34–36,41,46). In animal experiments, the positive effects of these immunomodulatory activities included enhancement of nonspecific resistance to infectious agents and induction of a relative refractory state to the effects of endotoxin.

Endotoxin tolerance can be induced by administrating a sublethal dose of endotoxin which renders experimental animals or human subjects refractory to subsequent endotoxin challenge. Greisman et al. (33,50,51) divided induction of endotoxin tolerance into early and late phases. Early-phase tolerance occurred within days of exposure to endotoxin, was relatively transient, and was dependent on the lipid A moiety of the endotoxin molecule. Late-phase endotoxin tolerance manifested several weeks after exposure to endotoxin and was related to the production of O-polysaccharide-specific antibodies (50,51). MLA was shown to induce early endotoxin tolerance in experimental animals (41–45).

Results of the present study provide evidence that a single dose of MLA can induce early-phase endotoxin tolerance in normal human subjects. Systemic responses to endotoxin (headache, chills, myalgias, fever, tachycardia, and increased circulating levels of TNF-α, IL-6, and IL-8) were attenuated in subjects pretreated with a single 20μg/kg dose of MLA. These effects were significant even though MLA was administered 24 h prior to endotoxin challenge. It is possible the tolerance induced by MLA may be greater if shorter intervals between dosing and endotoxin challenge are used.

The exact mechanisms by which MLA pretreatment attenuated human responses to endotoxin challenge in this study are unknown. Previous studies in animals related induction of endotoxin tolerance by MLA to activation of cells of the monocyte/macrophage line and to the cytokines released by these cells (34–36). In other studies, pretreatment of animals with TNF-α, IL-1, or a combination of TNF-α and IL-1 resulted in tolerance to lethal endotoxin doses (38,52,53). The role of TNF-α in endotoxin tolerance was further elucidated by Fraker et al. (54), who reported that endotoxin-tolerant rats were significantly protected against lethal doses of TNF-α. In the present study, a 20μg/kg dose of MLA used to induce tolerance resulted in significant increases in serum concentrations of TNF-α, IL-6, and IL-8. This observation supports the hypothesis that endotoxin tolerance is at least partly dependent on an autocrine mechanism involving cytokines released by activated monocytes and/or macrophages (55).

IL-1RA (56), IL-6 (57), IL-10 (58), and glucocorticoids (59,60) were also implicated in the induction of endotoxin tolerance. A tolerogenic dose of MLA in the present study resulted in measurable increases in serum levels of IL-1RA, IL-6, and cortisol. Therefore, these molecules may have contributed to MLA's ability to induce tolerance in normal volunteers. IL-10 responses to MLA were not measured in the current study.

It is also possible that other systems are involved in inducing endotoxin tolerance by pretreatment with MLA. For example, it was reported that pretreatment of human neutrophils with MLA significantly attenuated endotoxin priming for oxygen radical production in these cells (46). Modulation of the neutrophil response to endotoxin may be a component of endotoxin tolerance (61). Alteration in the affinity of CD14, a cell surface receptor for endotoxin, was implicated in tolerance induction (62). The effect of MLA on CD14 receptors is being studied at this time.

With respect to novel approaches to the clinical management of septic shock, the results of the present study demonstrate two important findings: (a) MLA is administered intravenously to normal human subjects in doses well tolerated as well as immunostimulatory; and (b) pretreatment with a single injection of MLA at a dose of 20 µg/kg attenuates many of the physical and biochemical responses to purified endotoxin; i.e., MLA pretreatment induces endotoxin tolerance in healthy human volunteers. While the concept of prophylactically inducing endotoxin tolerance with MLA in patients at high risk of sepsis and septic shock is intriguing, the question must be asked: Is this approach practical? Stated another way, what is minimally required for a tolerance-inducing product like MLA to be considered clinically acceptable? First, the product must be relatively safe, and side effects to an effective dose must be minimal. This requirement becomes more important as, even in high-risk cohorts, only a percentage of patients treated prophylactically will require protection against sepsis and septic shock. An infusion of 20 µg/kg of MLA which induced endotoxin tolerance appears relatively safe and has minimal side effects of short duration. Second, the product must be able to induce and maintain tolerance during the time the patient is at risk of developing septic shock. Depending on the cohort chosen, this period could be from 1 or 2 days to several weeks. The duration of endotoxin tolerance induced by MLA in humans is currently unknown. It is reasonable to predict from animal experiments that tolerance begins to wane between 24 and 48 h following a single injection of MLA. However, tolerance is readily maintained and even enhanced in animals dosed daily with MLA (63). The feasibility of repeat dosing with MLA is supported by the results of one clinical study in which multiple doses of MLA were administered safely to cancer patients (64). Third, induction of endotoxin tolerance should not suppress natural host resistance mechanism (e.g., phagocytosis), which might further render immunocompromised patients susceptible to infection. This possibility has not been tested in humans treated with MLA; however, mice made tolerant with either single-/or multiple-dose regimens of MLA actually have enhanced resistance to challenge with viable bacteria (63). Fourth, it is known that human septic shock is caused by a variety of different classes of microorganisms and microbial toxins (1). As a prophylactic, an acceptable product should be able to protect against most common causes of septic shock. It is encouraging to note that preclinical data shows MLA protects animals against a wide variety of septic shock-inducing agents, including gram-negative and gram-positive bacteria and their toxins, viruses, yeast, and at least one protozoan (63). Finally, the product must be effective. For MLA, proof of effectiveness must come from future clinical trials.

Prophylactic induction of endotoxin tolerance in humans represents a novel approach to the clinical management of septic shock. In light of the difficulties of successfully treating patients with septic shock, it seems wise to consider developing new products like MLA, which may prevent this serious problem in certain high-risk patient groups. Carefully designed and controlled clinical trials of prophylactic agents such as MLA are needed to demonstrate both the safety and efficacy of such agents in preventing septic shock.

ACKNOWLEDGMENTS

The author acknowledges the expert secretarial assistance of Ms. Penny Sullivan and technical editing assistance of Ms. Jennifer Laing.

The author would like to acknowledge that a manuscript describing the results of this clinical trial has been written by M. E. Astiz, et al. and has been accepted for publication in *Critical Care Medicine*.

REFERENCES

1. Bone RC. The pathogenesis of sepsis. Ann Int Med 1991; 115:457–469.
2. Parrillo JE, Parker MM, Natanson C. Septic shock in humans. Ann Int Med 1990; 113:227–242.
3. Suffredini AF, Fromm RE, Parker MM. The cardiovascular response of normal humans to the administration of endotoxin. N Engl J Med 1989; 321:280–287.
4. Rackow EC, Astiz ME. Pathophysiology and treatment of septic shock. JAMA 1991; 266:548–554.
5. Wolff SM. Biological effects of bacterial endotoxins in man. J Infect Dis 1973; 128(suppl):5251–5256.
6. Engelhardt R, Mackensen A, Galanos C, Andreesen R. Biological response to intravenously administered endotoxin in patients with advanced cancer. J Biol Resp Modif 1990; 9:480–491.
7. Mechanic RC, Frei E III, Landy M, Smith WW. Quantitative studies of human leukocytic and febrile response to single and repeated doses of purified bacterial endotoxin. J Clin Invest 1962; 41:162–172.
8. Haas JG, Baeuerle PA, Riethmüller G, Ziegler-Heitbrock HWL. Molecular mechanisms in down-regulation of tumor necrosis factor expression. Proc Natl Acad Sci USA 1990; 87:9563–9567.
9. Martich GO, Danner RL, Ceska M, Suffredini AF. Detection of interleukin 8 and tumor necrosis factor in normal humans after intravenous endotoxin: the effect of antiinflammatory agents. J Exp Med 1991; 173:1021–1024.
10. Fong Y, Moldawer LL, Marano M. Endotoxemia elicits increased circulating β_2-IFN/IL-6 in man. J Immunol 1989; 142:2321–2324.
11. Michie HR, Manogue KR, Spriggs DR. Detection of circulating tumor necrosis factor after endotoxin administration. N Engl J Med 1988; 318:1481–1486.
12. Bryan CS, Reynolds KL, Brenner ER. Analysis of 1,186 episodes of gram-negative

bacteremia in non-university hospitals: the effects of antimicrobial therapy. Rev Infect Dis 1983; 5:629–638.

13. Kreger BE, Craven DE, McCabe WR. Gram-negative bacteremia. IV. Reevaluation of clinical features and treatment in 612 patients. Am J Med 1980; 68:344–355.

14. Bone RC, Fisher CJ Jr, Clemmer TP. A controlled clinical trial of high-dose methylprednisolone in the treatment of severe sepsis and septic shock. N Engl J Med 1987; 317:653–658.

15. Hinshaw L, Peduzzi P, Young E. Effects of high-dose glucocorticoid therapy on mortality in patients with clinical signs of systemic sepsis. N Engl J Med 1987; 317:653–658.

16. Ziegler EJ, McCutchan JA, Fierer J. Treatment of gram-negative bacteremia and shock with human antiserum to a mutant *Escherichia coli*. N Engl J Med 1982; 307:1225–1230.

17. Ziegler EJ. Protective antibody to endotoxin core: the emperor's new clothes? J Infect Dis 1988; 158:286–290.

18. Greenman RL, Schein RMH, Martin MA. A controlled clinical trial of E5 murine monoclonal IgM antibody to endotoxin in the treatment of gram-negative sepsis. JAMA 1991; 266:1097–1102.

19. Ziegler EJ, Fisher CJ, Sprung CL. Treatment of gram-negative bacteremia and septic shock with HA-1A human monoclonal antibody against endotoxin. N Engl J Med 1991; 324:429–436.

20. J5 Study Group. Treatment of severe infectious purpura in children with human plasma from donors immunized with *Escherichia coli* J5: a prospective double-blind study. J Infect Dis 1992; 165:695–701.

21. Greenman RL, Schein RMH, Martin MA, et al. A controlled clinical trial of E5 murine monoclonal IgM antibody to endotoxin in the treatment of gram-negative sepsis. JAMA 1991; 266:1097–1102.

22. Stames HF Jr, Pearce MK, Tewari A, Yim JH, Zou J-C, Abrams JS. Anti-IL-6 monoclonal antibodies protect against lethal *Escherichia coli* infection and lethal tumor necrosis factor-α challenge in mice. J Immunol 1990; 145:4185–4191.

23. Wakabayashi G, Gelfand JA, Burke JF, Thompson RC, Dinarello CA. A specific receptor antagonist for interleukin 1 prevents *Escherichia coli*-induced shock in rabbits. FASEB J 1991; 5:338–543.

24. Bone RC. Monoclonal antibodies to tumor necrosis factor in sepsis: help or harm? Crit Care Med 1993; 21:311–312.

25. Cross AS, Sadoff JC, Kelly N, Bernton E, Gemski P. Pretreatment with recombinant murine tumor necrosis factor alpha/cachectin and murine interleukin-1 alpha protects mice from lethal bacterial infection. J Exp Med 1989; 169:2021–2027.

26. Fisher E, Marano MA, Van Zee KJ. Interleukin-1 receptor blockade improves survival and hemodynamic performance in *Escherichia coli* septic shock, but fails to alter host responses to sublethal endotoxemia. J Clin Invest 1992; 89:1551–1557.

27. Greisman SE, Hornick RB. Mechanisms of endotoxin tolerance with special reference to man. J Inf Dis 1973; 128 (suppl): S265–S276.

28. Beeson PB. Tolerance to bacterial pyrogens. II. Role of the reticulo-endothelial system. J Exp Med 1947; 86:39–44.

29. Morgan HR. Resistance to the action of the endotoxins of enteric bacilli in man. J Clin Invest 1948; 27:706–709.

30. Beeson PB. Tolerance to bacterial pyrogens. I. Factors influencing its development. J Exp Med 1947; 86:29–38.

31. Greisman SE, Hornick RB, Carozza FA Jr, Woodward TE. The role of endotoxin during typhoid fever and tularemia in man. I. Acquisition of tolerance to endotoxin. J Clin Invest 1963; 42:1064–1075.

32. Greisman SE, Hornick RB, Woodward TE. The role of endotoxin during typhoid fever and tularemia in man. III. Hyperactivity to endotoxin during infection. J Clin Invest 1964; 43:1747–1757.

33. Greisman SE, Wagner HN, Iio M, Hornick RB. Mechanisms of endotoxin tolerance. II. Relationship between endotoxin tolerance and reticuloendothelial system phagocytic activity in man. J Exp Med 1964; 119:241–264.

34. Madonna GS, Vogel SN. Early endotoxin tolerance is associated with alterations in bone marrow-derived macrophage precursor pools. J Immunol 1985; 135:3763–3771.

35. Freudenberg MA, Galanos C. Induction of tolerance to lipopolysaccharide (LPS)-D-galactosamine lethality by pretreatment with LPS is mediated by macrophages. Infect Immun 1988; 56:1352–1357.

36. Mathison JC, Virca GD, Wolfson E, Tobias PS, Glaser K, Ulevitch RJ. Adaptation to bacterial lipopolysaccharide controls lipopolysaccharide-induced tumor necrosis factor production in rabbit macrophages. J Clin Invest 1990; 85:1108–1018.

37. Henricson BE, Benjamin WR, Vogel SN. Differential cytokine induction by doses of lipopolysaccharide and monophosphoryl lipid A that result in equivalent early endotoxin tolerance. Inf Immun 1990; 58:2429–2437.

38. Vogel SN, Henricson B. Role of cytokines as mediators of endotoxin-induced manifestations: a comparison of cytokines induced by doses of LPS and MLA that elicit comparable early endotoxin tolerance. In: Nowotny A, Spitzer JJ, Zeigler EJ, eds. Cellular and Molecular Aspects of Endotoxin Reactions. Amsterdam: Elsevier, 1990:464–474.

39. Mengozzi M, Ghezzi P. Review. Cytokine down-regulation in endotoxin tolerance. Eur Cytokine Netw 1993; 4:89–98.

40. Ulrich JT, Cantrell JL, Gustafson GL. The adjuvant activity of monophosphoryl lipid A. In: Spriggs DR, Koff WC, eds. Topics in Vaccine Adjuvant Research. Boston: CRC Press, 1991:131–143.

41. Madonna GS, Peterson JE, Ribi EE, Vogel SN. Early-phase endotoxin tolerance: induction by a detoxified lipid A derivative, monophosphoryl lipid A. Infect Immun 1986; 52:6–11.

42. Chase JJ, Kubey W, Dulek MH. Effect of monophosphoryl lipid A on host resistance to bacterial infection. Infect Immun 1986; 53:711–712.

43. Rackow EC, Astiz ME, Kim YB, Weil MH. Monophosphoryl lipid A blocks the hemodynamic effects of lethal endotoxemia. J Lab Clin Med 1989; 113:112–127.

44. Astiz ME, Rackow EC, Kim YB, Weil MH. Monophosphoryl lipid A induces tolerance to lethal hemodynamic effects of endotoxin. Circ Shock 1991; 33:92–97.

45. Carpati CM, Astiz ME, Rackow EC, Kim J, Kim Y, Weil MH. Monophosphoryl lipid A attenuates the effects of endotoxic shock in pigs. J Lab Clin Med 1992; 119:346–352.

46. Heiman DF, Astiz ME, Rackow EC. Monophosphoryl lipid A inhibits neutrophil priming by lipopolysaccharide. J Lab Clin Med 1990; 116:237–241.

47. McMahon FG, Vargas R. A new clinical bioassay for antipyresis. J Clin Pharmacol 1991; 31:736–740.

48. Myers KR, Truchot AT, Ward J. A critical determinant of lipid A endotoxic activity. In: Nowotny A, Spitzer JJ, Zeigler EJ, eds. Cellular and Molecular Aspects of Endotoxin Reactions. Amsterdam: Elsevier, 1990:145–156.

49. Ribi E. Beneficial modification of the endotoxin molecule. J Biol Resp Modif 1984; 3:1–9.

50. Greisman SE, Young EJ, Corozza FA Jr. Mechanisms of endotoxin tolerance. V. Specificity of the early and late phases of pyrogenic tolerance. J Immunol 1969; 103:1223–1236.

51. Greisman SE. Induction of endotoxin tolerance. In: Nowotny A, ed. Beneficial Effects of Endotoxin. New York: Plenum, 1983:149–179.

52. Dinarello CA, Bodel PT, Atkins E. The role of the liver in the production of fever and in pyrogenic tolerance. Trans Assoc Am Phys 1968; 81:334–344.

53. Wallach D, Holtmann H, Engelmann H, Nophar Y. Sensitization and desensitization to lethal effects of tumor necrosis factor and IL-1. J Immunol 1988; 140:2994–2999.

54. Fraker DL, Stovroff MC, Merino MJ, Norton JA. Tolerance to tumor necrosis factor in rats and the relationship to endotoxin tolerance and toxicity. J Exp Med 1988; 168:95–105.

55. Fahmi H, Chaby R. Selective refractoriness of macrophages to endotoxin-induced production of tumor necrosis factor, elicited by an autocrine mechanism. J Leukocyte Biol 1993; 53:45–52.

56. Santos AA, Scheltinga MR, Lynch E. Elaboration of interleukin-1 receptor antagonist is not attenuated by glucocorticoids after endotoxemia. Arch Surg 1993; 128:138–143.

57. Barton BE, Jackson JV. Protective role of interleukin-6 in the lipopolysaccharide-galactosamine septic shock model. Infect Immun 1993; 61:1496–1499.

58. Gérard C, Bruyns C, Marchant A. Interleukin-10 reduces the release of tumor necrosis factor and prevents lethality in experimental endotoxemia. J Exp Med 1993; 177:547–550.

59. Wright LJ, Lipsett MB, Ross GT, Wolff SM. Effects of dexamethasone and aspirin on the responses to endotoxin in man. J Clin Endocrinol 1972; 34:13–17.

60. Evans GF, Zuckerman SH. Glucocorticoid-dependent and independent mechanisms involved in lipopolysaccharide tolerance. Eur J Immunol 1991; 21:1973–1979.

61. Solomkin JS, Bass RC, Bjornson HS, Tindal CJ, Babcock GF. Alterations of neutrophil responses to tumor necrosis factor alpha and interleukin-8 following human endotoxemia. Infect Immun 1994; 62:943–647.

62. Labeta MO, Durieux J-J, Spagnoli G, Fernandez N, Wijdenes J, Herrmann R. CD14 and tolerance to lipopolysaccharide: biochemical and functional analysis. Immunology 1993; 80:415–423.

63. Rudbach JA, Myers KR, Rechtman DJ, Ulrich JT. Prophylactic use of monophosph-
oryl lipid A in patients at risk for sepsis. In: Levin J, van Deventner SJH, van der
Poll T, Sturk A, eds. Bacterial Endotoxins. Basic Science to Anti-Sepsis Strategies.
New York: Wiley-Liss, 1994:107–124.
64. Vosika GJ, Barr C, Gilbertson D. Phase I study of intravenous modified lipid A.
Cancer Immunol Immunother 1984; 18:107–112.

10

Specific Lipid A Analog Which Exhibits Exclusive Antagonism of Endotoxin

Tsutomu Kawata
John R. Bristol
Jeffrey R. Rose
Daniel P. Rossignol
William J. Christ
Osamu Asano
Gloria R. Dubuc
Wendy E. Gavin
Lynn D. Hawkins
Michael D. Lewis
Pamela D. McGuinness
Maureen A. Mullarkey
Michel Perez
Andrea L. C. Robidoux
Yuan Wang
Yoshito Kishi
Eisai Research Institute
Andover, Massachusetts

Seiichi Kobayashi
Akifumi Kimura
Ieharu Hishinuma
Kouichi Katayama
Isao Yamatsu
Eisai Co. Ltd. Tsukuba Research Laboratories
Tsukuba, Japan

A variety of antisepsis therapies have aimed at blocking one or more cytokines produced by cells in response to lipopolysaccharide (LPS). A more effective means of antagonizing the effects of LPS would be through blocking the primary event of LPS-mediated cellular activation. We have targeted our design of a therapeutic drug toward antagonism of the toxic lipid A portion of the LPS molecule. Several possible lead structures and analogs, including lipid X, lipid IV$_A$, and lipid As from the nontoxic bacteria *Rhodobacter capsulatus* and *Rhodobacter sphaeroides* have been synthesized and biologically characterized. In-vitro and in vivo analyses using several animal models indicated that the lipid As from *R. capsulatus* and *R. sphaeroides* posessed the greatest antagonistic potencies without demonstrating LPS-like agonistic activity. Using the proposed structure of *R. capsulatus* lipid A, we have synthesized and characterized a fully stabilized endotoxin antagonist, designated E5531. E5531 potently antagonizes LPS-mediated cellular activation of human and murine cells in vitro. This inhibition results in dramatic suppression of release of a wide variety of cytokines and cellular mediators, tumor necrosis factor alpha (TNF-α), interleukin-1 (IL-1), interleukin-6 (IL-6), interleukin-8 (IL-8), interleukin-10 (IL-10), and nitric oxide. In in-vivo systems, E5531 protects mice from LPS-induced lethality and, when administered with antibiotic, blocks septic shock due to lethal infection of viable *Escherichia coli*. Based on these results, E5531 may be clinically useful for the treatment of gram-negative sepsis and septic shock in humans.

I. INTRODUCTION

Gram-negative bacterial sepsis and septic shock remain serious unsolved clinical problems (1,2). One current hypothesis for induction of septic shock suggests that while administration of antibiotics resolves bacterial infection, it is possible that their antimicrobial action may paradoxically contribute to the septic response by triggering release of LPS from the bacterial outer membrane (3–6). Septic shock is the severe consequence of the inflammatory response of the host to LPS and/or lipid A (7), which triggers release of cytokines and cellular mediators, including TNF-α, IL-1, IL-6, leukotrienes, thromboxane A2, and nitric oxide from monocytes and macrophages (8,9). At extreme levels, these cytokines and cellular mediators have been shown to initiate many pathophysiological events including fever, shock, disseminated intravascular coagulation (DIC), hypotension, and organ failure (10,11).

A variety of approaches have been taken to alleviate the morbidity and mortality of patients due to septic shock associated with gram-negative bacterial infection (12). These approaches have focused on blocking cellular response to LPS (LPS antagonist) or blocking one or more cytokines induced by LPS. In an attempt to block cellular responses to LPS, efforts have been directed toward development of anti-LPS antibodies with the hopes that they would neutralize or enhance LPS clearance (13,14). The alternative goal of antagonizing cytokines has been approached both by blocking cytokine release from LPS-activated cells (15) and by inhibiting cytokine activity using one of three methods: passive immunization [e.g., anti-TNF antibodies (16)], neutralization with soluble receptor (17), or blocking the cytokine cell-surface receptor with a specific receptor antagonist (18–20).

While these methodologies first held promise as therapeutic agents, none has yet proven clinically effective. A more promising strategy of antagonizing LPS-induced cellular activation has not been thoroughly pursued. Because the toxicophore of LPS has been identified as lipid A (7), antagonism of a cellular "receptor" for lipid A may halt the chain of events leading to acute inflammatory response and septic shock. Naturally derived molecules from *R. capsulatus* and *R. sphaeroides* are potent LPS antagonists (21,22). However, it is likely that difficulties involved in obtaining sufficient amounts of homogenous material with pharmaceutically acceptable purity and stability could severely limit the use of bacterially derived compounds as therapeutic antagonists for treatment of endotoxin-related diseases. For these reasons, organic synthesis was used to obtain a homogeneous, pure, and stable LPS antagonist that demonstrates in-vitro and in-vivo activity in a variety of model systems. Results from these studies indicate that E5531 demonstrates potential as a therapeutic clinical entity for ameliorating or preventing septic shock.

II. MATERIALS AND METHODS

A. Compounds

Synthesis of the proposed structures of the *R. capsulatus* lipid A (sRcLA; >85% pure), E5531 (>99% pure), and B1060 (>85% pure) were performed at Eisai Research Institute. Synthesis of the proposed structure of *R. sphaeroides* lipid A (sRsLA) has been described previously (23). All compounds were in the form of tetra-sodium salts. In addition, a tetra-lysine salt of sRcLA was also tested and yielded similar results. Compounds were sonicated in sterile water at 1 mM and diluted into Ca^{2+}-, Mg^{2+}-free Hanks' balanced salt solution. LPS from *E. coli* (0111:B4) was purchased from Sigma Chem. Co. (St. Louis, MO). Murine interferon-γ was purchased from Genzyme Corp. (Cambridge, MA). *Bacillus Calmette-Guérin* (BCG) was obtained from Japan BCG Inc. (Tokyo, Japan).

B. TNF-α Assays in Human Whole Blood and Monocytes

Fifty microliters of the indicated concentrations of antagonists were added to heparinized human blood (400 μL), followed by 50 μL of LPS (10 ng/mL final concentration). After a 3-h incubation at 37°C, 5% CO_2, plates were centrifuged at 1000 × g for 10 min at 4°C; then the plasma was removed and stored at −80°C. Plasma samples were analyzed for TNF-α by ELISA (R & D Systems, Minneapolis, MN, or Genzyme Corp., Cambridge, MA). All compounds were tested at least three times and in triplicate.

Human monocytes were isolated from heparinized whole blood by the Leuco Prep system for mononuclear cell isolation (Becton Dickinson, Lincoln Park, NJ), suspended in serum-free RPMI 1640, washed twice by centrifugation at $600 \times g$, 5 min, 4°C, and plated at $1-2 \times 10^6$ cells/well in 0.5 mL. After allowing adherence of cells for 3 h in RPMI 1640/10% heat-inactivated human AB serum, nonadherent cells were removed by two gentle washes with serum-free RPMI 1640. Antagonist and LPS (10 ng/mL, final concentration) were added to cells in 400 µL of RPMI/1% human AB serum and incubated for 3 h at 37°C, 5% CO_2. Supernatants were removed, stored at -80°C, and later assayed for TNF-α as described above.

C. Induction of Nitric Oxide in Murine Macrophage Cells

Induction of nitric oxide in murine macrophages has been described (24). RAW 264.7 cells (ATCC) were cultured in Ham's F12/10% fetal calf serum and plated at 2×10^5/well in 200 µL of DMEM/10% fetal calf serum. In some cases, interferon-γ was added along with agonist (25). After 18–24 h, nitrite was quantitated by adding 100 µL of Greiss reagent, as described (26), to 100 µL of culture supernatant and then absorbance was measured at A_{540} on an ELISA microplate reader.

D. In-Vivo Efficacy

Male C57BL/6 mice (5–6 weeks old) were primed (27) by tail-vein injection of 0.2 mL of a BCG suspension (10 mg/mL), then used in experiments 10–14 days later. Pyrogen-free 5% glucose (0.4 mL) containing the indicated amount of LPS with or without E5531 was injected intravenously into the tail vein. One hour later, mice were ether-anesthetized and 30 µL of blood was drawn from the retro-orbital vein using a heparinized hematocrit tube. Plasma TNF-α levels were determined by ELISA using rabbit anti-murine TNF-α polyclonal antiserum and recombinant mouse TNF-α standard (Genzyme Corp., Cambridge, MA). Protection from LPS-induced lethality in BCG-primed mice was studied after intravenous (tail-vein) injection of 3 µg of LPS mixed with the indicated amount of E5531. Incidence of death was monitored for 48 h.

III. RESULTS AND DISCUSSION

A. Chemistry

To identify potential endotoxin antagonists, we synthesized and evaluated three types of compounds and analogs: lipid X, lipid IV_A, and lipid As from two non-toxic bacteria. Lipid X is a monosaccharide biosynthetic precursor of lipid A that was first isolated from a variant of *E. coli* (28,29). In in vitro systems, it antagonizes LPS activity (30) and has been reported to protect mice and sheep from LPS-induced lethality (31,32). However, efforts to develop a monosaccharide-based endotoxin antagonist by us and others (33) have met with limited success, yielding only compounds with low antagonistic potency. In addition, more recent work has shown lipid X to be ineffective in vivo in a canine sepsis model (34).

Lipid IV_A is a diphosphodisaccharide, biosynthetic precursor of LPS (35). It has been previously shown that lipid IV_A is an LPS antagonist in human in-vitro assays (36). Studies on the diether analog of lipid IV_A (B1060) lead to the same conclusion (vide infra), but also confirm that these materials demonstrate LPS-like agonistic activity in murine systems (vide infra; 36).

Our most promising potential lead came from the proposed structure of the lipid A from *R. capsulatus* (37). It was hoped that the synthetic lipid A would possess the potent antagonistic activity previously attributed to the nontoxic LPS from which it was derived (21). This hypothesis was supported by antagonism studies done by us and others using *R. sphaeroides* lipid A and LPS (22,36,38,39).

As shown in Fig. 1, the proposed structures of the nontoxic lipid As from *R. sphaeroides* and *R. capsulatus* differs from toxic *E. coli* lipid A by the length of their fatty-acid side chains, the presence of unsaturation on the acyloxyacyl moiety, and the presence of a 3-ketoamide(s) functionalities at the C.2 and C.2′ positions. A synthetic route to lipid As of the *E. coli* type has been established by seminal contributions of Shiba and co-workers (40). However, Shiba's route was incompatible with the 1,3-ketoamido and olefinic functionalities that may be necessary for antagonistic activity. To overcome this problem, we have successfully developed a general, flexible, and convergent synthetic method (41). Synthesis of the proposed structures of both RsLA and RcLA has enabled us to firmly establish structural information on the bacterially derived products, and has also provided us with the unique opportunity to evaluate the biological properties of structurally homogeneous preparations with high purity. Using the synthetic material of the proposed structure for *R. sphaeroides* lipid A, we have determined that bacterially derived RsLA is not identical to its proposed structure (23). In addition, the synthetic material possessed antagonistic activity approximately equivalent to bacteria-derived material, but was devoid of the agonistic properties observed in the bacteria-derived material (39). This biological information, together with the development of a practical synthetic route to the structure proposed for *R. capsulatus* lipid A, served as the basis for the design and synthesis of our lead compound.

Synthetic material of the proposed structure of RcLA (sRcLA) potently antagonized the release of TNF-α induced by LPS in human whole blood and monocytes (Figs. 2 and 3). In these systems, sRcLA was devoid of LPS-like agonistic activity when tested at concentrations up to 100 μM. However, stability studies indicated that, upon storage, hydrolytic cleavage of the C.3 and/or C.3′ acyl

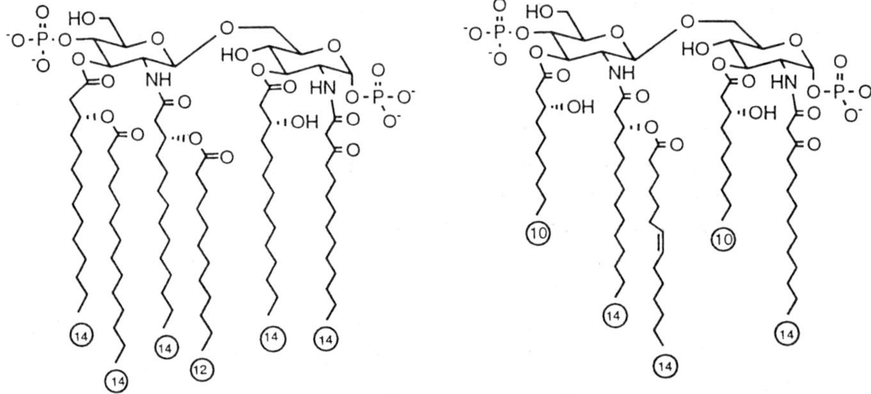

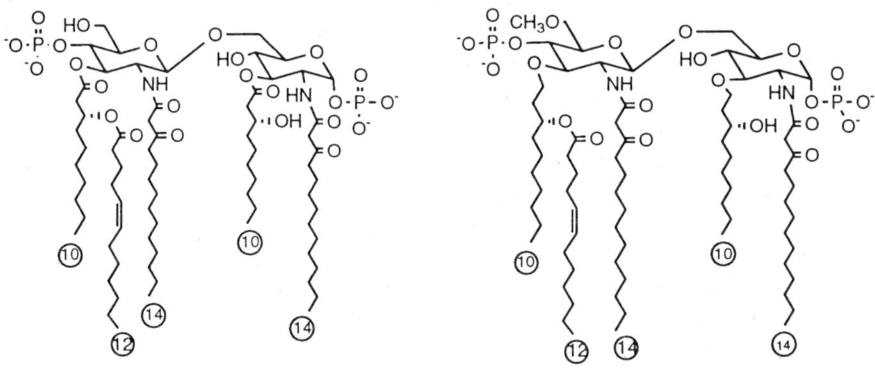

Figure 1   Structures of *E. coli* lipid A, RsLA proposed structure, ReLA proposed structure, and E5531. E5531 is an ether-stabilized form of sReLA, lipid IV_A is a biosynthetic precursor of lipid A that lacks the tetradecanoic and dodecanoic acid moieties acylated on the C.2′ and C.3′ β-hydroxy fatty acids. B1060 is a lipid IV_A-like molecule containing ether-stabilized linkages at the C.3 and C.3′. The structural elucidation of bacteria-derived RSLA has been described (38), but the R/S configurations of the C.3 substituents of the fatty-acid side chains were not assigned in the natural product.

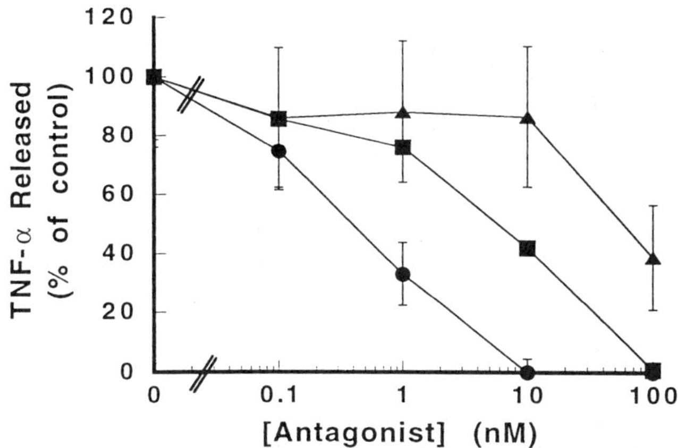

Figure 2 Inhibition of LPS-induced release of TNF-α in human whole blood. Human whole blood was incubated with the indicated concentration of E5531 (●), sRcLA (■), or B1060 (▲) along with 10 ng/mL of LPS for 3 h. Plasma was obtained and TNF-α assayed as described in the Materials and Methods section. Results are representative of three assays, with control values ranging from 1525 to 2330 pg/mL TNF-α.

groups produced agonistic by-products, making this material unsuitable as a drug candidate.

To overcome this problem, a series of hydrolytically stable analogs bearing ether linkages in place of the naturally occurring acyl linkages at the C.3 and/ or C.3′ positions were synthesized. The C.3, C.3′ diether analog demonstrated antagonistic potency equivalent to synthetic *R. capsulatus* lipid A (data not shown), but the C.3 and C.3′ side chains no longer hydrolyzed to produce agonistic by-products. However, small amounts of contaminants, possibly due to chemical interactions involving the C.6′ hydroxyl group, were found in some preparations making it difficult to obtain analogs with a satisfactory level of purity. This problem was overcome by blocking the C.6′ hydroxyl with a methyl group. Thus, the fully stabilized endotoxin antagonist, E5531, was created (Fig. 1). It contains ether linkages in both the C.3 and C.3′ positions in place of the more labile ester linkages and is derivatized by methylation at the C.6′ position. This material now demonstrated long-term stability during storage, purity greater than 99%, and sufficient water solubility. Insofar as these characteristics met our desired chemical properties, E5531 was subjected to rigorous in-vitro and in-vivo evaluation as a potential drug candidate.

In order to compare agonistic and antagonistic properties of E5531 to other lipid A-like molecules, similar structural modifications involving ester-to-ether

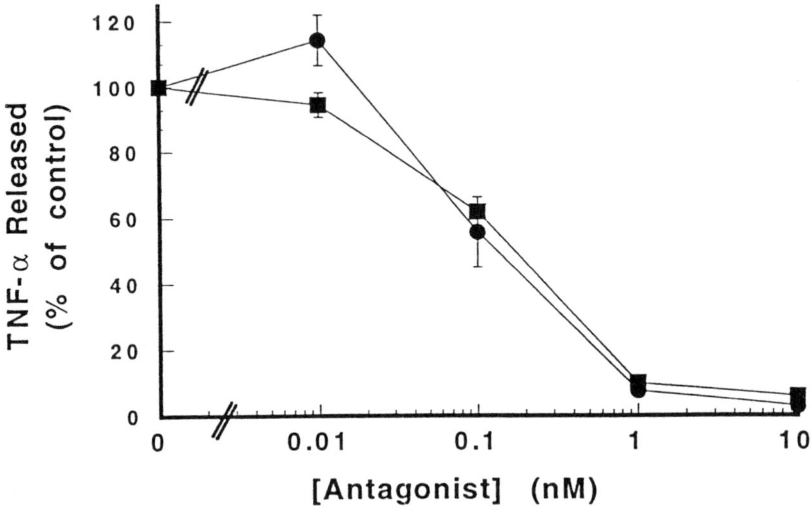

Figure 3 Inhibition of LPS-induced release of TNF-α in human monocytes. Human monocytes were incubated with the indicated concentration of E5531 (●) or sRcLA (■) along with 10 ng/mL of LPS for 3 h. Supernatants were harvested and assayed for TNF-α as described in the Methods and Materials section.

conversions at C.3 and C.3′ were made to lipid IV_A, resulting in a tetra-substituted di-alkyl lipid IV_A analog (B1060).

B. Biology

1. Analysis in Human In-Vitro Systems

Insofar as sepsis can be considered a consequence of a blood-borne bacterial infection, LPS stimulation of human whole blood provides a relevant and convenient assay system. Three hours of incubation of fresh whole blood with 10 ng/mL of LPS results in a vigorous cellular response which can be measured by quantitating cytokines such as TNF-α, IL-1, IL-6, IL-8, and IL-10. Routinely, stimulation by 10 ng/mL of LPS was measured by release of TNF-α which averaged 2422 ± 149 pg/mL (n = 25). As shown in Fig. 2, E5531 potently inhibited this response (in more than 20 assays the IC_{50} was 2.6 ± 0.2 nM), and concentrations greater than 10 nM completely inhibited the LPS-induced responses. The initial lead compound, sRcLA, was slightly less active (IC_{50} = 5.9 ± 1.9 nM), and the lipid IV_A analog B1060 was considerably less active (IC_{50} = 48 ± 6 nM).

Antagonistic activity of these analogs was also measured in primary cultures of human monocytes/macrophages. As shown in Fig. 3, the response of cultured monocytes to 10 ng/mL of LPS was potently inhibited by sRcLA, as well as by E5531. Again, total inhibition of TNF-α release was observed at < 10 nM, while the IC_{50}s of both compounds were between 0.05 and 0.3 nM (n = 8 or more for each compound).

It is important to note that similar antagonistic potencies were obtained for E5531 when other indicators of LPS stimulation such as IL-1, IL-6, IL-8, and IL-10 were used to assess drug activity in whole blood or monocytes. In all cases, E5531 demonstrated IC_{50}s between 1.8 and 5.2 nM (data not shown), similar to the IC_{50}s observed for inhibition of TNF-α release.

These results indicate that the potent antagonistic activity observed with the synthetic lipid A proposed structures (sRcLA and sRsLA; Ref.39) were preserved in the fully stabilized analog, E5531.

2. Spectrum and Specificity of Action of E5531

The spectrum of specificity of antagonistic action of E5531 was determined through the use of different agonists. First, LPSs from different gram-negative bacteria were used as agonists in the human monocyte system. In these assays, E5531 potently antagonized the release of TNF-α induced by LPS from *Klebsiella pneumonia*, *Pseudomonas aeruginosa*, and *Salmonella minnesota*. In all cases, the IC_{50}s ranged from 0.14 to 2.7 nM, comparable to those seen against *E. coli* LPS (1.2 nM). These results indicate that directing synthesis toward antagonism of the highly conserved lipid A portion of LPS resulted in a molecule that antagonizes LPSs from a broad range of gram-negative bacteria.

Specificity of antagonism of E5531 was evaluated by the use of alternative agonists. E5531 was ineffective at inhibiting interferon-γ-induced generation of nitric oxide in murine macrophages (data not shown). In addition, while E5531 blocked superoxide production induced by LPS synergism with N-formyl-methionyl-leucyl-phenylalanine in human neutrophils, it was ineffective against superoxide production stimulated by phorbol 12-myristate 13-acetate alone (42). These results indicated that the antagonistic activity of E5531 is specific for LPS.

3. In Vitro Antagonism of LPS in Murine Model Systems

Nontoxic lipid As and analogs inhibited LPS-induced cellular activation as measured by release of TNF-α and nitric oxide (NO) in murine systems. As in human systems, sRcLA and E5531 inhibited LPS-induced release of TNF-α in primary cultures of murine macrophages (IC_{50} = 11 ± 2.9 for sRcLA, and 2.6 ± 0.93 nM for E5531; data not shown).

Potent antagonistic activity was also observed when compounds were tested for inhibition of LPS-induced generation of NO in murine macrophage (RAW 264.7) cells. Treatment of these cells with 10 ng/mL of LPS results in vigorous induction of nitric oxide synthase (NOS) mRNA and release of NO (24,25). As shown in Fig. 4, E5531 effectively antagonized LPS-mediated release of NO in these cells (IC_{50} = 2.6 ± 0.9 nM), while B1060 was less effective, with an IC_{50} greater than 1 µM (data not shown). More important, however, B1060 was found to be highly agonistic in interferon-γ-primed RAW 264.7 cells. While E5531 did not induce measureable NO release, 1 µM B1060, in the presence of 5 U/mL interferon-γ, induced 34 µM nitrite. In contrast, 4 µM nitrite seen with interferon-γ alone. This response to B1060 is approximately equivalent to that seen with 10 ng/mL LPS in the presence of 5 U/mL interferon-γ. This finding is consistent with that describing tetra-substituted lipid IV_A as an antagonist in human in vitro systems and an agonist in murine systems (36).

4. Studies on Mechanism of Action of E5531

Several lines of evidence indicate that E5531 antagonizes LPS at its receptor, or prior to signal transduction. First, inhibitory activity of E5531 was dependent on the dose of LPS used as an agonist, since higher doses of LPS required greater concentrations of E5531 for efficacy (42). Second, inhibition by E5531 was specific for LPS-/and lipid A-mediated induction of cellular activation (42).

Measurement of ^{125}I-labeled LPS binding to human monocytes, monocyte-derived macrophages, and murine macrophages indicated that E5531 was a more potent competitor for cell-surface LPS binding than *E. coli* lipid A (42,43). However, other experiments indicate that LBP-mediated LPS binding is difficult to inhibit quantitatively (44,45). Inhibition of binding did not correlate with inhibition of cellular activation (data not shown). These results support previously

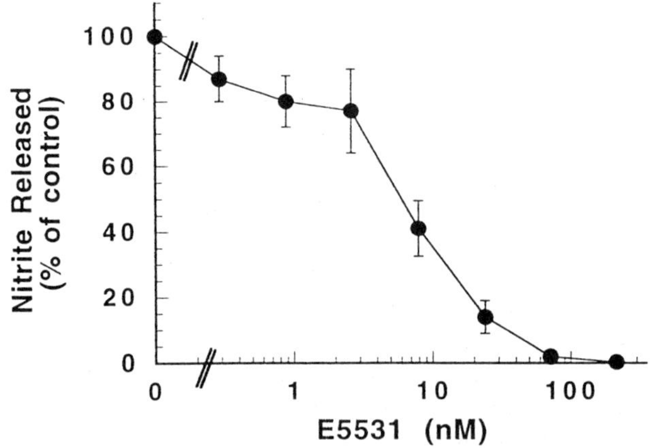

Figure 4   Inhibition of LPS-induced NO in murine macrophages. RAW 264.7 cells were treated with the indicated concentrations of E5531 (●) along with ng/mL of LPS. The supernatants assayed for nitrite as described in the Materials and Methods section. Data (average ± SEM) are derived from three experiments and plotted as percent of control (LPS only), which varied from 21.7 to 33.7 µM nitrite.

obtained results aguing that inhibition of activity and binding are not closely correlated (44,45). Other experiments focused on the study of LPS-mediated signal transduction (NF-κB) indicate that E5531 inhibition occurs at or near the point of signal initiation. In human promonocytic cells (U38; Ref. 46) stimulated with 33 ng/mL LPS, E5531 (333 nM) completely blocked NF-κB activation and translocation to the nucleus (manuscript in preparation). Taken together, these results suggest that E5531 may antagonize LPS activity at its cell surface receptor, leading to inhibition of transmembrane signal transduction.

5. In Vivo Evaluation of LPS Antagonism

LPS activates fixed macrophages in the liver and other organs as well as those in circulation, making it likely that antagonism of LPS in vivo is more complicated than in in vitro systems. Evaluations of E5531 and B1060 in vivo were performed using a BCG-primed murine model (47). Approximately 1 h after intravenous injection, as little as 100 ng of *E. coli* LPS induces a rapid increase in plasma TNF-α levels, while a larger dose of LPS (3 μg) is lethal (Fig. 5). Co-injection of E5531 with 3 μg of LPS suppressed this increase in plasma TNF-α and its associated lethality (Fig. 5). Other results from this laboratory indicate that co-administration of E5531 with LPS also blocks induction of interferon-γ and IL-1α. These results indicate that E5531 effectively blocks LPS-mediated activation of "fixed" macrophages as well as circulating cells. More convincingly, protection from lethality by E5531 indicates that it effectively antagonizes a broad spectrum of potentially deadly cytokines and cellular mediators induced by LPS.

Analysis of the activity of E5531 together with an antibiotic in an infection model utilized intraperitoneal injection of viable *E. coli* into BCG-primed mice. In this model, either E5531 or the β-lactam antibiotic latamoxef gave noticeable yet transient protection (Table 1). However, co-treatment with antibiotic and E5531 provided long-lasting, significant protection against lethality (Table 1). The inability of the antibiotic alone to cause sustained suppression of lethality in this model is likely due to the deleterious host inflammatory response to endotoxin released from bacteria killed by antibiotic (48). While administration of antibiotic decreased blood bacterial counts by approximately 2-log orders, plasma endotoxin levels concomitantly increased in these animals from 1735 pg/ mL to greater than 10,000 pg/mL (Table 1; Ref. 49). This intraperitoneal infection model may be representative of the clinical situation associated with human sepsis (3–6).

6. Analysis of LPS-like Agonistic Activity

E5531 has been extensively tested for agonistic activity in a variety of human and murine systems. In all the above assays, E5531 and sRcLA were completely devoid of agonistic activity, even when used at concentrations 10,000-fold higher

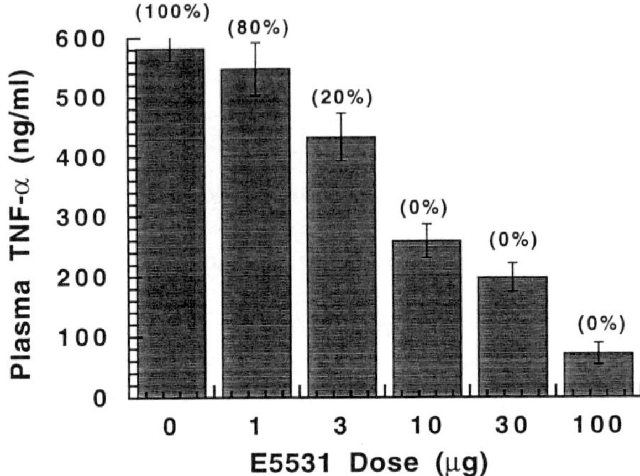

Figure 5 E5531 inhibition of LPS-induced increases in plasma TNF-α and lethality. BCG-primed mice were intravenously injected with 3 μg of *E. coli* LPS plus the indicated amount of E5531. After 1 h, plasma samples were obtained and assaysed for TNF-α as described in the Materials and Methods section. Lethality was assessed in a separate experiment using 10 BCG-primed mice per dose and observing lethality for 48 h after intravenous injection of 3 μg/kg of *E. coli* LPS plus the indicated amount of E5531. Values are shown in parentheses as percent of control lethality. Statistical significance for the 10-, 30-, and 100-μg treated groups were $p < 0.01$ versus control ($\chi^{2/}$ test).

than those required for antagonistic efficacy. In addition, we have assayed for potentially weak agonistic activity in vitro and in vivo in systems that have been "primed" to enhance their sensitivity to agonism. For example, LPS activation is enhanced by the addition of interferon-γ in murine macrophage (RAW 267.4) cells (25,50) or phorbol myristate acetate in human U937-derived cells (U38; Ref. 46). In all assays, E5531 was devoid of measurable agonistic activity at concentrations up to 100 μM. In contrast, the tetra-substituted lipid IV_A analog, B1060, was a potent LPS-like agonist when added to RAW cells in the presence of interferon-γ. Bacteria-derived RsLA was weakly to moderately agonistic in both human and murine cell assays (39).

E5531 was not agonistic when administered to BCG-primed mice at doses as high as 300 μg, (approximately 40 times higher dose than its IC_{50} for suppression of TNF-α). Similar analysis of B1060 indicates that it was agonistic in this system. At a dose of 300 μg, B1060 induced a 100- to 500-fold increase in plasma TNF-α over control basal levels, which was up to 95% of the stimulation seen after challenge with 200 ng of LPS. These results indicate that the strong

Table 1 E5531 and Antibiotic Cooperate to Protect Mice from a Lethal Infection of Viable *E. coli*

Treatment	Lethality at 48 h (%)[a]	Blood bacterial counts at 4 h (CFU/mL)[b]	Endotoxin level (pg/mL)[c]
None	87	117,500 ± 22,900	1,734 ± 344
Latamoxef (600 μg)	70	40 ± 10	11,487 ± 1,837
E5531 (100 μg)	87	122,500 ± 68,000	NT
Latamoxef plus E5531	13***	8 ± 5	NT

[a]BCG-primed mice ($n = 30$) were infected by intraperitoneal (i.p.) injection of *E. coli*. (2.0 × 10^7 CFU). One hour later, the indicated treatment or 5% glucose solution alone was intravenously injected (tail vein), and the incidence of death was monitored at the times for 48 h. Statistical significance: ***, $p < 0.001$ versus control (two-sided Fisher exact test). Seven days after i.p. infection with *E. coli*, only 4 of 30 mice co-treated with E5531 and latamoxef died, whereas 26/30 (no treatment), 26/30 (E5531 alone), and 21/30 (latamoxef alone) died.
[b]BCG-primed mice ($n = 4$) were infected intraperitoneally with 8.6 × 10^6 CFU of *E. coli*. One hour later, mice were intravenously administered drug(s) or 5% glucose alone, and blood bacterial counts were measured 2 and 4 h after administration of antibiotic by plating plasma dilutions on modified Drigalski agar (BTB agar E-MA84, Eiken Chemical Co. Tokyo, Japan). Prior to administration of antibiotic, blood bacterial counts were 205,000 ± 6455 CFU/mL.
[c]BCG-primed mice ($n = 4$) were infected intraperitoneally with 2.3 × 10^7 CFU of *E. coli* and peak endotoxin levels, 1 h after administration of antibiotic, were determined by an endotoxin-specific colorimetric limulus test (Toxicolor System-ENDOSPECY: ES-TEST, Seikagaku Kogyo Tokyo, Japan). NT = not tested.

agonistic activity of B1060 seen in murine in-vitro systems is also seen in vivo, making it an unsuitable candidate for pharmaceutical development.

IV. SUMMARY AND CONCLUSIONS

E5531 is an extraordinarily potent endotoxin antagonist with no agonistic properties. In-vitro studies demonstrated that E5531 is specific for LPS, while in vivo experiments demonstrated that E5531 protected BCG-primed mice from lethality induced by LPS and viable *E. coli* infection. These remarkable protective effects suggest that E5531 may be clinically useful in the treatment of gram-negative sepsis and septic shock in humans.

REFERENCES

1. Bone RC. Gram negative sepsis: background, clinical features, and intervention. Chest 1991; 100:802–808.

2. Parrillo JE. Pathogenetic mechanisms of septic shock. N Engl J Med 1993; 328:1471–1477.

3. Prins JM, van Deventer SJH, Kuijper EJ, Speelman P. Clinical relevance of antibiotic-induced endotoxin release. Antimicrob Agents Chemother 1994; 38: 1211–1218.

4. Dofferhoff ASM, Esselink MT, de Vreis-Hospers HG, et al. The release of endotoxin from antibiotic-treated *Escherichia coli* and the production of tumor necrosis factor by human monocytes. J Antimicrob Chemother 1993; 31:373–384.

5. Endo S, Inada K, Inoue Y, et al. Two types of septic shock classified by the plasma levels of cytokines and endotoxin. Circ Shock 1992; 38:264–274.

6. Crosby HA, Bion JF, Penn CW, Elliott TSJ. Antibiotic-induced release of endotoxin from bacteria in vitro. J Med Microbiol 1994; 40:23–30.

7. Galanos C, Lüderitz O, Rietschel ET, et al. Synthetic and natural *E. coli* free lipid A express identical endotoxic activities. Eur J Biochem 1985; 148:1–5.

8. Billiau A, Vandekerckhove F. Cytokines and their interactions with other inflammatory mediators in the pathogenesis of sepsis and septic shock. Eur J Clin Invest 1991; 21:559–573.

9. Glauser MP, Heumann D, Baumgartner JD, Cohen J. Pathogenesis and potential strategies for prevention and treatment of septic shock: an update. Clin Infect Dis 1994; 18(suppl 2): S205–S216.

10. Welbourn CRB, Young Y. Endotoxin, septic shock and acute lung injury: neutrophils, macrophages and inflammatory mediators. Br J Surg 1992; 79:998–1003.

11. Bone RC. Gram-negative sepsis: a dilemma of modern medicine. Clin Microbiol. Rev 1993; 6:57–68.

12. Corriveau CC, Danner RL. Antiendotoxin therapies for septic shock. Inf Agents Dis 1993; 2:44–52.

13. Ziegler EJ, Fisher CJ, Sprung CL, et al. Treatment of Gram-negative bacteremia and septic shock with HA-1A human monoclonal antibody against endotoxin. N Engl J Med 1991; 324:429–436.

14. Young LS, Gascon R, Alam S, Bermudez LEM. Monoclonal antibodies for treatment of Gram negative infections. Rev Infect Dis 1989; 11(suppl 7):S1562–S1571.

15. Zabel P, Schade FU, Schlaak M. Modulating effects of pentoxyfylline on cytokine release syndromes. In: Levin J, Alving CR, Munford RS, Stütz PL, eds. Bacterial Endotoxin: Recognition and Effector Mechanisms. Amsterdam: Elsevier, 1993:413–421.

16. Beutler B, Milsark IW, Cerami AC. Passive immunization against cachectin/tumor necrosis factor protects mice from lethal effects of endotoxin. Science 1985; 229:869–871.

17. Peppel K, Beutler B. Biological properties of a recombinant tumor necrosis factor inhibitor. In: Levin J, Alving CR, Munford RS, Stütz PL, eds. Bacterial Endotoxin: Recognition and Effector Mechanisms. Amsterdam: Elsevier, S 1993:447–454.

18. Dinarello CA, Gelfand JA, Wolff SM. Anticytokine strategies in the treatment of the systemic inflammatory response syndrome. JAMA 1993; 269:1829–1835.

19. Redmond HP, Chavin KD, Bromberg JS, Daly JM. Inhibition of macrophage-

activating cytokines is beneficial in the acute septic response. Ann Surg 1991; 214:502–509.

20. Natanson C, Hoffman WD, Suffredini AF, Eichacker PQ, Danner RL. Selected treatment strategies for septic shock based on proposed mechanisms of pathogenesis. Ann Intern Med 1994; 120:771–783

21. Loppnow H, Libby P, Freudenberg M, Krauss JH, Weckesser J, Mayer H. Cytokine induction by lipopolysaccharide (LPS) corresponds to lethal toxicity and is inhibited by non-toxic *Rhodobacter capsulatus* LPS. Infect Immun 1990; 58:3743–3750.

22. Takayama K, Qureshi N, Beutler B, Kirkland TN. Diphosphoryl lipid A from *Rhodopsuedomonas sphaeroides* ATCC 17023 blocks induction of cachectin in macrophages by lipopolysaccharide. Infect Immun 1989; 57:1336–1338.

23. Christ WJ, McGuinness PD, Asano O, et al. Total synthesis of the proposed structure of *Rhodobacter sphaeroides* lipid A resulting in the synthesis of new potent lipopolysaccharide antagonists. J Am Chem Soc 1994; 116:3637–3638.

24. Wang SC, Rossignol DP, Christ WJ, et al. Suppression of LPS-induced macrophage nitric oxide and cytokine production *in vitro* by a novel LPS antagonist. Surgery 1994; 116:339–347.

25. Lorsbach RB, Murphy WJ, Lowenstein CJ, Snyder SH, Russell SW. Expression of the nitric oxide synthase gene in mouse macrophages activated for tumor cell killing: molecular basis for the synergy between interferon-γ and lipopolysaccharide. J Biol Chem 1993; 268:1908–1913.

26. Stuehr DJ, Nathan CF. Nitric oxide—a macrophage product responsible for cytostasis and respiratory inhibition in tumor target cells. J Exp Med 1989; 169:1543–1555.

27. Vogel SN, Moore RN, Sipe JD, Rosenstreich DL. BCG-induced enhancement of endotoxin sensitivity in C3H/HeJ mice. J Immunol 1980; 124:2004–2009.

28. Ray BL, Painter G, Raetz CRH. The biosynthesis of Gram-negative endotoxin: formation of lipid A disaccharides from monosaccharide precursors in extracts of *Escherichia coli*. J Biol Chem 1984; 259:4852–4859.

29. Bulawa CE, Raetz CRH. The biosynthesis of Gram-negative endotoxin: identification and function of UDP-2,3-diacylglucosamine in *Escherichia coli*. J Biol Chem 1984; 259:4846–4851.

30. Danner RL, Joiner KA, Parrillo JE. Inhibition of endotoxin-induced priming of human neutrophils by Lipid X and 3-Aza-Lipid X. J Clin Invest 1987; 80:605–612.

31. Proctor RA, Will JA, Burhop KE, Raetz CRH. Protection of mice against lethal endotoxemia by a lipid A precursor. Infect Immun 1986; 52:905–907.

32. Golenbock DT, Will JA, Raetz CRH, Proctor RA. Lipid X ameliorates pulmonary hypertension and protects sheep from death due to endotoxin. Infect Immun 1987; 55:2471–2476.

33. Danner RL, Van Dervort AL, Doerfler ME, Stuetz P, Parrillo JE. Antiendotoxin activity of lipid A analogues: requirements of the chemical structure. Pharm Res 1990; 7:260–263.

34. Danner RL, Doerfler ME, Eichacker PQ, et al. A therapeutic trial of lipid X in a canine model of septic shock. J Infect Dis 1993; 167:378–384.

35. Raetz CRH. Biochemistry of endotoxins. Ann Rev Biochem 1990; 59:129–170.

36. Golenbock DT, Hampton RY, Qureshi N, Takayama K, Raetz CRH. Lipid A-like molecules that antagonize the effects of endotoxins on human monocytes. J Biol Chem 1991; 266:19490–19498.

37. Krauss JH, Seydel U, Weckesser J, Mayer H. Structural analysis of the nontoxic lipid A of *Rhodobacter capsulatus* 37b4. Eur J Biochem 1989; 180:519–526.

38. Qureshi N, Honovich JP, Hara H, Cotter RJ, Takayama K. Location of fatty acids in lipid A obtained from lipopolysaccharide of *Rhodopseudomonas sphaeroides* ATCC 17023. J Biol Chem 1988; 263:5502–5504.

39. Rose JR, Christ WJ, Bristol JR, Kawata T, Rossignol DP. Agonistic and antagonistic activities of bacterially-derived *Rhodobacter sphaeroides* lipid A; comparison to synthetic material of the proposed structure and analogs. Infect Immun 1995; 68:833–839.

40. Imoto M, Yoshimura H, Sakaguchi N, Kusumoto S, Shiba T. Total synthesis of *Escherichia coli* lipid A. Tetrahedron Lett 1985; 26:1545–1548.

41. Christ WJ, Kawata T, Hawkins LD, Asano O, Kobayashi S, Rossignol DP. Anti-endotoxin compounds and related molecules and methods. U.S. Patent 1992; application no. 935050.

42. Kawata T, Bristol J, McGuigan L, et al. Anti-endotoxin activities of E5531, a novel synthetic derivative of lipid A. Abstracts of the 1992 ICAAC, 1992:337.

43. Rossignol D, Ackermann K, Kawata T, et al. Role of lipopolysaccharide binding protein (LBP) in lipopolysaccharide binding and activation of murine macrophage cells; inhibition by E5531. Abstracts of the 1992 ICAAC, 1992:337.

44. Kitchens RL, Ulevitch RJ, Munford RS. Lipopolysaccharide (LPS) partial structures inhibit responses to LPS in a human macrophage cell line without inhibiting LPS uptake by a CD 14-mediated pathway. J Exp Med 1992; 176:485–494.

45. Ulmer AJ, Feist W, Heine H, et al. Modulation of endotoxin-induced monokine release in human monocytes by lipid A partial structures that inhibit binding of ^{125}I-lipopolysaccharide. Infect Immun 1992; 60:5145–5152.

46. Felber BK, Pavlakis GN. A quantitative bioassay for HIV-1 based on trans-activation. Science 1988; 239:184–187.

47. Kobayashi S, Kimura A, Hishinuma I, et al. Protection from lethal bacteremia by E5531, a novel synthetic lipid A derivative in mice primed with *Bacillus Calmette-Guerin* (BCG). Abstracts of the 1992 ICAAC, 1992:338.

48. Røkke O, Revhaug A, Østerud B, Giercksky KE. Increased plasma levels of endotoxin and corresponding changes in circulatory performance in a porcine sepsis model: the effect of antibiotic administration. Prog Clin Biol Res 1988; 272:247–262.

49. Christ WJ, Asano O, Robidoux ALC, et al. E5531, a pure endotoxin antagonist of high potency. Science 1995; 268:80–83.

50. Wang M-H, Flad H-D, Feist W, et al. Inhibition of endotoxin-induced interleukin-6 production by synthetic lipid A partial structures in peripheral blood mononuclear cells. Infect Immun 1991; 59:4655–4664.

11

The Efficacy of Recombinant CD14 in Preventing LPS-Induced Shock

Sanna M. Goyert, Jack Silver, and Alain Haziot
North Shore University Hospital
Cornell University Medical College
Manhasset, New York

I. INTRODUCTION

Endotoxin shock is a potentially lethal consequence of gram-negative bacteremia. The cascade of events leading to death appears to be initiated by the interaction of LPS (lipopolysaccharide, endotoxin) with CD14, a myeloid cell surface glycoprotein expressed strongly by monocytes and weakly by neutrophils (1–7). Several lines of evidence suggest that membrane CD14 (mCD14) is required for the myeloid cell response to LPS: (a) anti-CD14 antibodies inhibit the secretion of TNF-tumor necrosis factor-α by myeloid cells (7–10); (b) CD14-negative cells transfected with CD14 respond to LPS at least 1000 times better than non-transfected cells (11,12); (c) transgenic mice expressing high levels of human CD14 are hypersensitive to LPS (13); and (d) CD14-deficient mice produced by homologous recombination are at least 1000 times less sensitive to LPS than normal mice (A. Haziot, E. Ferrero, C. Stewart, and S. M. Goyert, in preparation).

These observations, documenting a central role for CD14 in the response to endotoxin, led us to hypothesize that a soluble form of the CD14 receptor might be a potent inhibitor of LPS and thus might serve as an effective therapeutic for endotoxin shock. To test this hypothesis we produced a recombinant (r) form of the soluble (s) receptor (rsCD14) using a Baculovirus expression system and tested it for its effects on the response to LPS both in vitro and in vivo.

II. CHARACTERISTICS OF RECOMBINANT HUMAN CD14 PRODUCED BY INSECT CELLS

Cell surface CD14 is normally anchored to the membrane through a glycosylphosphatidylinositol (GPI) group. However, mammalian cells which express CD14 spontaneously shed some of it from the cell surface. This material can be recovered from the culture media of monocytes/macrophages and neutrophils in a soluble form. In addition, other cells which are normally CD14 negative but which have been genetically engineered to express CD14 on their surface (3,13) also release a soluble form of CD14 into the culture media and/or blood. The release of a soluble form of CD14 appears to involve a proteolytic cleavage event which occurs close to the C terminus of the GPI-anchored protein, resulting in the removal of the GPI anchor (3,14). This property of CD14 in eukaryotic cells was very useful for the production of a soluble form of recombinant CD14 (rsCD14).

To produce a recombinant form of CD14 in high quantities, the Baculovirus system, which utilizes the expression of recombinant proteins in insect cells, was chosen. Insect cells (High 5 or SF9) transformed with a recombinant Baculovirus containing the complete human CD14 cDNA coding region (15–17) express both a GPI-anchored form of human CD14 on their surface as well as a soluble form lacking the GPI anchor which is released into the tissue culture media (17). The release of a soluble form of CD14 even by insect cells suggests that the enzyme(s) involved in the release (shedding) of CD14 from the cell surface are not cell type or species specific and are probably evolutionarily conserved. The human rsCD14 produced by the Baculovirus-infected insect cells was isolated from the culture media by affinity chromatography using an anti-human CD14 mAb. The recombinant protein shows a heterogeneous pattern on SDS-PAGE, with the bands having an average molecular weight of 43 kDa (Fig. 1). However, digestion of this protein with N-glycanase, an enzyme that removes N-linked glycoprotein, leads to the reduction of this complex pattern to a single homogenous band with a molecular weight of approximately 35 kDa; this is similar in molecular weight to the size predicted, on the basis of its nucleotide sequence, for a nonglycosylated CD14 protein (Fig. 1, Refs. 15, 16). These results strongly suggest that the molecular-weight heterogeneity of soluble CD14 produced by insect cells is due to differences in glycosylation.

III. BIOLOGICAL PROPERTIES OF rsCD14

To ascertain that the rsCD14 was fully functional, a number of different assays were used to measure its biological properties.

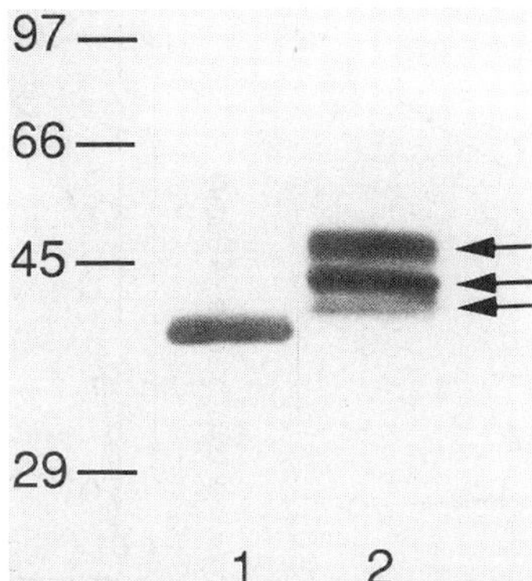

Figure 1   SDS-PAGE profiles of rsCD14 imunoprecipitated from the culture media of High 5 insect cells 3 days after infection with the human CD14 recombinant Baculovirus. Lane 1, rsCD14 digested with N-glycanase; lane 2, rsCD14. The samples were electrophoresed under nonreducing conditions. The migration of molecular-weight markers is noted on the left. Arrows indicate the individual bands.

A. Binding of LPS to rsCD14

To examine the ability of the rsCD14 to bind LPS specifically, a solid-phase binding assay was developed. Briefly, rsCD14 was used to coat the wells of a polystyrene microtiter plate and serial dilutions of biotinylated-LPS (bLPS) were added. After a period of incubation, the amount of bound bLPS was measured by ELISA. As can be seen in Fig. 2A, bLPS binds directly in a dose-dependent manner. The specificity of this binding is demonstrated by the fact that bLPS does not bind to an immobilized irrelevant protein (murine lg) (Fig. 2A). In addition, the binding of bLPS to rsCD14 is saturable (Fig. 2B). Furthermore, a 15-fold excess of unlabeled autologous LPS inhibits 90% of the binding of bLPS to rsCD14 (Fig. 3). Finally, the addition of increasing amounts of rsCD14 but not murine lg inhibits the binding of bLPS to immobilized rsCD14 (Fig. 3). In this regard it is interesting to note that a natural form of soluble CD14 (nsCD14) isolated from the urine of nephrotic patients inhibits the binding of bLPS to immobilized CD14 only slightly less efficiently than rsCD14 (Fig. 3). These studies document that LPS binds to our rsCD14 whether it is immobilized on a surface or free in solution.

   To further confirm the biological activity of our rsCD14, we measured the ability of the serum protein, LBP (LPS-binding protein) to enhance the binding of LPS to it. Previous studies have shown that the activation of cells by low levels of LPS (<10 ng/mL) can be significantly enhanced by the addition of

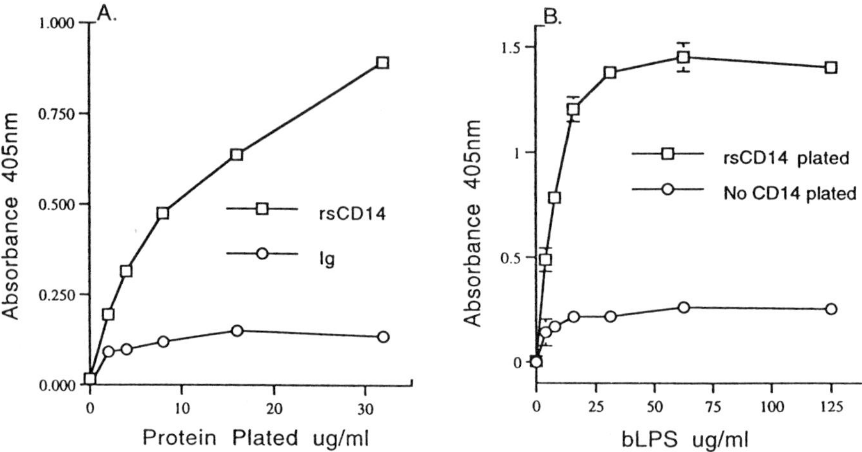

Figure 2   Binding of biotinylated LPS to immobilized rsCD14. (A) bLPS binds directly to rsCD14. Wells of a microtiter plate were coated with increasing amounts of rsCD14 (open square) or murine lg (open circle), and bound bLPS was measured using a streptavidin-alkaline phosphatase detection system (17). Results are representative of four experiments. (B) The binding of bLPS to rsCD14 is saturable. rsCD14 (16 μg/mL, open square) or coating buffer (0.2 M acetate buffer, pH 5.0, open circle) was plated in the wells of a microtiter plate and residual sites were blocked with gelatin (0.5%). Increasing concentrations of bLPS were added to the wells and bound bLPS was measured as above. When error bars are not seen, they fall within the symbol.

LBP (7,8). This effect of LBP is believed to be due to its ability to accelerate the binding of LPS to membrane CD14 (18). Accordingly, the effects of LBP on the binding of bLPS to immobilized rsCD14 were measured. As can be seen in Fig. 4, the addition of purified rabbit LBP enhances the binding of bLPS to immobilized rsCD14 by 5- to 10-fold, whereas the addition of an irrelevant protein (BSA) has no effect.

B.   Activation of Endothelial Cells by rsCD14

Experiments by Frey et al. (19) suggested that soluble CD14 found in serum might be required for LPS-induced activation of endothelial cells. We examined endothelial cell responses to LPS in the presence and absence of rsCD14 (20) and found that LPS-induced up-regulation of ICAM-1 expression (an indicator of activation) by human umbilical vein endothelial cells (HUVEC) requires the presence of rsCD14 (Fig. 5). Under these conditions where LPS is present in a high concentration (50 ng/mL), LBP does not influence the response (20); how-

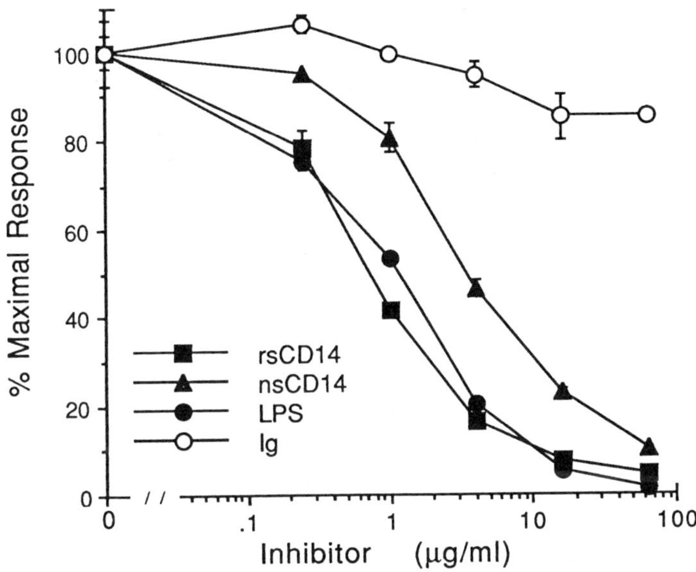

Figure 3   Inhibition of bLPS binding to immobilized rsCD14 in the presence of LBP by increasing amounts of unbound rsCD14, unbound nsCD14, unlabeled LPS, or unbound murine IgG. Plates were coated with rsCD14 at 64 μg/mL. Increasing concentrations of rsCD14, nsCD14, or murine IgG were preincubated with bLPS (1 μg/mL) and LBP (350 ng.mL) and then added to the rsCD14-coated wells. For the inhibition with unlabeled LPS, increasing concentrations of LPS were preincubated with the immobilized rsCD14 in the presence of LBP (350 ng/mL) before addition of bLPS (1 μg/mL). Specific binding was calculated by subtraction of the amount of bLPS bound to wells coated with PBS-gelatin (0.5%). Filled square, unbound rsCD14; filled triangle, unbound nsCD14; filled circle, unlabeled LPS (and LBP); open circle, unbound murine IgG.

ever, when the concentration of LPS is low (<10 ng/mL), LBP potentiates the response to LPS-rsCD14 (20). These studies further confirm that rsCD14 is functional and document its role in inducing endothelial cell responses to LPS. Furthermore, they suggest that rsCD14 is an agonist for endothelial cell responses to LPS.

C.   Inhibition of TNF-α Secretion by Human Cells

The potential use of rsCD14 as a therapeutic requires that it be able to inhibit the LPS-induced activation of cells. Since many studies have implicated TNF-

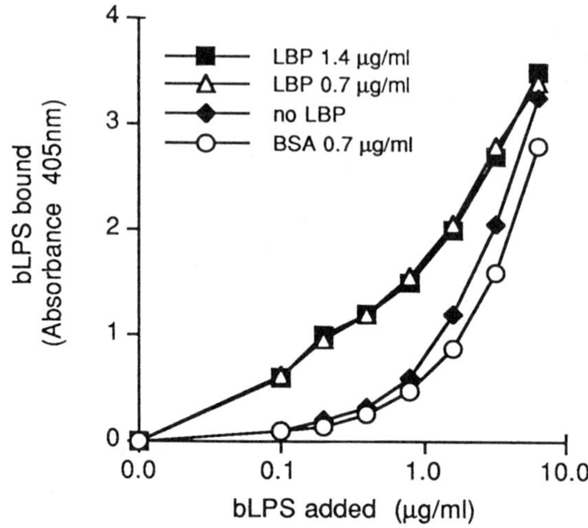

Figure 4 Effect of LBP on the binding of bLPS to immobilized rsCD14. Wells were coated with rsCD14 (32 µg/mL) and blocked with gelatin (0.5%). Increasing concentrations of bLPS were preincubated with or without purified rabbit LBP or BSA and added to the wells. Filled square, LBP (1.4 µg/mL); open triangle, LBP (0.7 µg/mL); filled diamond, no LBP; open circle, BSA (0.7 µg/mL).

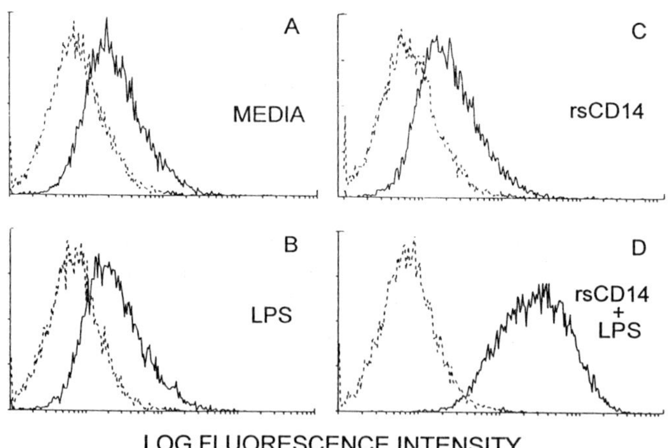

Figure 5 Up-regulation of ICAM-1 expression by HUVEC in the presence of LPS and rsCD14. Solid line, FITC-conjugated anti-ICAM-1; dotted line, isotype control.

α as a primary mediator of the cascade of events occurring during endotoxin shock, inhibition of its release during LPS-induced activation is a convenient way to assess the therapeutic potential of rsCD14. Accordingly, the ability of rsCD14 to inhibit the LPS-induced secretion of TNF-α by human peripheral blood mononuclear cells (PBMC) was measured in vitro (17). Briefly, increasing amounts of rsCD14 were added to purified human mononuclear cells exposed to several different doses of LPS and rabbit LBP. As can be seen in Fig. 6A, the addition of increasing amounts of rsCD14 inhibits the LPS:LBP-induced secretion of TNF-α by human mononuclear cells isolated from peripheral blood. No similar inhibition was observed when globulin-free (gf) BSA was used as a control. This inhibition requires large amounts of rsCD14 as indicated by the fact that 100 μg of rsCD14/mL is required to inhibit 82% of the secretion of TNF-α in the presence of 0.5 ng LPS/mL.

A similar degree of inhibition was observed when whole human blood (a more relevant in-vitro model of endotoxin shock) was used instead of purified

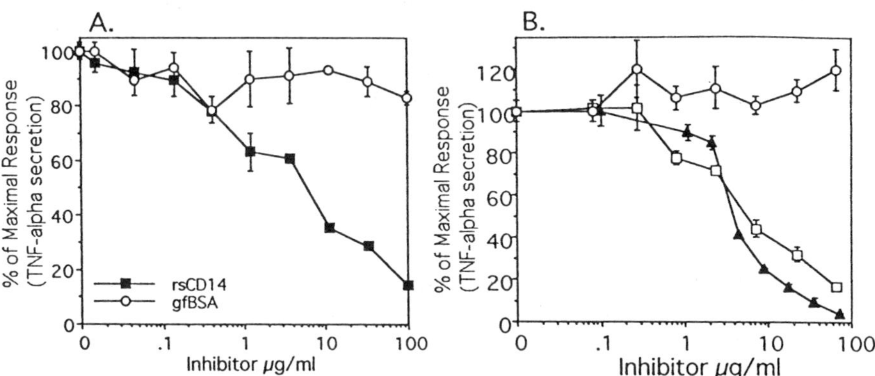

Figure 6 Inhibition of LPS-induced TNF-α production by human cells. (A) PBMC: cells (8 × 10^5) were incubated in the presence of LPS (0.5 ng/mL) and increasing concentrations of rsCD14 or globulin-free BSA (gfBSA) in 1% autologus plasma for 3 h. TNF-α was measured in cell-free supernatants by ELISA. In the absence of inhibitor, the TNF-α concentration was 1.24 ng/mL. Filled square, rsCD14; open circle, gfBSA. (B) Whole blood: increasing concentrations of rsCD14 or gfBSA were added to whole blood immediately before adding LPS at 0.25 ng/mL (squares and circles) or 0.1 ng/mL (triangles). After incubation at 37°C for 3 h, the cells were pelleted and the supernatants assayed for TNF-α by ELISA. In the absence of inhibitor, the TNF-α concentrations were 1.72 (LPS 0.25 ng/mL) and 0.65 ng/mL (LPS 0.1 ng/mL). LPS at 0.25 ng/mL with rsCD14 (open square), gfBSA (open circle); LPS at 0.1 ng/mL with rsCD14 (filled triangle).

PBMC. As seen in Fig. 6B, the addition of increasing amounts of rsCD14 to cells exposed to 0.25 ng/mL of LPS inhibited as much as 82% of the secretion of TNF-α, while the addition of 71 μg/ul of rsCD14 to cells exposed to 0.1 ng LPS/mL almost completely inhibited (96%) the secretion of TNF-α. Thus, a very large excess of rsCD14 is required to completely inhibit the response of cells in whole blood to LPS. This concentration of rsCD14 is probably 20–40 times the concentration of endogenous rsCD14 normally present in the blood of most individuals (21).

D.   Inhibition of TNF-α Secretion by Murine Cells

Before considering the possibility of testing the therapeutic effects of rsCD14 in an in-vivo model such as mice, it was first necessary to determine whether rsCD14 could similarly inhibit the activation of murine PBMC in vitro. Since the human and murine CD14 proteins show a high degree of homology (66% identity at the amino acid level [13]), it was not unreasonable to hypothesize that their active site might be conserved and that human rsCD14 might be able to inhibit the LPS-induced stimulation of murine cells. Accordingly, the ability of human rsCD14 to inhibit the LPS-induced release of TNF-α by murine PBMC was determined. As seen in Fig. 7, the addition of rsCD14 to murine PBMC exposed to LPS inhibits TNF secretion in a dose-dependent fashion, with similar levels of human rsCD14 being required to inhibit the murine response as was observed for human cells. These encouraging results prompted us to further explore the possibility that rsCD14 might function as a therapeutic for endotoxic shock.

IV.   THERAPEUTIC EFFECTS OF rsCD14 IN A MURINE ENDOTOXIC SHOCK MODEL OF LPS-INDUCED LETHALITY

The results obtained above, in a murine in-vitro model of endotoxic shock, suggested that rsCD14 might also be effective in vivo. Accordingly, we examined the effects of rsCD14 in a murine in-vivo model of LPS-induced mortality. Briefly, LPS [12 μg/g body weight (gbw), *Salmonella minnesota*, wild type] was given intraperitoneally (i.p.) to mice (C57BL/6J), followed immediately by an i.p. administration of rsCD14 (12μg/gbw) or an equivalent volume of saline, and the effects on mortality were recorded. As can be seen in Fig. 8, the administration of rsCD14 prevented death in 100% of the mice, whereas nearly 60% of the control mice treated only with saline died (Fig. 8A). Similarly, when the rsCD14 was administered i.p. 10 min after the LPS was administered, all of the mice receiving LPS and rsCD14 survived (Fig. 8A). To eliminate the possibility that the therapeutic effects of rsCD14 were due to neutralization of

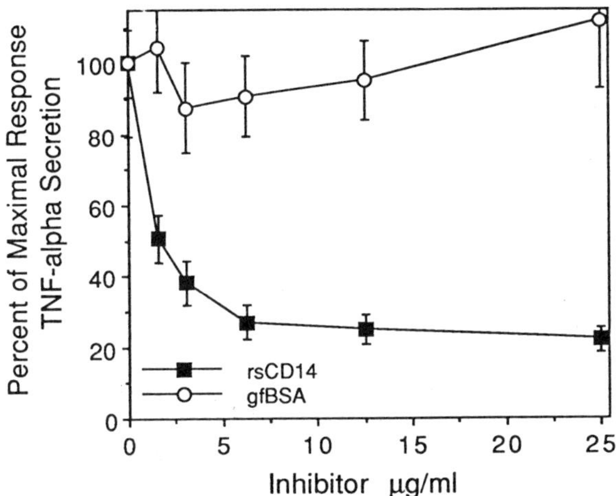

Figure 7 Inhibition of LPS-induced TNF-α production by murine PBMC. Murine PBMC (1 × 10⁵mL) were incubated for 3 h at 37°C with LPS (0.5 ng/mL) and increasing concentrations of rsCD14 (filled square) or gfBSA (open circle) in the presence of 1% autologous serum. Cell-free supernatants were assayed for TNF-α production by the MTT cytotoxicity assay using WEHI 2F cells (7). The 100% response represents a TNF-α concentration of 121 U/mL.

the LPS in the peritoneal cavity, these experiment were repeated except that the LPS was injected i.p. while the rsCD14 was administered intravenously (i.v.), immediately following the LPS injection. Again, administration of rsCD14 was therapeutic (Fig. 8B). In both types of experiments, the mice treated with LPS and rsCD14 showed signs of a response to the LPS which were similar to the symptoms seen in the control mice, including ruffled fur and exudate in the eyes of some animals. However, the mice treated with rsCD14 recovered completely within a 24-h period.

To confirm that the therapeutic effects of rsCD14 were indeed due to its ability to inhibit the activation of myeloid cells and, correspondingly, the release of TNF-α, mice were injected with LPS and rsCD14 as before and blood samples obtained at various times following the injection were assayed for the presence of TNF-α. As can be seen in Fig. 9, treatment of mice with 50 µg of rsCD14/gbw shows a significant reduction of TNF in serum taken 90 min following the injections; at 135 min, little or no TNF is detected in contrast to the control mice. Treatment with 35 µg rsCD14/gbw also resulted in a decreased secretion of TNF-α, although the difference was not as pronounced.

In summary, these results suggest that the injected rsCD14 binds to LPS and

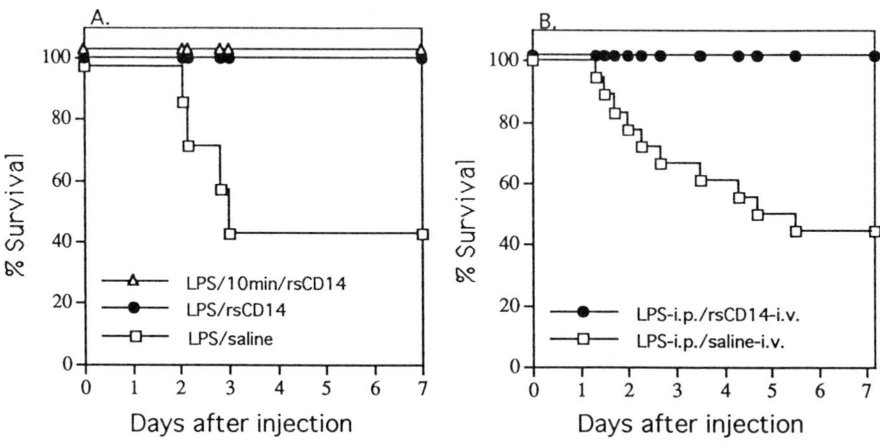

Figure 8 Therapeutic effect of rsCD14 on LPS-induced lethality. (A) Mice were injected i.p. with LPS [12 μg/g body weight (gbw) in 0.1 mL saline], followed either immediately with an i.p. injection of rsCD14 (12 μg/gbw in 0.1 mL saline, filled circle) or 10 min later (open triangle). Control animals were injected with an equivalent volume of saline (open square). Each group consisted of 7 mice. $p = 0.0175$ by the two-tailed Fisher exact test. (B) Mice were injected i.p. with LPS (13 μg/gbw in 0.2 mL saline), followed immediately by an i.v. injection of rsCD14 (12 μg/gbw in 0.2 mL saline). $p = 0.0039$ by the two-tailed Fisher exact test.

inhibits the ability of LPS to activate myeloid cells, the primary producers of TNF-α. This effect on myeloid cells, in turn, prevents death in this model of endotoxin shock. It is surprising, however, that although a large excess of rsCD14 was required to inhibit the activation of cells in vitro (see Figs. 6 and 7), a molar ratio of approximately 1:5 of rsCD14 to LPS, was found to be therapeutic in vivo. Furthermore, since humans normally have a large amount of circulating sCD14 (2–4 μg/mL) (21), one would expect that this amount of sCD14 should already be ample for inhibiting the effects of LPS in the bloodstream. One way of reconciling these discrepancies is to propose that, in vivo, only a small fraction of the injected LPS is functional, due to other mechanisms that may be operational in decreasing the effective concentration of LPS. Furthermore, although sCD14 has been detected by ELISA in humans, it is not clear that this circulating sCD14 is functional. In any event, our observations with rsCD14 support the contention that rsCD14 may represent a new therapeutic for endotoxin shock and warrant further investigation in a large animal model.

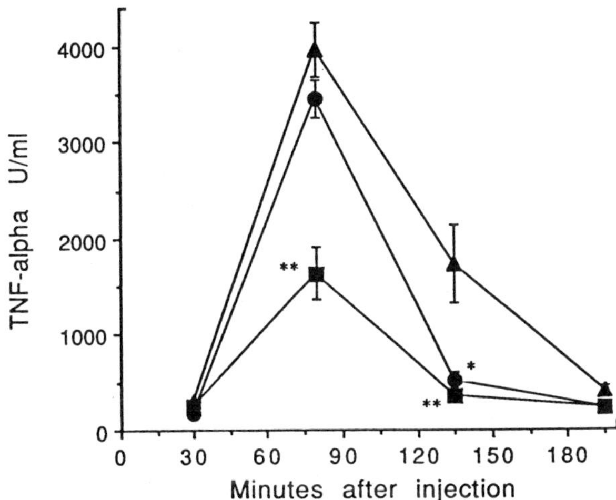

Figure 9 Serum levels of TNF-α in mice injected with LPS (13 μg/gbw, i.p.) and rsCD14 (i.p.). Filled square, rsCD14 at 50 μg/gbw, $n = 6$; filled circle, rsCD14 at 35 μg/gbw, $n = 6$; filled triangle, saline control, $n = 5$. Mice were injected as in Fig. 8A. At 30, 80, and 135 min following the injections, the mice were bled from the tail vein (30 μL), and the serum concentration of TNF-α was measured. Bars indicate ± SEM. *, $p < 0.001$ and **, $p < 0.0001$ by the Mann-Whitney test.

ACKNOWLEDGMENTS

This work was supported by National Institutes of Health grants AI23859 and GM47175 to S.M.G. and The Council for Tobacco Research grant #2218. S.M.G. is a Leukemia Society of America Scholar. This is publication #40 from the Division of Molecular Medicine.

REFERENCES

1. Griffin JD, Ritz J, Nadler LM, Schlossman SF. Expression of myeloid differentiation antigens on normal and malignant myeloid cells. J Clin Invest 1981; 68:932–941.
2. Todd RF, Nadler LM, Schlossman SF. Antigens on human monocytes identified by monoclonal antibodies. J Immunol 1981; 126:1435–1442.
3. Haziot A, Chen S, Ferrero E, Low MG, Silber R, Goyert SM. The monocyte differentiation antigen, CD14, is anchored to the cell membrane by a phosphatidylinositol linkage. J Immunol 1988; 141:547–552.
4. Rigby WF, Shen L, Ball ED, Guyre PM, Fanger MW. Differentiation of a human

monocyte cell line by 1,25-dihydroxyvitamin D3 (Calcitriol); a morphologic, phenotypic, and functional analysis. Blood 1984; 64:1110–1115.

5. Goyert SM, Ferrero EM, Seremetis SV, Winchester RJ, Silver J, Mattison AC. Biochemistry and expression of myelomonocytic antigens. J Immunol 1986; 137:3909–3914.

6. Ball ED, Graziano RG, L Shen, Fanger MW. Monoclonal antibodies to novel myeloid antigens reveal human granulocyte heterogeneity. Proc Natl Acad Sci USA 1982; 79: 5374–5378.

7. Haziot A., Tsuberi B-Z, Goyert SM. Neutrophil CD14: biochemical properties and role in the secretion of TNFα in response to LPS. J Immunol 1993; 150:5556–5565.

8. Wright SD, Ramos RM, Tobias PS, Ulevitch RJ, Mathison JC. CD14, a receptor for complexes of lipopolysaccharide (LPS) and LPS binding protein. Science 1990; 249:1431–1433.

9. Goyert SM, Haziot A, Jiao D, et al. CD14 cluster workshop report. In: Schlossman S, et al., eds. Leukocyte Typing V. Oxford: Oxford University Press, 1994: in press.

10. Haziot A, Katz IR, Jiao D, Rong G-W, Goyert, SM. Functional epitopes of CD14. In: Schlossman S, et al., eds. Leukocyte Typing V. Oxford: Oxford University Press, 1994: in press.

11. Lee JD, Kato K, Tobias PS, Kirkland TN, Ulevitch RJ. Transfection of CD14 into 70Z/3 cells dramatically enhances the sensitivity to complexes of lipopolysaccharide (LPS) and LPS binding protein. J Exp Med 1992; 75:1697–1705.

12. Golenbock DT, Liu Y, Millham FH, Freeman MK, Zoeller RA. Surface expression of human CD14 in chinese hamster ovary fibroblasts imparts macrophage-like responsiveness to bacterial endotoxin. J Biol Chem 1993; 268:22055–22059.

13. Ferrero E, Jiao D, Tsuberi B, et al, Transgenic mice expressing human CD14 are hypersensitive to LPS. Proc Natl Acad Sci USA 1993; 90:2380–2384.

14. Bazil V, Strominger JL. Shedding as a mechanism of down-modulation of CD14 on stimulated human monocytes. J Immunol 1991; 147:1567–1574.

15. Goyert SM, Ferrero E, Rettig WJ, Yenamandra AK, Obata F, LeBeau MM. The CD14 monocyte differentiation antigen maps to a region encoding growth factors and receptors. Science 1988; 239:497–239.

16. Ferrero E, Goyert SM. Nucleotide sequence of the gene encoding the monocyte differentiation antigen, CD14. Nuclsic Acids Res 1988; 16:4173.

17. Haziot A, Rong G-W, Bazil V, Silver J, Goyert SM. Recombinant soluble CD14 inhibits LPS-induced tumor necrosis factor -α production by cells in whole blood. J Immunol 1994; 152:5868–5876.

18. Hailman E, Lichenstein HS, Wurfel MM, et al. Lipopolysaccharide (LPS)-binding protein accelerates the binding of LPS to CD14. J Exp Med 1994; 179:269–277.

19. Frey EA, Miller DS, Jahr TG, et al. Soluble CD14 participates in the response of cells to lipopolysaccharide. J Exp Med 1992; 176:1665–1671.

20. Haziot, A, Rong G-W, Silver J, Goyert SM. Recombinant soluble CD14 mediates the activation of endothelial cells by LPS. J Immunol 1993; 51:1500–1507.

21. Grunwald U, Kruger C, Westermann J, Lukowsky A, Ehlers M, Schutt C. An enzyme-linked immunosorbent assay for the quantification of solubilized CD14 in biological fluids. J Immunol Meth 1992; 155:225–232.

12

Selective Inhibition of Phosphatidic Acid Synthesis: A Novel Approach to the Treatment of Sepsis and the Systemic Inflammatory Response Syndrome

Stuart L. Bursten, Ward E. Harris, and Glenn C. Rice
Cell Therapeutics, Inc.
Seattle, Washington

I. INTRODUCTION

Lipid A, the major active component of lipopolysaccharide (LPS: bacterial endotoxin), has numerous in-vitro biological effects, including cytolysis of endothelial cells, polyclonal induction of B-lymphocyte mitogenesis, and stimulation of inflammatory cytokine and eicosanoid release by many types of cells (1–8). Lipid A effects on glomerular mesangial cells (GMC), for example, are profound, inducing the synthesis and release of interleukin-1β (IL-1β) within 8–12 h (9,10). In addition, lipid A potently induces tumor necrosis factor α (TNF-α) mRNA expression and synthesis in a variety of cell types (11–15). The induction of TNF-α and IL-1β, in combination with the presence of lipid A in the serum, is felt to be the primary initiating and mediating event for the diffuse organ injury referred to as systemic inflammatory response syndrome (SIRS) (12).

A number of studies involving direct infusion or, conversely, the use of cytokine-specific inhibitors in animal models have suggested that the primary endogenous initiators of SIRS are TNF-α and IL-1β (13–17). These primary endogenous inflammatory mediators are synergistic (14,15) and para- and autostimulatory (16,17). Lipid A may mimic the actions of both IL-1β and TNF-α (18,19), as well as inducing these cytokines. Each of these primary inflammatory mediators in turn stimulates release of a succession of additional inflammatory signals including interleukin-6 (IL-6) (20), interferon-γ (IFN-γ) (21), platelet-activating factor (PAF) (22), interleukin-8 (IL-8) (23), macrophage inflammatory protein-1α (MIP-1α) (24), and nitric oxide (25). In some cases, these proinflammatory mediators can act in an additive as well as synergistic manner to further amplify the inflammatory cascade and its deleterous consequences (21,23,26).

Most therapeutic interventions developed for sepsis and SIRS have targeted only single components of the monokine cascade, and in preclinical models require administration either prior to or within 1–2 h following endotoxin for significant protection (16,20,27,28). The observation that inhibitors of IL-1β, TNF-α, or IL-6 block enodotoxin-induced mortality only if given before or shortly after LPS or lipid A suggests that the inflammatory cascade contains significant redundancy. Recently interleukin 10 (IL-10) has been shown to efficiently protect mice from endotoxin-induced lethality (29), and most likely does so by blocking LPS-induced release of several primary and secondary inflammatory monokines including TNF-α, IL-6, and IFN-γ (30). This suggests that, for an optimal anti-SIRS effect, a multitargeted approach is advantageous. Besides the relative high cost and difficulty of administration of biological, IL-10 suffers from the potential clinical disadvantage of costimulating B cells and mast cells (30).

An alternative approach to biological agents is to pharmacologically suppress intracellular signal transduction pathways used by several inflammatory mediators involved in SIRS. Recent studies have shown that IL-1β (31), TNF-α (32), PAF (33), as well as bacterial cell wall products such as lipid A or LPS (18,19,34), may activate and signal through at least one common lipid intracellular signaling pathway. Activation of this pathway occurs within seconds of exposure of cells to a stimulus and leads to rapid increases in intracellular levels of specific species of phosphatidic acid (PA) and diacylglycerol (DG). One species of interest is PA produced by a membrane-associated enzyme acyl CoA: lysophosphatidic acid acyl transferase and converted to 1,2-sn-DG via phosphatidate phosphohydrolase (18,19,31,34). Subtypes of DG stimulate several secondary signaling processes such as activation of protein kinase C and acidic sphingomyelinase (35). Besides functioning as lipid second-messenger intermediates, PA species and PA precursors stimulate Ca^{2+} flux (36), phospholipase C activity (36), induce expression of several protooncogenes and growth factors (37), are mitogenic for certain cell types (38), and inhibit GAP-*ras* interactions (39).

CT-1501R [(R)-1-(5-hydroxyhexyl)-3,7-dimethylxanthine; lisofylline: LSF] is a novel metabolite of the rheological agent pentoxifylline (PTX). This compound was detected in patients treated with PTX in conjunction with the antibiotic and P450 IA2 inhibitor, ciprofloxacin (40). LSF was not detectable in patients treated with PTX alone. Increasing levels of LSF in patients treated with PTX and ciprofloxacin appeared to correlate with the ability to prevent multiorgan dysfunction in patients treated with IL-2 (40). When tested in a mouse monoblastic leukemia cell line, P388, stimulated with LPS, LSF was 800-fold more potent at inhibiting PA and DG generation than was PTX [the IC_{50} for inhibition of PA by LSF was approximately 0.6 μM] (34). This is in contrast to LSF's minimal effects on cAMP phosphodiesterases, where the IC_{50} has varied from 200 μM to 1 mM (34).

Our interests have therefore centered around studies of the effects of LSF in in-vitro and in-vivo systems relevant to SIRS. These studies demonstrate that, by its ability to block a redundant second messenger associated with inflammatory cytokines and mediators, LSF shows promise as a therapeutic in a wide spectrum of clinical disorders associated with increased production of specific PA species.

II. PHOSPHATIDIC ACID SIGNALING INDUCED BY LIPID A

Mechanisms by which bacterial endotoxin moieties alter the functional properties of cells remain incompletely understood. It is known that endotoxin readily inserts into cellular membranes, and it has been postulated that this event induces alterations in the physicochemical properties of the membrane to initiate cellular activation (41). However, evidence exists for specific LPS-receptor proteins in splenic lymphocytes to which lipid A binds (42,43). In addition, a serum LPS-binding protein which attaches to and activates macrophages through the CD14 molecule has been described (11,44,45). Considering the broad range of biochemical responses induced by LPS in cells not possessing the CD14 receptor, such as endothelial or mesangial cells, it is unclear as to which membrane events are primary inducers of cellular activation.

The monosaccharyl form of lipid A (lipid X: 2,3-diacylglucosamine 1-phosphate) has previously been shown to bear a close formal structural resemblance to PA (46–49; Fig. 1). Given the structural similarities, we postulated that lipid A might induce cellular activation by functioning as a biological mimetic of PA. The structural and functional mimicry of biologically active lipids by lipid A may account for the diverse range of cellular responses ascribed to this pathophysiologically important substance. It is important to note that lipid A resembles a number of other putative lipid mediators in addition to PA, including glycosylated phosphatidylinositol (PI), particularly species of the latter containing acylated myo-inositol (cf. Fig. 1). Energy-minimized three-dimensional representations of lipid A demonstrate how it may mimic both saturated PA molecules and myristoyl-containing glycosylated PI (Fig. 1). The forward portion of the lipid A molecule containing one glucosamine ring with a phosphate and a myristoyl/beta-hydroxy-myristoyl linkage demonstrates the similar orientation of the carbonyl oxygen atoms to the phosphate oxygen atoms (49). The mirror-image orientation of the glycosylated PI molecule to lipid A shows a similar orientation of glucosamine nitrogens and the terminal nonglucosaminyl acyl chain of the

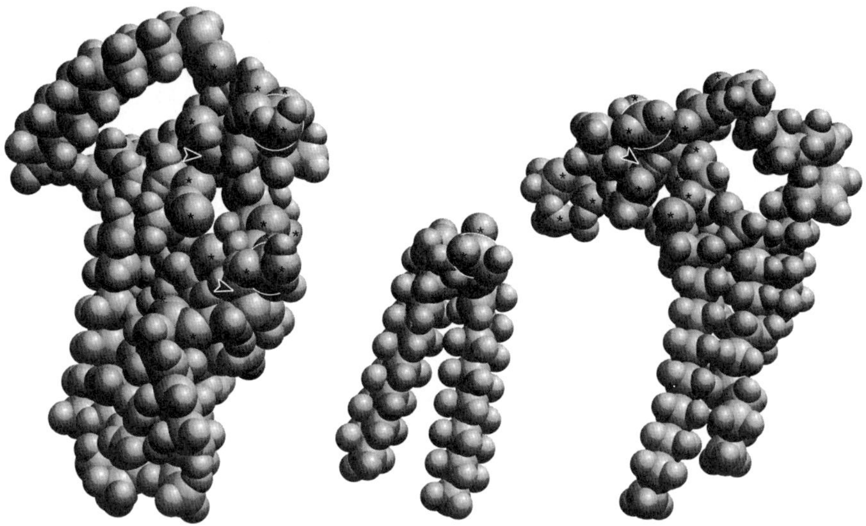

Figure 1   Comparative space-filling structures of diphosphoryl lipid A molecule from *S. minnesota* R595, phosphatidic acid (PA: dimyristoyl), and glycosylated phosphatidylinositol (ethanolaminephosphatidylmannosityl glucosaminyl acyl PI, dimyristoyl: glycosyl PI). Space-filling structures are energy minimized, and oriented so that similar structures within PA and glycosyl PI may correspond to areas within diphosphoryl lipid A. (Glycosyl PI appears in mirror image relative to lipid A molecule.) Phosphorus atoms are indicated by white circles around gray, oxygen atoms are indicated by stars, and nitrogen atoms are indicated with black arrows. Note similar relationships of charged phosphates to acyl carbonyl groups between lipid A and PA. Also note similarities, not only of charged phosphate:acyl carbonyl relations between glycosyl PI and lipid A, but also similarity in orientation of glycan structures and substituted glucosamine rings between glycosyl PI and lipid A.

lipid A to the glucosamine and 2′-inosityl acyl chain of the glycosylated PI (Fig. 1).

A. Fluorescence and Mass Spectrometric Studies of Lipid A Effects on Glomerular Mesangial Cells

GMC response to lipid A was first studied using uptake of *cis*-parinaric acid (9,11,13,15-*all cis-* octadecatetraesnoic acid: *cis*-PnA) in whole cells. *cis*-PnA is a naturally fluorescent fatty acid which is used as a substrate by acyltransferases and transacylases in isolated microsomal and whole-cell plasma membranes (49,50). As transacylation of the acyl chain results in transference to an environment that is much less polar, fluorescence is enhanced. In addition, chain translation motion constraint of *cis*-PnA results in an increase in polarization of fluorescence (Fig. 2A). Incubation of 4 μM *cis*-PnA with glomerular mesangial cell (GMC) microsomes enriched in plasma membranes (19,31,49,51) results in a steady increase in polarization of fluorescence over the first 3–4 min of incubation, followed by stabilization of the rate, reflecting a saturable system (49). Removal of co-factors for CoA ligase or acyltransferases, including Mg^{+2}, coenzyme CoA, or ATP, or heating at 60°C for 30 min, results in abrogation of increase in polarization of fluorescence, reflecting dependence of uptake on an active, enzyme-mediated processes. These processes are stimulated by addition of 100 ng/mL lipid A (Fig. 2B). Under these conditions, the initial velocity of the reaction, as well as the total *cis*-PnA uptake into the membrane, is stimulated. The observation that the initial velocity of the reaction is accelerated by lipid A is reinforced by closer analysis of initial rates of uptake (Fig. 2C), which demonstrates stimulation of *cis*-PnA uptake as early as 5 s after addition of lipid A, and an overall rate increase of >50%.

The target of acylation in the cell membrane was studied using high-performance liquid chromatography (HPLC) separation of lipids extracted from whole GMC incubated with lipid A and *cis*-PnA for 30 s, with fluorescence analysis in series to detect covalently labeled fluorescent (*cis*-PnA-labeled) lipids. The results of this experiment are seen in Fig. 3. The upper tracing shows ultraviolet absorbance, reflecting unsaturated acyl chain mass in lipids. The lower tracing shows relative fluorescence intensity for *cis*-PnA incorporated into lipids, delayed ~1.5 min from the associated peak. Under these conditions, several PA peaks are highly labeled, with little label entering other phospholipid fractions. There is some labeling of 1,2-sn-diacylglycerol fractions with retention times (R_f) around 4–5 min. These were subsequently shown to originate from the *cis*-PnA-labeled PA (19,31,49).

The large PA peak (Fig. 3: R_f 7–11 min) isolated from GMC whole-cell membranes was collected and analyzed by fast atom bombardment mass spectrometry (FAB-MS). FAB-MS negative-ion spectrometry (FAB-NI) verified this peak as PA (31,49: cf. Fig. 5). The peak was shown to have two separable components. The first, which appeared within 5 s of lipid A stimulation and oscillated in concentration during the first 5 min after stimulation, was derived from the activity of lyso-phosphatidate acyltransferase (LPAAT), as suggested from the *cis*-PnA data. This was characterized by masses (FAB-NI M-H/z) in the 695–701 range (also cf. Fig. 5). These LPAAT-derived PA species were shown by radioactive labeling, linked scan (tandem mass spectrometry), and gas–liquid chromatography (GLC) to be highly enriched in linoleate, both in the sn-1 and sn-2 positions (19,31,49). Further verification for the provenance of this PA species was provided by fatty acyl competition experiments, in which incubation with a variety of unsaturated fatty acids, particularly linoleate or linolenate, inhibited both fluorescence uptake and formation of the specific PA,

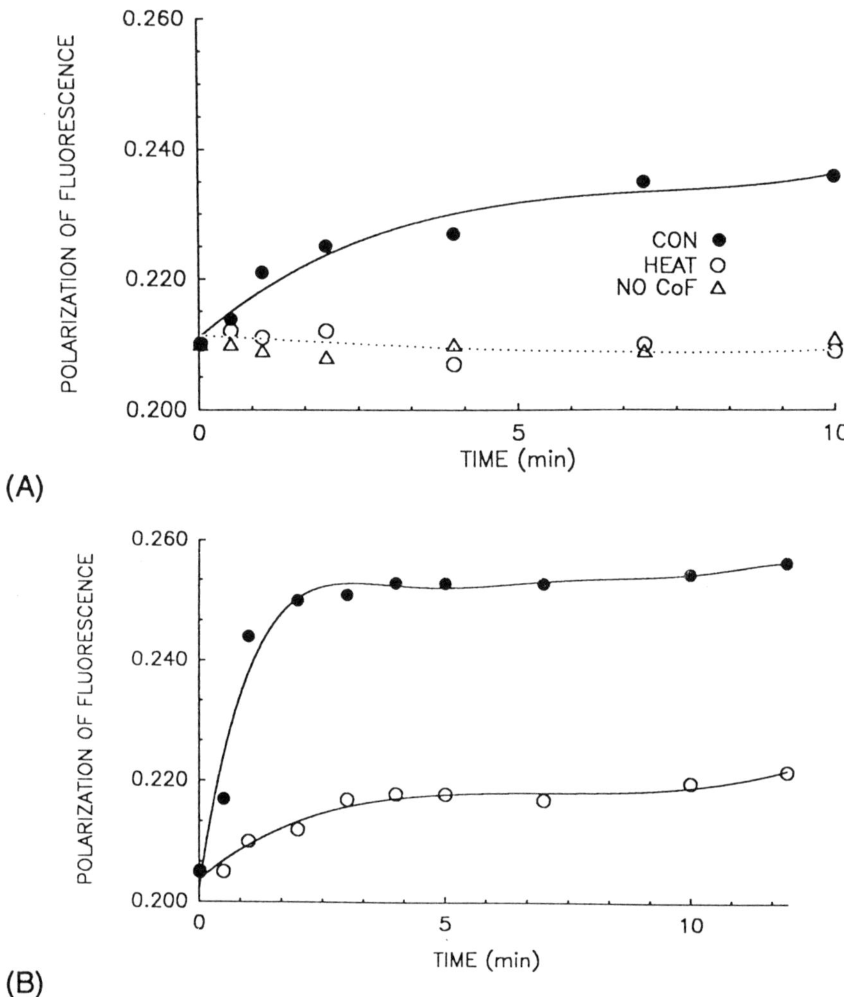

Figure 2 Changes in polarization of fluorescence of *cis*-parinaric acid (*cis*-PnA) in plasma membrane-enriched microsomes from glomerular mesangial cells (GMC). *cis*-PnA (4 μM) was added to 100 μg GMC microsomes in the presence of 5 mM $MgCl_2$, 5 mM ATP, and 0.1 mM coenzyme A (CoA). Polarization of fluorescence was determined as reported (19). Identity of curves are as indicated in part A, and are given below for parts B and C. (A) Time kinetics of *cis*-PnA uptake in GMC microsomes and after removal of co-factors, or after heating at 60°BC for 20–30 min. (B, C) ○, controls; ●, lipid A treated. (B) time kinetics of lipid A-mediated increases in microsomal polarization of fluorescence ranging from 0 to 60 s. (C) early time kinetic analysis of lipid A-mediated changes in polarization of fluorescence ranging from 0 to 60 s. (From ref. 49.)

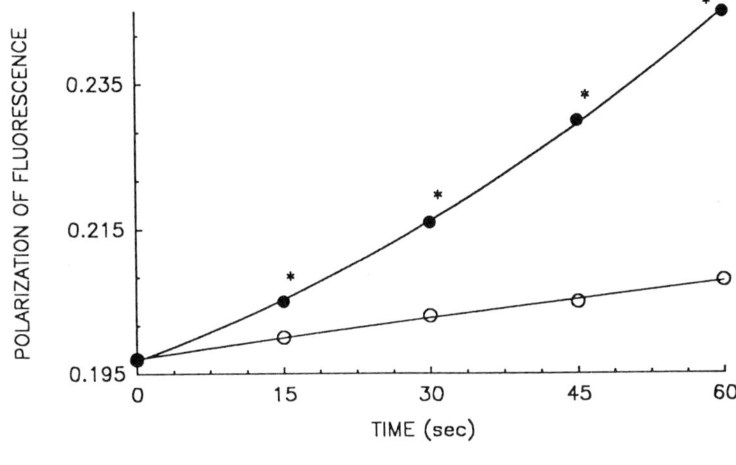

(C)

strongly supporting the observation that these PA species resulted from the activity of LPAAT (order of inhibitory strength: C18:2 ω-6 = C18:3 ω-3 > C20:3 ω-3 = C20:5 ω-3 >> C20:4 (arachidonate) > C18:1 ω-9 (oleate) >>>> palmitate or stearate: 49). The second PA species observed in this peak was synthesized later in GMC membranes after stimulation with lipid A (>60–90 s). It was derived from the activity of a phospholipase D (PLD) directed against phosphatidylethanolamine (PE), and was characterized by masses (FAB-NI M-H/z) in the 705–737 range, enriched in 1-alkyl/alkenyl (sn-1 ether and vinyl ether) species, and had significant C20 and C22 unsaturated species content (52). The provenance of this PA species was verified by the formation of phosphatidylethanol when GMC were stimulated with lipid A in the presence of ethanol (transphosphatidylation: cf. Ref. 52). In summary, lipid A stimulation of GMC resulted in the activation of several mechanisms for the synthesis of PA species, including the enzymes LPAAT and PE-directed PLD, of which the primary response, occurring very rapidly, was activation of LPAAT.

B. Structural Considerations in the Similarity Between Lipid A and Phosphatidic Acid

Lipid X resembles PA in that both are phosphomonoesters and can assume planar conformations facilitating membrane insertion. The respective 2-acyl carbonyl groups bear similar relationships to the charged phosphate groups, and the con-

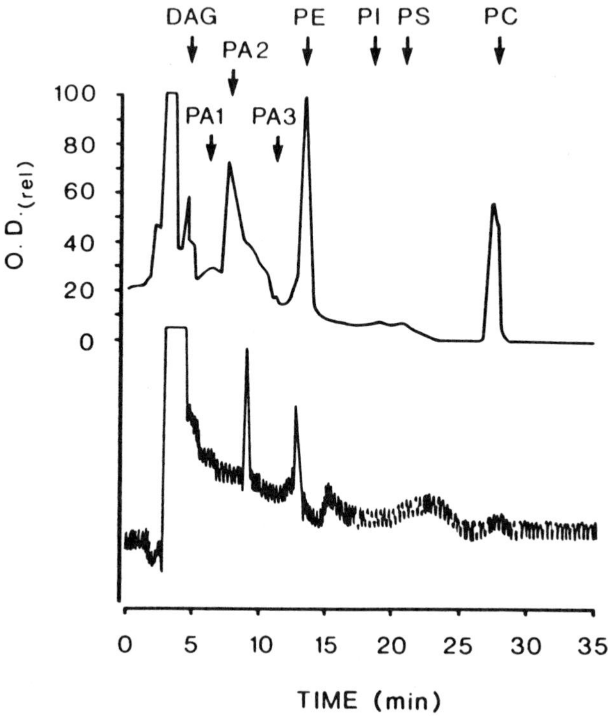

Figure 3 High-pressure liquid chromatography (HPLC) analysis of lipids from GMC microsomes incubated with *cis*-PnA for 30 s in presence of 100 ng/mL lipid A. Upper tracing represents phospholipid mass as measured at 206 nm with elution times of major phospholipid species denoted. Lower tracing shows relative fluorescence due to incorporation of *cis*-PnA. Three discrete PA peaks are denoted PA1-3. 1,2-sn-diacylglycerol is denoted as DAG. Fluorescence was determined in series after detection by ultraviolet optical density of sample, and hence fluorescent peaks are staggered 1.5 min after UV206 OD peaks. (From Ref. 19.)

straints imposed on acyl carbonyl movement would be expected to be similar (cf. Fig. 1, lipid A versus disaturated PA). Lyso-phosphatide acyltransferases demonstrate end-product stimulation (19,31,51,53,54) which is dependent upon incorporation of unsaturated fatty acids into acceptor lyso-phospholipids, and may be the result of membrane fluidity changes affecting acyltransferase activity (31,51,53,54). Specific structural requirements for feedback stimulation of LPAAT are present. Removal of the phosphate moiety from lipid X or from PA congeners results in loss of acyltransferase stimulation (49). Other researchers have reported that structural similarities between lipid A and PA may be responsible for monocyte activation (55,56). In monocytes, metabolic dephosphorylation of lipid A results in loss of biological activity. Nishijima and colleagues (55) have demonstrated that lipid A dephosphorylation is associated with loss of effect on glycerolipid metabolism. These studies suggest that lipid A has a profound effect on membrane metabolism and structure, and can rapidly effect phenotypic changes in cells independent of specific receptor binding or gene induction. The similarities in effects of lipid A and PA on membrane-active enzymes may be explained by phosphate–acyl chain interactions with specific proteins which, in the case of cells such as GMC, are not specific receptor–lipid A interactions (49).

III. PHOSPHATIDIC ACID SIGNALING INDUCED BY INTERLEUKIN-1β (IL-1β)

Studies in GMC had suggested that lipid A mimicry of membrane lipid reorganization and restructuring was related to inflammatory activation of these cells. It was observed that exogenous stimulation of GMC with either lipid A or IL-1β resulted in production of eicosanoids, and stimulated expression, synthesis, and myristylization of IL-1β itself (57,58). The similarities of response between IL-1β and lipid A in these cells prompted us to inquire as to whether a similar initial effect on PA remodeling was present.

A. Fluorescence, Linoleate Labeling, and Mass Spectrometric Studies in Human GMC

Stimulation of human GMC (whole cells or microsomes) with IL-1β in the presence of *cis*-PnA resulted in a pattern of uptake similar to that observed for rat GMC stimulated with lipid A (31). Preincubation of microsomes or whole GMC with anti-IL-1β antibodies, or the monoclonal antibody M-15 directed against the IL-1-type I receptor found on T cells and GMC, resulted in abrogation of this response (31). Analysis of *cis*-PnA fluorescence labeling of human GMC lipids using HPLC and fluorescence detection demonstrated baseline uptake of *cis*-PnA into PA fractions much greater than that into other lipids (Fig. 4A), and significant stimulation in PA mass and *cis*-PnA content in PA within 5 s of IL-1β addition (Fig. 4B). We also observed that *cis*-PnA-labeled 1,2-sn-DG was again increased (cf. DG1,DG2 in Fig. 4B). Rapid time kinetic studies demonstrated that *cis*-PnA was taken up into PA before it entered DG, and that the DG kinase inhibitor R59022 did not prevent formation of labeled PA (31). These studies suggested that IL- 1β stimulation of human GMC resulted in activation of an LPAAT, resulting in synthesis of diunsaturated PA species. IL-1β also activated phosphatidate phosphohydrolase (PAPh), which resulted in synthesis of diunsaturated DG from the PA species. PA species synthesized from DG were not seen after IL-1β stimulation of GMC.

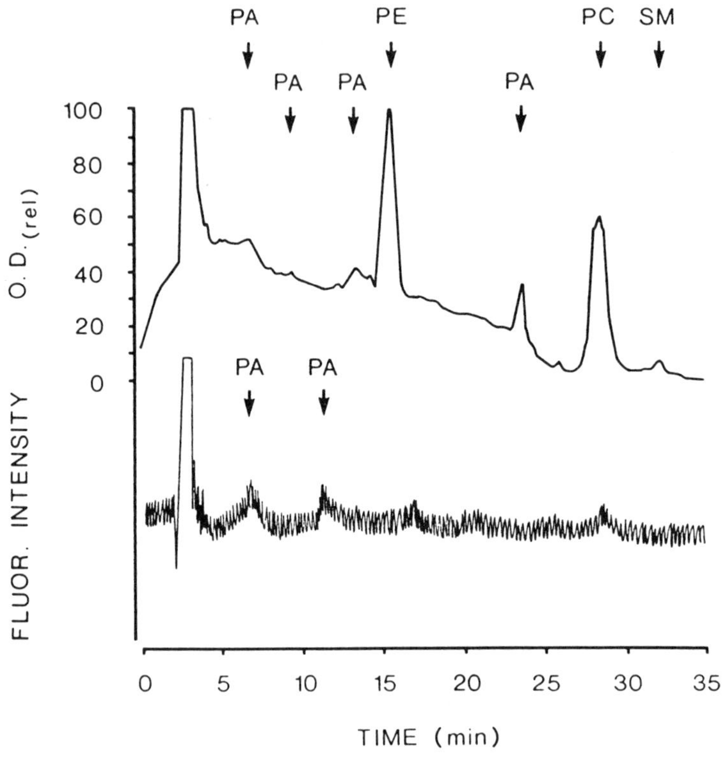

(A)

Figure 4 HPLC analysis of lipids from human GMC incubated with 4 μM *cis*-PnA in the presence or absence of 10^{-10} M IL-1β. 50 nM 1-oleoyl lyso-PA and 50 nM 1-palmitoyl lyso-PA were present. The microsomal phospholipids were extracted and separated by HPLC as detailed in (19,31). The upper tracing represents relative phospholipid mass as measured by OD at 206 nm; the lower tracing represents fluorescence due to incorporation of *cis*-PnA. Labeled PA fractions represent HPLC separation of 1-palmitoyl 2-unsaturated PA species from 1-oleoyl 1-linoleoyl/2-linoleoyl and alkyl 2-unsaturated species. A, HPLC profile of lipids from control HMC microsomes incubated for 5 s with *cis*-PnA; B, HPLC profile of microsomal lipids after treatment with IL-1β, 10^{-10} M, 5 s, with *cis*-PnA. (From Ref. 31.)

Radioactive labeling of both whole human GMC and plasma membrane-enriched microsomes with linolenate (C18:3 ω-3) and linoleoyl CoA (C18:2 ω-6) resulted in selective entry of label into PA which was significantly stimulated by IL-1β (31). This further reinforced the similarity between lipid A and IL-1β-stimulation of GMC LPAAT and PAPh (31,49,51), and the similarity in

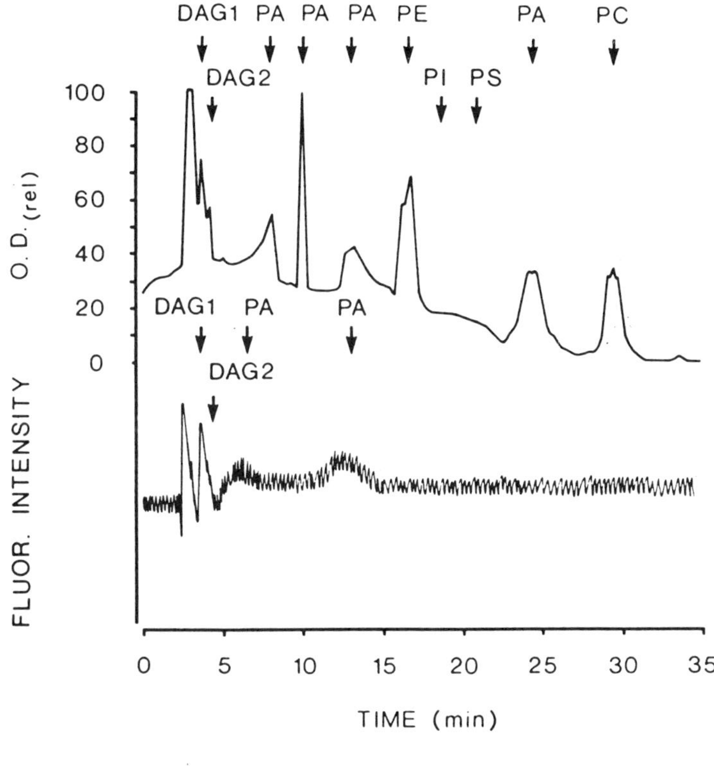

(B)

LPAAT substrate specificity. Gas–liquid chromatography of fractionated PA species revealed that >60% of all acyl side chains were unsaturated. More than 67% of these acyl groups were C18 unsaturated (oleate, linoleate, and linolenate) (31). FAB-NI of this fraction confirmed the PA species acyl content, as seen in Fig. 5. The predominant molecular species observed was 1,2-sn-dilinoleoyl PA (M-H/z 695), with other sn-2 linoleoyl species (e.g., M-H/z 697: 1-oleoyl 2-linoleoyl and 699: 1-stearoyl 2-linoleoyl PA) also well represented.

B. Similarities Between Lipid A and Interleukin-1β Signaling

The data described above suggest significant redundancy in the lipid A and IL-1β signaling pathways. Both phlogogens appear to stimulate activity in LPAAT within 5 s of entering the membrane or binding to an appropriate receptor. This induces an immediate change in the biophysical characteristics of the membrane,

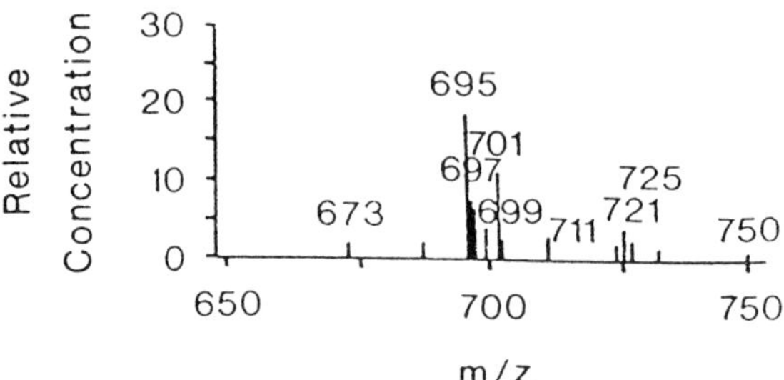

Figure 5 FAB-MS of PA fraction from human GMC. HMC were stimulated with IL-1β as in fig. 4, followed by fixation in cold methanol, lipid extraction in 2:1 chloroform:methanol, and fraction separation by HPLC. HPLC-isolated and repurified fractions were split and analyzed using GLC and FAB-MS as described for Fig. 4. The FAB-NI spectrum shown from 650 to 750 mass units is taken from the combined R_f 9.5–13 min mass peaks shown in Fig. 4B. Major peaks are identified in the text. (From Ref. 31.)

secondary to the presence of significant amounts of the membrane-disrupting acyl chain linoleate (C18:2 ω-6). These membrane alterations are associated with significant changes in enzyme activities, including positive feedback increases in lyso-phosphatide acyltransferases (54). Both phlogogens also increase activity in a pertussis toxin-sensitive PAPh, which converts dilinoleoyl PA to 1,2-sn-dilinoleoyl DG: Blockade of this conversion with pertussis toxin results in inhibition of phenotypic changes induced by both lipid A and IL-1β in cell shape and actin stress fiber formation (31,49). Furthermore, both lipid A and IL-1β, in stimulating dilinoleoyl PA synthesis, cause activation of a PE-directed PLD which results in formation of yet another PA species, enriched in alkyl PA (plasmanate: sn-1 ether) and alkenyl PA (plasmenate: sn-1-vinyl ether) (52,59). These effects are separable from induction of phospholipase A2 and formation of extracellular lyso-PA (59). The internal amplification of PA species induced by IL-1β and lipid A strongly suggest a permissive mechanism in the plasma membrane for the development of acute inflammatory response, similar to that seen in T lymphocytes (54), which requires importation of unsaturated acyl chains into selected membrane fractions within 30 min–1 h after initial stimulation of the cell.

IV.   EFFECT OF LISOFYLLINE (CT-1501R) ON LIPID A SIGNALING AND IN ANIMAL MODELS OF SEPSIS

A.   Lipid Studies in Murine P388 cells

To extend the observations on the lipid effects of lipid A or LPS, we examined lipid intermediates by HPLC, with subsequent FAB-MS analysis of the HPLC-derived lipid fractions, in the murine monoblastic leukemia cell line P388 (34). LPS stimulation of P388 cells induced synthesis of new PA species (Figs. 6B, 6C, Fig. 7A) within 5–15 s after stimulation, with an increase in PA of 250–400% [mean, 325%: Figs. 6B–6D,7A (34)]. These species included significant amounts of linoleoyl-containing plasmenate (1-O-'en-octadece-9,12-dienyl 2-linoleoyl PA: M-H/z 679), plasmanate (1-O-octadecanyl 2-linoleoyl PA: M-H/z 685) and diacyl PA (1-stearoyl/1-oleoyl 2-linoleoyl PA: M-H/z 698–699). Hence, the response in P388 cells was quite similar to that observed in GMC.

In addition, there was simultaneous formation of two separable DG species (Figs. 6B–6D; Fig. 7A), one of which derived from sn-2-arachidonoyl-containing phosphatidylinositol (PI: 1-stearoyl 2-arachidonoyl DG = M-H/z 643, 1-stearoyl 2-eicosatrienoyl (C20:3) DG = M-H/z 645) and the other of which derived from the PA observed above [1-O-'en-octadece-9,12-dienyl 2-linoleoyl DG, M-H/z 599; 1-O-octadecanyl 2-linoleoyl DG, M-H/z 605; 1-stearoyl/1-oleoyl 2-linoleoyl DG, M-H/z 617,619 (34)]. We also observed hydrolysis of N-palmitoyl sphingo-myelin (SM) into N-palmitoyl ceramide, beginning 30–60 s after stimulation with LPS and continuing at all of the times examined to 5 min (34). This argued for a rich and diffuse stimulation of membrane second-messenger metabolism by endotoxin species.

PTX, which inhibits some LPS and TNF-α-mediated activation in certain cell types (cf. Ref. 34) and has antiinflammatory effects in some animal models (60) was shown to be ineffective at inhibiting inflammatory cytokine-mediated disorders in a clinical setting such as regimen-related complications after bone marrow transplantation (61). This may correlate with the inability of PTX to suppress PA and PA-related DG synthesis in P388 cells at clinically achievable concentrations (3–5 μM; Figs. 6B–6D). The synthesis of PA and PA-related DG is suppressed completely in P388 cells only by concentrations of ⩾1 mM PTX (Fig. 6E), with the IC_{90} around 0.9–1 mM [Fig. 7C (34)]. In contrast, the unusual metabolite of PTX produced in the presence of ciprofloxacin, LSF, is 100–800 times more potent than PTX at suppression of the LPS-induced PA and DG synthesis following preincubation with P388 cells, as illustrated in Figs. 6E and 7C, with an IC_{90} of 1–10 μM. This may correlate with clinical benefit in patients treated with ciprofloxacin and PTX (40). Neither PTX nor LSF inhibited PI hydrolysis to DG [Fig. 6 (34)] or SM hydrolysis to ceramide (34). Thus, LSF has a specific effect on a single lipid metabolite, PA, rather than a diffuse membrane effect. The data suggest that LSF acts as a functional inhibitor of LPAAT activation.

When LSF is preincubated for 30 min with P388 cells, it not only suppresses PA and PA-derived DG synthesis as seen previously (summarized in Fig. 7B), but also causes the proportionate accumulation of lyso-PA (Fig. 6F; summarized in Fig. 7B) Lyso-PA accumulation also occurs with LSF treatment of IL-1β-, LPS-, or lipid A-stimulated GMC and human U-937 monoblastic cells. The

Bursten et al.

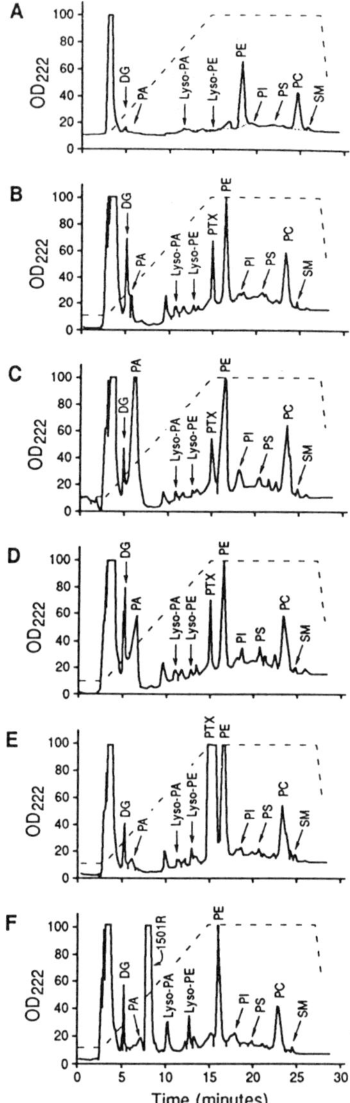

Figure 6 HPLC analysis of changes in mass and composition of cell activation-associated lipids in P388 cells following stimulation with LPS. (A) Unstimulated control cells without LPS, PTX, or LSF. (B–D) Cells incubated with LPS and 10 μM PTX (indistinguishable from cells stimulated with LPS alone) for 5, 15, or 30 s, respectively. (E) Cells stimulated with LPS in the presence of 1 mM PTX for 15 s. (F) Cells stimulated with LPS in the presence of 10 μM LSF for 120 s. No PA activation was found at any surveyed time point from 5 to 300 s when either 1mM PTX or 10 μM LSF was present. (From Ref. 34.)

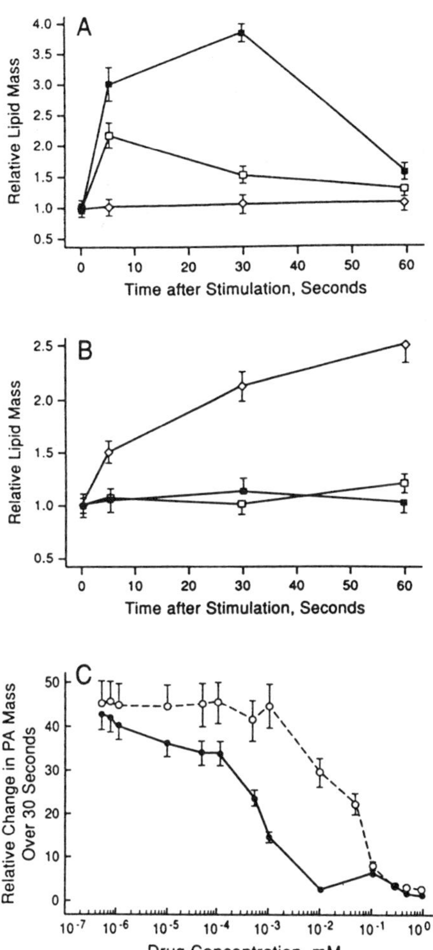

Figure 7   Time course of PA and DG induction in P388 cells following LPS treatment and blocking of the increase by LSF or PTX. Cells were stimulated and treated as described previously, and lipids were extracted for HPLC separation. Mass was determined by evaporative light scattering in series with UV absorption. Estimates of initial PA mass (cells at rest) for the indicated number of cells ran from 250 to 500 pmol. These initial masses were set as 1.0, and the increase in mass following stimulation with LPS is expressed as multiples of this mass. (A) P388 cells were treated with LPS for various times, fixed, and analyzed by HPLC. Shown are mass levels of PA (■), DG (□), and lyso-PA (◇) as measured by HPLC. (B) P388 cells were treated with LPS as in A, but with the addition of 10 μM LSF added 1 h prior to LPS stimulation. (C) Dose response of the inhibition of PA generation in P388 cells measured at 30 s following LPS treatment, in the presence of PTX (○) or LSF (●). (From Ref. 34.)

lyso-PA species observed are consistent with the PA species observed in the absence of LSF [e.g., 1-stearoyl and 1-O-octadecanyl and octadece-9-enyl lyso-PA species (34,62)]. LSF is a weak inhibitor of cAMP phosphodiesterase (PDE) activity, with an IC_{50} in ex-vivo or cellular assays in RAW 264.7 cells ranging from 300 μM to 1 mM. Therefore, any observed clinical effects at concentrations under 100 μM are unlikely to result from inhibition of PDE. We have concluded that LSF activities result from its effects on LPAAT activation.

B. Effects of Lisofylline on Mice in *S. abortus* LPS Models

If the PA derived from lyso-PA is an important intracellular activating molecule or amplification factor for LPS- or IL-1β-induced cellular activation, then inhibitors of PA formation may protect against endotoxic shock or SIRS. Moreover, a more active inhibitor of PA formation (LSF) should demonstrate greater in-vivo activity than a less active inhibitor (PTX). To test these hypotheses, BALB/c mice were treated with an approximate LD_{100} dose of *S. abortus* endotoxin and mortality was measured at 72 h. Mice were treated with either LSF or PTX at 100 μg/g intraperitoneally three times a day for 3 days beginning either immediately (0 h) or 2 or 4 h after administration of the endotoxin. PTX and LSF have similar pharmacokinetic profiles at these doses in mice. For instance, for a dose of 100 μg/g, the peak plasma concentrations were 65.7 and 77.6 μg/mL, half-lives were 0.067 and 0.103 h, and area-under-the-curve values were 9.23 and 11.6 μg·h/mL for LSF and PTX, respectively (34). The survival data from 10 independent experiments are summarized in Fig. 8A. LSF conferred significant protection when administered up to 4 h after LPS. Survival was 68% when LSF was given simultaneously, 55% when LSF was started after 2 h, and 37% when LSF was started after 4 h, compared with 3% for the LPS-treated mice not given LSF ($p < 10^{-4}$, 10^{-4}, and 10^{-3} for 0, 2 h, and 4 h, respectively; two-tailed Fisher's exact test). In contrast to LSF, PTX was unable to protect mice when administered beginning 4 h after LPS ($p < 10^{-3}$ compared with LSF; $p = 0.318$ compared with control).

To determine whether the observed protective effects of LSF resulted from secondary inhibition of proinflammatory cytokines, levels of TNF-α were measured in the plasma of mice after LPS administration. TNF-α levels peaked at 1 h (Fig. 8B) and gradually declined for the next 5 h. Treatment of the mice with LSF or PTX equivalently decreased TNF-α at all time points measured. Peak levels of TNF-α were decreased approximately 2.5- and 2.6-fold in the LSF- and the PTX-treated mice, respectively. Thus, even though PTX reduced circulating levels of TNF-α to an equivalent degree compared to LSF, it failed to protect against death when administered starting 4 h after LPS. These data suggest that inhibition of TNF-α is not the sole determinant of outcome in sepsis,

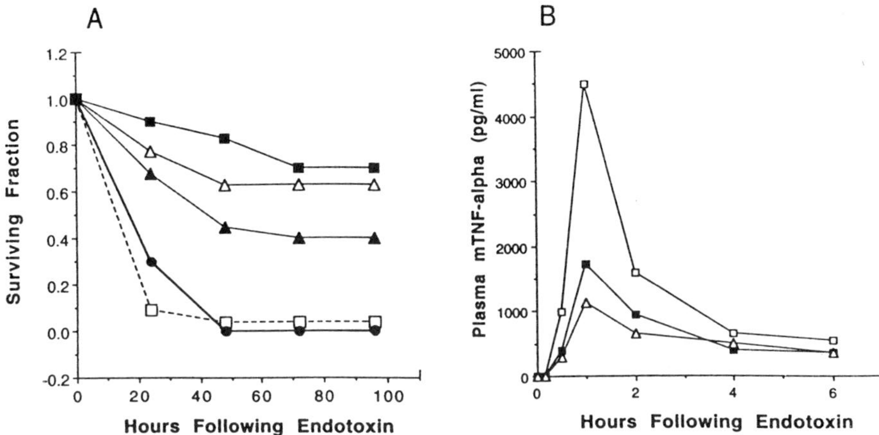

Figure 8 (A) Inhibition of LPS-induced lethality in mice by LSF. Shown is a cumulative percent survival of mice from up to 10 independent experiments. Mice were treated with LPS (10 μg/g, i.v.) (□). Mice received their first treatment of LSF immediately following the LPS (■) or 2 h (△) or 4 hr (▲) later. The mice were treated with LSF three times per day thereafter and survival was monitored. Also shown are data for mice treated with PTX 4 h after LPS (●); these mice were treated like the LSF-treated mice with the substitution of PTX for LSF. LPS only, n = 10/ 105 mice; t = 0 h, n = 7/65 mice; t = 2 h, n = 3/20 mice; t = 4 h, n = 4/35 mice; PTX, n = 2/20 mice (where n is the number of experiments and t is the time of drug administration following endotoxin in hours). (B) Plasma levels of TNF-α in mice treated with LPS only (□) or LPS plus either LSF (■) or PTX (△). The drugs were given as a single i.p. injection (100 μg/g) immediately following injection of the LPS. (From Ref. 34.)

particularly if initiation of therapy is significantly delayed. It can be argued that delayed onset of intervention is more relevant to the clinical situation in humans than is simultaneous or prophylactic administration of a cytokine inhibitor. In fact, using the same model system, but an approach that targets only a single cytokine, others have observed 20% survival of mice given a TNF-α receptor-IgG chimeric molecule 1 h after a lethal dose of LPS, but 0% survival when administration was delayed for 2 h (27).

V. EFFECT OF LISOFYLLINE ON EX-VIVO INDUCTION OF CYTOKINES BY LPS, TNF-α, AND IL-1β

The efficacy of LSF in blocking induction of cytokines relevant to SIRS was measured in an ex-vivo human whole-blood assay (63). In addition, other exogenous microbial inflammatory mediators such as zymosan and *S. aureus*-derived protein A were also examined. Release of TNF-α in whole blood was measured after stimulation with varying levels of *S. abortus equi* LPS, LPS, 0113 (smooth), LPS R595 (Re: rough), lipid A R595 (monophosphoryl), lipid A K12 (diphosphoryl), zymosan A, or protein A in the absence and presence of LSF. Preincubation or simultaneous incubation of 200 μM LSF inhibited 66% of TNF-α release, with IC_{50} noted at 100 μM. The magnitude of the inhibitory effect was nearly constant across the concentration range of the stimuli despite large differences in magnitude of TNF-α induction (63). At 50 μM, LSF inhibited release of TNF-α by 21% with 0113, 21% with LPS R595, 40% with *S. abortus equi*, 28% with zymosan, 34% with protein A, 32% with lipid A K12 (diphosphoryl), and 31% with lipid A R595 (monophosphoryl).

As IL-1β is implicated as a synergistic cytokine with LPS in SIRS, and has a parallel PA-producing mechanism, IL-1β release from whole blood induced by LPS and related compounds was measured 6 h following stimulation with *S. abortus equi* LPS, *E. coli* O113 LPS, protein A, or zymosan A [Fig. 9 (64)]. As shown in the figure, LSF inhibited IL-1β release with all stimuli and at all concentrations (Figs. 9A,9B). The effect was generally constant both at low and high concentrations of stimulus, even when large amounts of IL-1β were released. Figures 9C and 9D show the dose–effect curves of LSF on IL-1β release in whole blood stimulated with LPS, zymosan, or protein A. At 200 μM, LSF blocked 37–75% of the maximal IL-1β released by each of the stimuli. Inhibition was greatest for LPS, which was a less potent inducer of IL-1β than zymosan or protein A. LSF inhibited 75% of IL-1β stimulated by *S. abortus equi* (251 to 62 pg/mL), 60% of that stimulated by *E. coli* O113 (184 to 73 pg/mL), 42% for zymosan (392 to 227 pg/mL), and 37% for protein A (502 to 317 pg/mL).

IL-1 itself induces expression of TNF-α in monocytes and macrophages (14,15). Whole blood was stimulated with various concentrations of either IL-1α or IL-1β, and assayed for TNF-α by enzyme-linked immunosorbent assay (ELISA) 6 h later (63). As shown in Fig. 10A, LSF completely inhibited IL-1-induced TNF-α release at all concentrations of IL-1α or β tested. As IL-1 potentiates the lethal and hypothermic effects of TNF-α in mice, and shock and organ failure in rabbits (14,15), we also tested the effects of LSF on stimulation of IL-1β or TNF-α release in whole blood by combined TNF-α and IL-1α (63). Stimulation of whole blood with the two cytokines together induced a moderate increase in IL-1β (Fig. 10B). Treatment with 200 μM LSF inhibited release of IL-1β at all levels of stimulation with TNF-α and hIL-1α. LSF inhibited IL-1β release by 60% at 100 ng/mL TNFα and IL-1α, and 40% at 400 ng/mL. Thus LSF inhibited the synergistic response to stimulation of IL-1 by the two cytokines. Stimulation of whole blood with TNFα and IL-1α together also induced significant release of hTNF-α (Fig. 10C). Addition of LSF at 200 μM significantly attenuated the release of hTNF-α by 89% at 50 ng/mL stimulus and 63% at 400 ng/mL (Fig. 10C). Hence, LSF was shown capable of inhibiting synergistic and/

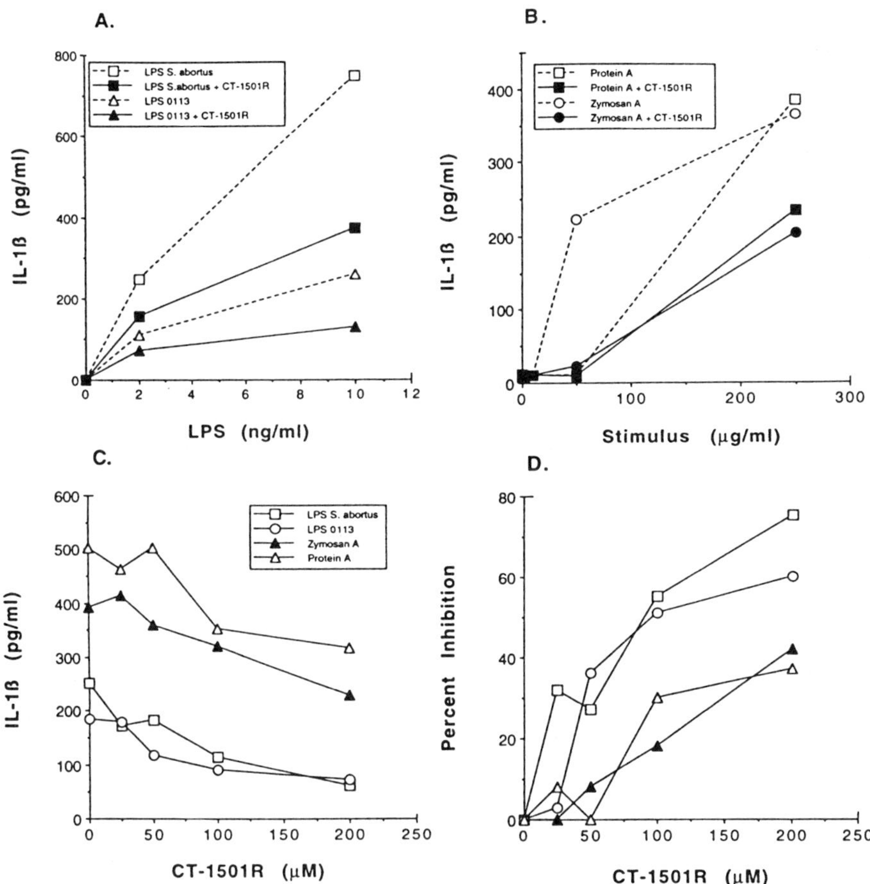

Figure 9 (A) IL-1β release by stimulation of human whole blood with either LPS derived from *S. abortus equi* or *E. coli*-derived 0113 and the effect of addition of 200 μM LSF. Drug was added 1 h prior to addition of LPS and IL-1β measured by ELISA at 6 h. (B) IL-1β release by stimulation of human whole blood by protein A or zymosan and the effect of 200 μM LSF. (C) Dose response of LSF for IL-1β release in the human whole blood ex-vivo assay in response to various stimuli. Cells were treated with either zymosan (25 μg/mL), *S. aureus*-derived protein A (25 μg/mL), *E. coli* 0113 LPS (smooth; 10 ng/mL), or *S. abortus equi* LPS (10 ng/mL). LSF was added to the blood 1 h prior to addition of the stimuli and monokine levels assayed by ELISA 6 h following addition of stimulus. (D) Shows the data from C plotted as the percent inhibition. (From Ref. 63.)

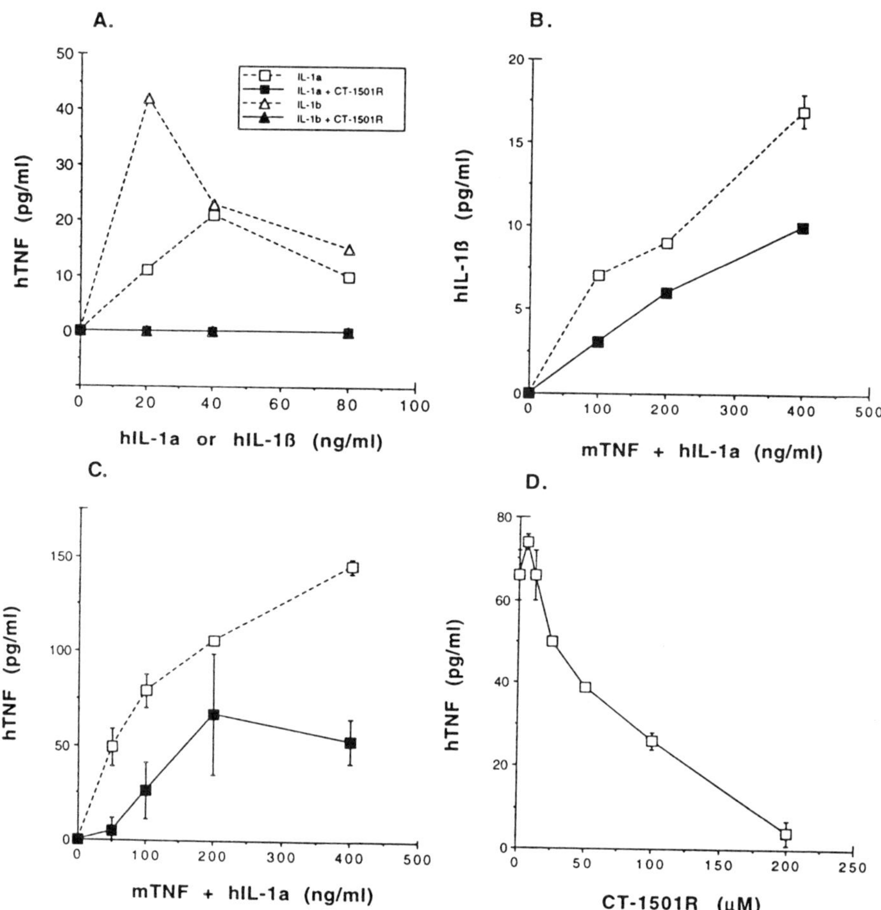

Figure 10 (A) induction of TNF-α release in whole blood by treatment with either IL-1α or IL-1β and the inhibition of TNF-α release by LSF. Human whole blood was stimulated with various concentrations of IL-1α or IL-1β for 6 h with or without 200 µM LSF. Supernatants were collected and assayed for TNF-α by ELISA. (B) stimulation of hIL-1β release from the whole-blood ex-vivo assay induced with mTNFα and IL-1α. Blood was incubated for 24 h with equal concentrations of mTNF-α and hIL-1α together. Blood was incubated for 24 h with equal concentrations of TNF-α and hIL-1α with (■) or without (□) the addition of 200 µM LSF 1 h prior to addition of the stimuli. (C) stimulation of hTNF-α release by induction with TNF-α and hIL-1α with (■) or without (□) the addition of 200 µM LSF. (D) dose response of LSF with a synergistic combination of mTNF-α and hIL-1α in the human whole-blood ex-vivo assay. Blood was stimulated for 24 h with 100 ng/mL mTNF-α and 100 ng/mL hIL-1α with or without the addition of various concentrations of LSF added 1 h prior to the monokines. At these concentrations, stimulation with either TNF-α or hIL-1α alone did not give any detectable released hTNF-α. Supernatants were collected and assayed by ELISA for hTNF-α. (From Ref. 63.)

or amplificatory cytokine induction; this also further supports the possibility that phosphatidic acid serves as a shared amplificatory signal in inflammation.

An LSF dose response for inhibition of TNF-α-and IL-1β-stimulated hTNF-α release was determined (Fig. 10D). For these experiments the concentrations of TNF and IL-1 were kept constant at 100 ng/mL. At this concentration, neither TNF-α nor hIL-1α alone induced any detectable hTNF-α release. Thus, TNF-α and IL-1α were acting in a synergistic manner to induce hTNF-α. LSF at 200 μM blocked 94% of this response, and 50 μM inhibited 40% (Fig. 10D). LSF was thus observed to have very potent blocking effects on both LPS-induced release of cytokines, and synergistic release of monokines in response to each other. Thus, LSF had a tendency to damp the entire multiplicative and redundant response to endotoxin, which has been implicated as the major factor contributing to sepsis and SIRS (1–15).

IL-8 is a chemokine involved primarily in neutrophil chemotaxis and activation, and is released by blood monocytes following stimulation by LPS or lipid A, TNF-α, or IL-1 (23). IL-8 levels are markedly increased in endotoxemia, and therefore this monokine likely plays an important role in the neutrophil response to infection. IL-8 may also be involved in the neutrophil-associated pathological changes associated with sepsis (23). *S. abortus equi*, *E. coli* 0113, zymosan, and protein A stimulation induced large amounts of IL-8 in the ex-vivo assay, with maximal levels of 5600–5800 pg/mL with zymosan or protein A stimulation (Figs. 11A and 11B). In contrast to LSF's inhibitory effects on TNF-α, and IL-1β release, IL-8 release was not appreciably inhibited even at 200 μM LSF, suggesting that its induction is controlled by a separate signaling pathway. In addition to the latter observation, LSF had no inhibitory effect on release of IL-1 receptor antagonist, a naturally occurring IL-1 antagonist that binds to both IL-1 type 1 and type 2 receptors with no demonstrable agonistic activity (63). Thus, the signaling pathways that direct release of first-order inflammatory cytokines (e.g., IL-1,TNF) may be separated from those that direct release of negative feedback substances (IL-Ira) or that act to stimulate white blood cell function (IL-8). LSF does not interfere with critical functions that naturally dampen the inflammatory response or that allow response to infectious agents.

Further evidence also exists that parallel and divergent pathways derive from the same receptor. IL-1 is known to stimulate prostaglandin E_2 (PGE$_2$) production in human foreskin fibroblasts through binding to the type I receptor, with subsequent activation of cAMP synthesis (34). IL-1α at concentrations up to 100 pg/mL increases release of PGE$_2$ in a dose-dependent manner (63). Under these conditions, treatment of fibroblasts with 100 nM dexamethasone blocked 94% of released PGE$_2$. In contrast, treating the fibroblasts with LSF at 8, 40, or 200 μM had no appreciable inhibitory effect on IL-1α-induced PGE$_2$ release, nor was there an increase in PGE$_2$ production. Thus, whereas LSF may act to inhibit

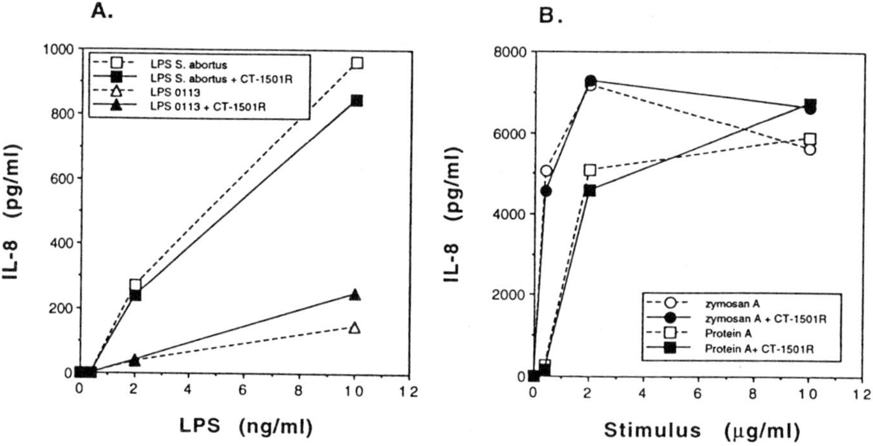

Figure 11   (A) IL-8 release by stimulation of human whole blood with either LPS derived from *S. abortus equi*- or *E. coli*-derived 0113 and the effect of addition of 200 μM LSF. Drug was added 1 h prior to addition of the LPS and IL-8 measured by ELISA at 6 h. (B) IL-8 release by stimulation of human whole blood by protein A or zymosan and the effect of 200 μM LSF. Drug was added 1 h prior to addition of the stimulus and IL-8 assayed 6 h following addition of stimulus by ELISA. (From Ref. 63.)

PA production induced by IL-1, the parallel induction of cAMP production (and subsequent activation of protein kinase A) are clearly not inhibited. It is also possible that, even at 200 μM LSF, the PDE inhibitory effects of the xanthine core are not sufficient to greatly enhance the cAMP effect (i.e., prostaglandin release is neither stimulated nor inhibited).

VI.   THE CONCEPTS OF REDUNDANCY AND OVERLAP IN SIGNALING

It is well known that specific receptors can elicit multiple biological effector functions, depending on the cellular context of expression. For instance, cells can respond to TNF α by entering the cell cycle, differentiating to a new phenotype, elaborating cytokines, undergoing apoptosis, demonstrating chemotaxis, priming for a second stimulus, or remodeling the extracellular matrix. Interestingly, many of these responses are shared by structurally very divergent receptors such as IL-1 type I, or by molecules without receptors in each cell, such as lipid A or LPS. There are therefore likely to be both multiple signal transduction mechanisms to account for such a large number of potential biological responses as well as a significant degree of redundancy in intracellular signal transduction mechansism triggered by structurally unrelated receptors.

A large number of receptor signal transduction mechanisms have been defined that are involved in effecting biological responses. As detailed above, lipid A or LPS stimulation of P388 cells results in hydrolysis of 1-stearoyl 2-arachidonoyl PI to the corresponding diacylglycerol by PI-directed phospholipase C (PLC), synthesis of highly unsaturated PA species by LPAAT, hydrolysis of PA species to DG by PAPh, and hydrolysis of sphingomyelin to ceramide by sphingomyelinase. In GMC and B lymphocytes, evidence exists for subsequent amplificatory stimulation by 1,2-sn-dilinoleoyl PA or lipid A of a PE-directed phospholipase D (31,34,64). There is good evidence that these multiple signal transduction or activating pathways may operate in a divergent manner, i.e., without direct linkage, as demonstrated by the selective blockade by LSF of LPAAT-generated PA and the resultant DG, with correlative blockade of selected biological effects while others are not blocked. Signal transduction pathways may also be convergent and amplifying, as with PA stimulation of phospholipase D. Furthermore, depending on the cell type, there may in fact be more than one pathway to a given biological effect. For example, TNF and fas antigen-induced apoptosis may be mediated by more than a single pathway (64).

Receptors with divergent molecular structures can activate shared second-messenger pathways. For instance, receptors with a seven-transmembrane-spanning domain such as IL-8 can elicit many, though not all, of the same signaling pathways elicited by intrinsic tyrosine kinase-containing receptors such as the platelet-derived growth factor (PDGF) receptor. As an example, both PDGF and IL-8 mobilize intracellular calcium via inositol phosphate breakdown and activate PI-3′-kinase (65). Thus, shared biological responses may result from activation of the same second-messenger or lipid activation pathways by structurally divergent cellular receptors.

PA is apparently one such shared activating molecule which is regulated by several enzymatic pathways, including LPAAT and phospholipases D directed against a variety of phospholipid precursors, particularly the zwitterionic lipids PC and PE, and DG kinase. As shown here and elsewhere, PA is a remarkably pleiotropic and redundant lipid activating molecule, induced by a number of divergent inflammatory stimuli and/or by a number of structurally unrelated receptors (18,19,31–40,49,51,52). Specific blockade of one form of this PA, occurring following incubation at a particular concentration of LSF, correlates with profound suppression of many but not all effects of LPS and IL-1β, and suggests that PA is indeed a pleiotropic intermediate in the inflammatory response. In addition, that this species of PA contains a particular sn-2-enriched content of linoleate may account for two previous observations: (a) The particular inflammatory potency of the essential fatty acids (linoleate and linolenate) over and above their contribution to synthesis of arachidonate (66); and (b) potentiation of both inflammatory and cytokinetic responses previously observed with linoleate (67). This further argues that structural considerations for phospholipid classes, i.e., type of sn-1 bond (ether versus ester), and saturated versus unsaturated content and number of unsaturated bonds in the sn-1 and sn-2 positions, are relevant considerations in analysis of membrane activity. These structural considerations would appear to apply to the mechanism of action of a number of inflammatory cytokines and mitogenic phlogogens (19,31,49,51,63).

The suppression of amplificatory membrane mechanisms of inflammation as a means of treatment of human disease thus presents itself as both a viable and powerful option. In addition to suppression of a single class of linoleate-enriched PA, suppression of other classes of PA molecules induced by other inflammatory mediators (i.e., IL-2 and myristoyl DG and PA), is proving to be a possible means of treatment (68). It is our contention that efforts to address issues of human inflammatory pathology in future years will center on modulation of membrane activity, as well as on direct suppression of genetic expression.

ACKNOWLEDGMENT

The authors gratefully acknowledge the superb technical contributions of Lisa Grimm, Jody Rosen, Rob Chaney, Tim Michnick, and Tana Wilson. We would also like to acknowledge Jack Singer and Jody Rosen for helpful discussions and critical reading of the manuscript.

REFERENCES

1. Aderem AA, Cohen DS, Wright SD, Cohn ZA. Bacterial lipopolysaccharides prime macrophages for enhanced release of arachidonic acid metabolites. J Exp Med 1986; 164:165–179.

2. Bottoms GD, Johnson MA, Lamar CH, Fessler JF, Turek JJ. Endotoxin-induced eicosanoid production by equine vascular endothelial cells and neutrophils. Circ Shock 1985; 15:155–162.

3. Harlan JM, Harker LA, Reidy MA, Gajdusek CM, Schwartz SM, Striker GE. Lipopolysaccharide-mediated bovine endothelial cell injury in vitro. Lab Invest 1983; 48:269–274.

4. Jakway JP, deFranco AL. Pertussis toxin inhibition of B cell and macrophage responses to bacterial lipopolysaccharide. Science 1986; 234; 743–746.

5. Libby P, Ordovas JM, Akuger KR, Robbins LS, Birinyi LK, Dinarello CA. Endotoxin and tumor necrosis factor induce interleukin 1 gene expression in adult human vascular endothelial cells. Am J Pathol 1986; 124:179–186.

6. Loppnow H, Brade L, Brade H, et al. Induction of human interleukin-1 by bacterial and synthetic lipid A. Eur J Immunol 1986; 16:1263–1267.

7. Morrison DC, Ryan JL. Bacterial endotoxins and host immune responses. Adv Immunol 1979; 28:293–450.

8. Lovett DH, Bursten SL, Gemsa D, Bessler W, Resch K, Ryan JL. Activation of glomerular mesangial cells by gram negative bacterial cell wall components. Am J Pathol 1988; 133:472–484.

9. Lovett DH, Resch K, Gemsa D. Interleukin 1 and the glomerular mesangium. II. Monokine stimulation of mesangial cell prostanoid secretion. Am J Pathol 1987; 129:543–551.

10. Lovett DH, Szamel M, Ryan JL, Sterzel RB, Gemsa D, Resch K. Interleukin 1 and the glomerular mesangium. I. Purification and characterization of a mesangial cell-derived autogrowth factor. J Immunol 1986; 13:3700–3705.

11. Mathison JC, Wolfson E, Ulevitch RJ. Participation of tumor necrosis factor in the mediation of gram negative bacterial lipopolysaccharide-induced injury in rabbits. J Clin Invest 1988; 81:1925–1937.

12. Bone RC, Balk RA, Cerra FB, et al. Definitions for sepsis and organ failure, and guidelines for the use of innovative therapies in sepsis. Chest 1992; 101:1644–1655.

13. Beutler B. Tumor necrosis, cachexia, shock, inflammation: a common mediator. Ann Rev Biochem 1988; 57:505–518.

14. Okusawa S, Gelfand JA, Ikejima T, Connolly RJ, Dinarello CA. Interleukin 1 induces a shock-like state in rabbits. J Clin Invest 1988; 81:1162–1172.

15. Waage A, Espevik T. Interleukin 1 potentiates the lethal effect of tumor necrosis factor-α/cachectin in mice. J Exp Med 1988; 167:1987–1992.

16. Alexander HR, Doherty GM, Buresh CM, Venzon DJ, Norton JA. A recombinant human receptor antagonist to interleukin 1 improves survival after lethal endotoxin in mice. J Exp Med 1991; 173:1029–1032.

17. Dinarello CA, Ikejima T, Warner SJ, et al. Interleukin-1 induces interleukin-1: induction of circulating interleukin 1 in rabbits in vivo and in human mononuclear cells in vitro. J Immunol 1987; 139:1902–1910.

18. Chen T-Y, Lei M-G, Suzuki T, Morrison DC. Lipopolysaccharide receptors and signal transduction pathways in mononuclear phagocytes. Curr Top Microbiol Immunol 1992; 181:169–188.

19. Bursten SL, Harris WE. Rapid activation of phosphatidate phosphohydrolase in mesangial cells by lipid A. Biochemistry 1991; 30:6195–6203.

20. Starnes HF Jr, Pearce MK, Tewari A, Yim JH, Zou J-C, Abrams JS. Anti-IL-6 monoclonal antibodies protect against lethal *Escherichia coli* infection and lethal tumor necrosis factor alpha challenge in mice. J Immunol 1990; 145:4185–4191.

21. Doherty JM, Lange JR, Langstein HN, Alexander HR, Buresh CM, Norton JA. Evidence for IFN-γ as a mediator of the lethality of endotoxin, tumor necrosis factor α. J Immunol 1992; 149:1666–1670.

22. Toth PD. The biological effects of PAF antagonists on endotoxinemia. In: Handley DA, Houlihan WJ, Saunder RN, Tomesch JC, eds. Platelet Activating Factor in Endotoxin and Immune Diseases. New York: Marcel Dekker, 1990:509–608.

23. Van Zee KJ, DeForge LE, Fisher E, et al. IL-8 in septic shock, endotoxinemia, and after IL-1 administration. J Immunol 1991; 146:3478–3482.

24. Schall TS. Biology of the RANTES/SIS cytokine family. Cytokine 1991; 3:165–183.

25. Zhang X, Morrison DC. Pertussis toxin-sensitive factor differentially regulates tumor necrosis factor-α and nitric oxide production in mouse peritoneal macrophages. J Immunol 1993; 150:1011–1018.

26. Myers AK, Robey JW, Price RM. Relationships between tumor necrosis factor, eicosanoids, platelet-activating factor as mediators of endotoxic shock in mice. Br J Pharmacol 1990; 99:499–502.

27. Ashkenazi A, Marsters SA, Capon DJ, et al. Protection against endotoxic shock by a tumor necrosis factor receptor immunoadhesin. Proc Natl Acad Sci USA 1991; 88:10535–10539.

28. Mohler KM, Torrance DS, Smith CA, et al. Soluble tumor necrosis factor (TNF) receptors are effective therapeutic agents in lethal endotoxinemia, and function simultaneously as both TNF carriers and TNF antagonists. J Immunol 1993; 151:1548–1561.

29. Howard M, Muchamuel T, Andrade S, Menon S. Interleukin 10 protects mice from lethal endotoxemia. J Exp Med 1993; 177:1205–1208.

30. Moore KW, O'Garra A, Waal Malefyr R, Vieira P, Mosmann TR. Interleukin 10. Annu Rev Immunol 1990; 11:165–190.

31. Bursten SL, Harris WE, Bomsztyk K, Lovett DH. Interleukin-1 rapidly stimulates lysophosphatidate acyltransferase and phosphatidate phosphohydrolase activities in mesangial cells. J Biol Chem 1991; 266:20732–20743.

32. Bursten SL, Harris WE, Bianco JA, Singer JW. CT-1501R (LSF) inhibits rapid synthesis of specific phosphatidic acid (PA) species following stimulation of tumor necrosis factor (TNF) type I but not type II receptors (abstr). Blood 1993; 82:363a.

33. Hanahan DJ, Kumar R. Platelet activating factor: chemical and biochemical characteristics. Prog Lipid Res 1987; 26:1–28.

34. Rice GC, Brown PA, Nelson RJ, Bianco JA, Singer JW, Bursten SL. Protection from endotoxic shock in mice by pharmacologic inhibition of phosphatidic acid. Proc Natl Acad Sci USA 1994; 91:3857–3861.

35. Nishizuka Y. Intracellular signaling by hydrolysis of phospholipids and activation of protein kinase C. Science 1992; 258:607–611.

36. Jalink K, van Corven EJ, Moolenaar WH. Lyso-phosphatidic acid, but not phosphatidic acid, is a potent Ca^{+2} mobilizing stimulus for fibroblasts. J Biol Chem 1990; 265:12232–12239.

37. van Corven J, van Rijswijk A, Jalink K, van der Bend RL, van Blitterwijk WJ, Moolenaar WH. Mitogenic action of lyso-phosphatidic acid and phosphatidic acid on fibroblasts. Biochem J 1992; 281:163–169.

38. Moolenaar WH, Kruijer W, Tilly BC, Verlaan I, Bierman AJ, deLaat SW. Growth factor-like action of phosphatidic acid. Nature (Lond) 1986; 323:171–173.

39. Tsai M-H, Yu C-L, Wei F-S, Stacey DW. The effect of GTPase activating protein upon ras is inhibited by mitogenically responsive lipids. Science 1989; 243:522–525.

40. Thompson JA, Bianco JA, Benyunes MC, Neubauer MA, Slattery JT, Fefer A.

Phase Ib trial of pentoxifylline and ciprofloxacin in patients treated with interleukin-2 and lymphokine-activated killer cell therapy for metastatic renal carcinoma. Semin Oncol 1993; 20:46–51.

41. Carr C, Morrison DC. Lipopolysaccharide interaction with rabbit erythrocyte membranes. Infect Immun 1984; 43:600–606.

42. Lei M-G, Morrison DC. Specific endotoxic LPS-binding protein on murine splenocytes. I. Detection of LPS-binding sites on splenocytes and splenocyte subpopulations. J Immunol 1988; 141:996–1005.

43. Lei MG, Morrison DC. Specific endotoxic LPS-binding proteins on murine splenocytes. II. Membrane localization and binding characteristics. J Immunol 1988; 141:1006–1011.

44. Schumann RR, Leong SR, Flaggs GW, et al. Structure and function of lipopolysaccharide binding protein. Science 1990; 249:1429–1431.

45. Wright SD, Ramos RA, Tobias PS, Ulevitch RJ, Mathison JC. CD14, a receptor for complexes of LPS and LPS binding protein. Science 1990; 249:1431–1433.

46. Bulawa CE, Raetz CR. The biosynthesis of gram negative endotoxin. Identification and function of UDP-2,3-diacylglucosamine in *Escherichia coli*. J Biol Chem 1984; 259:4846–4851.

47. Ray BL, Painter G, Raetz CR. The biosynthesis of gram negative endotoxin. Formation of lipid A disaccharides from monosaccharide precursors in extracts of *Escherichia coli*. J Biol Chem 1984; 259:4852–4859.

48. Zoeller RA, Wightman PD, Anderson MS, Raetz CRH. Accumulation of lysophosphatidylinositol in RAW 264.7 macrophage tumor cells stimulated by lipid A precursors. J Biol Chem 1987; 262:17212–17219.

49. Bursten SL, Harris WE, Resch K, Lovett DH. Lipid A activation of glomerular mesangial cells: mimicry of the bioactive lipid, phosphatidic acid. Am J Physiol (Cell Physiol) 1992; 262:C328–C338.

50. Harris WE, Stahl WL. Use of the fluorescent probe *cis*-parinaric acid to examine function of acyltransferases. Biochim Biophys Acta 1983; 736:79–91.

51. Lovett DH, Martin M, Bursten SL, Szamel M, Gemsa D, Resch K. Interleukin 1 and the glomerular mesangium. III. IL-1-dependent stimulation of mesangial cell protein kinase activity. Kidney Int 1988; 3:26–35.

52. Harris WE, Bursten SL. Lipid A stimulates phospholipase D activity in rat mesangial cells via a G-protein. Biochem J 1992; 281:675–682.

53. Bursten SL, Stevenson F, Torrano F, Lovett DH. Mesangial cell activation by bacterial endotoxin: induction of rapid cytoskeletal reorganization and gene expression. Am J Pathol 1991; 139:371–382.

54. Szamel M, Resch K. Modulation of enzyme activities in isolated lymphocyte plasma membranes by enzymatic modification of phospholipid fatty acids. J Biol Chem 1981; 256:11618–11623.

55. Nishijima M, Amano F, Akamatsu Y, Akagawa K, Tokunaga T, Raetz CRH. Macrophage activation by monosaccharide precursors of *E. coli* lipid A. Proc Natl Acad Sci USA 1985; 82:282–286.

56. Prpic V, Weiel JE, Somers SD, et al. Effects of bacterial lipopolysaccharide on

the hydrolysis of phosphatidylinositol-4,5-bisphosphate in murine peritoneal macrophages. J Immunol 1987; 239:526–533.

57. Lovett DH, Larsen A. Cell cycle-dependent gene expression of Interleukin 1 by cultured human glomerular mesangial cells. J Clin Invest 1988; 82:115–122.

58. Bursten SL, Locksley RM, Ryan JL, Lovett DH. Acylation of monocyte and glomerular mesangial cell proteins: myristyl acylation of the interleukin 1 precursors. J Clin Invest 1988; 82:1479–1488.

59. Bursten SL, Harris WE. Interleukin-1 stimulates phosphatidic acid-mediated phospholipase D activity in human mesangial cells. Am J Physiol (Cell Physiol) 1994; 266:C1093–C1104.

60. van Leenan D, van der Poll T, Levi M, et al. Pentoxifylline attenuates neutrophil activation in experimental endotoxemia in chimpanzees. J Immunol 1993; 151:2318–2325.

61. Clift RA, Bianco JA, Appelbaum FR, et al. A randomized controlled trial of pentoxifylline for the prevention of regimen-related toxicities in patients undergoing allogeneic marrow transplantation. Blood 1993; 82:2025–2030.

62. Bursten SL, Weeks R, West J, et al. A potential role for phosphatidic acid in mediting the inflammatory responses to TNF-α and IL-1β. Cire Shock. In press.

63. Rice GC, Rosen J, Weeks R, et al. CT-1501R selectively inhibits induced inflammatory monokines in human whole blood ex vivo. Shock 1994; 1:254–266.

64. Wong GHW, Goeddel DV. Apoptosis mediated by fas antigen and p55 tumor necrosis factor receptor is through distinct pathways. Eur Cyto Net 1994; 5:114.

65. Holmes WE, Lee J, Kuang W-J, Rice GC, Wood WI. Structure and functional expression of a human interleukin 8 receptor. Science 1991; 253:1278–1283.

66. Docherty JC, Wilson TW. Indomethacin increases the formation of lipoxygenase products in calcium ionophore-stimulated human neutrophils. Biochem Biophys Res Commun 1987; 148:534–538.

67. Glasgow WC, Eling TE. Epidermal growth factor stimulates linoleic acid metabolism in BALB/c 3T3 fibroblasts. Mol Pharmacol 1990; 38:503–510.

68. Singer JW, Bursten SL, Rice GC, Gordon WP, Bianco JA. Inhibitors of intracellular phosphatidic acid production: novel therapeutics with broad clinical applications. Exp Opin Invest Drugs 1994; 3:631–643.

13

Adenine Nucleotides Prevent Endotoxicity and Can Influence LPS Signal Transduction

Loren C. Denlinger, Philip L. Fisette, Kristen A. Garis, Steven K. Daugherty, Paul J. Bertics, and Richard A. Proctor
University of Wisconsin Medical School
Madison, Wisconsin

I. INTRODUCTION AND MODELS OF LPS SIGNAL TRANSDUCTION

Despite advances in antibiotic and intensive supportive therapy of gram-negative sepsis, there still remains a need for a new therapeutic approach due to unacceptably high mortality rates (1,2). Several novel therapeutic venues focus on lipopolysaccharide (LPS) neutralization, competition of endotoxin receptors with LPS derivatives, and cytokine inhibition. These developments arose from recent advances regarding LPS structure, the relation between LPS structure and bioactivity, and the identification of mediators important to the pathogenesis of septic shock, including tumor necrosis factor-α (TNF-α) and interleukin-1α (IL-1α) (reviewed in ref. 3). In contrast, relatively little is known about the events required for LPS-induced cellular activation, in comparison with the field of growth factor biology. Recently, while defining some of the details of LPS-induced signal transduction in macrophages, we found that adenine nucleotides can modulate the immunotoxic response that follows endotoxin challenge. Research in the area of LPS signaling offers potentially exciting therapeutic opportunities for the development of specific signal transduction inhibitors of LPS-mediated macrophage activation. This review will therefore focus on LPS signal transduction, the influence of adenine nucleotides on these pathways, and the advantages of potential therapeutics directed at inhibiting LPS signal transduction.

As GTP-binding proteins are involved in several signal transduction pathways (4), it was not surprising that studies of the early events in LPS-induced macrophage activation led to our observation that inhibition of a macrophage GTPase, which has the characteristics of a G protein, by a new class of drugs, namely, substituted adenine nucleotides, correlated with a reduction in murine endotoxicity (5). We showed that 2-methylthio-ATP (2-MeS-ATP) and 2-MeS-ADP, but not 2-MeS-AMP, were able to protect mice from endotoxic death (5). These results paralleled a significant reduction in the serum levels of TNF-α at 1 h and IL-1α at 4 h, but not interleukin-6 (IL-6) at 4-h, after the mice were challenged with LPS and treated with 2-MeS-ATP (5). Thus, the reduced mortality probably comes from the selective inhibition of cytokine release, indicating that 2-MeS-ATP acts as an immunomodulator, and not a nonspecific inhibitor, of host responses to LPS.

We have generated two working models of LPS signal transduction based on our in-vitro results and the work of others (Fig. 1). A cellular amplification system involving receptors, G proteins, and kinases is suggested by the observation that minute quantities of LPS induce disease (6,7). Initial binding of LPS to macrophages probably occurs via CD14 (8). LPS is believed to be transferred to CD14 by LPS-binding protein (LBP) found in the serum (8). One molecule of LBP is able to stimulate the formation of multiple LPS-CD14 complexes, hence LBP is a lipotransferase (9).

Several independent studies have characterized cellular effects of LPS on macrophages (Table 1). The tyrosine kinases p56[lyn], p58[hck], and p59[c-fgr] are activated in their association with LPS-CD14 (10). These events seem particularly important for LPS-mediated responses at low concentrations of endotoxin. However, others have documented that high concentrations of LPS can activate macrophages independently of CD14 (11), and that CD14 knockout mice are still susceptible to endotoxic death, although higher challenge doses are required for lethality (12). Treatment of rat type II pneumocytes, which are epithelial cells and therefore probably do not express CD14, with high concentrations of endotoxin results in LPS distribution to several subcellular compartments (13).

After initial LPS association with macrophages, our two models diverge. Model A (Fig. 1) depicts the interaction of CD14 with p56[lyn], p58[hck], and p59[c-fgr] as an event required for transport of low concentrations of LPS to the appropriate subcellular location necessary for potent activation, as suggested by others (8). In support of this idea is the observation that CD14 is a glycosyl-phosphatidyl inositol (GPI)-linked protein with no homology to classic transmembrane receptors (14), but with similarities to GPI-linked transport systems for large molecules via caveolae (15). If this is the case, LPS could be internalized and directed to interact with a GTP-binding protein. This type of interaction is possible given that lipids are known to influence the function of both heterotrimeric and small-molecular-weight G proteins (16,17). Based on our in-vitro results (5,18,19),

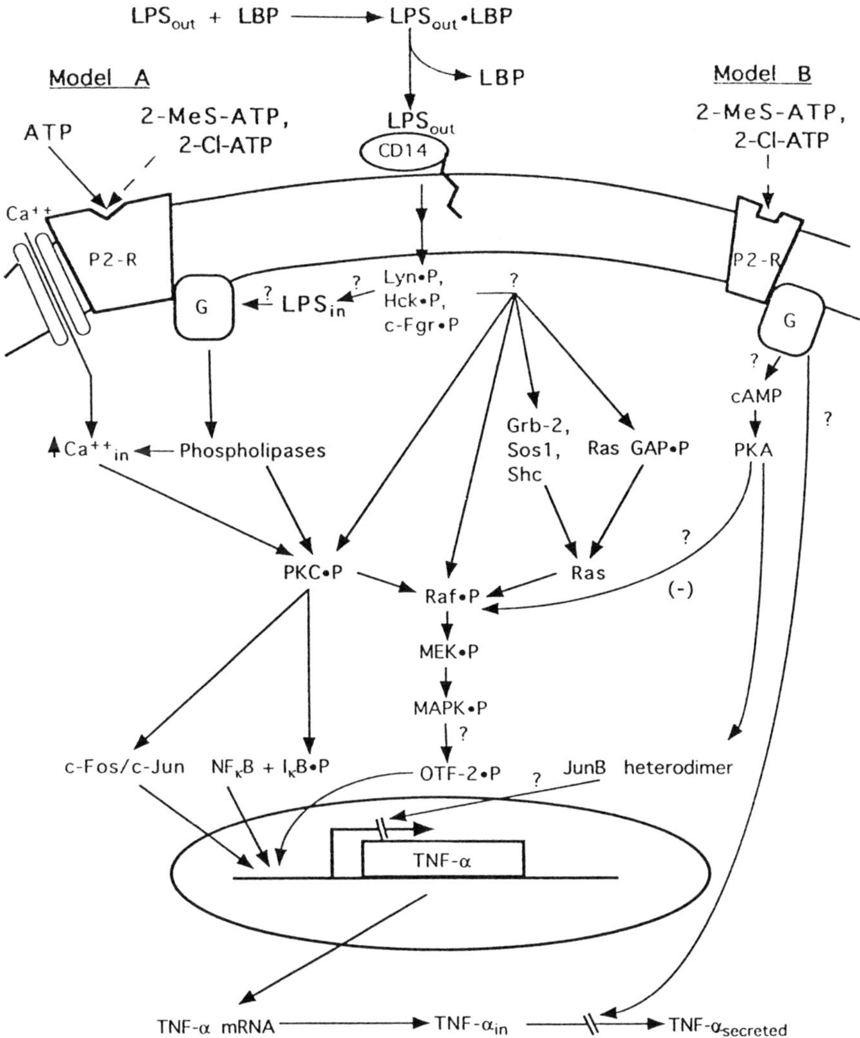

Figure 1 Proposed signaling pathways regulating TNF-α expression and secretion as influenced by LPS and adenine nucleotide derivatives. Model A depicts the potential outcomes of ATP and LPS interactions with the membrane and how the 2-substituted ATP derivatives may compete with ATP. Model B illustrates an alternative pathway through which 2-MeS- and 2-Cl-ATP might influence the regulation of TNF-α production. For details of individual steps, see references in Table 1.

Table 1 Signal Transduction Events Influenced by LPS or ATP Activation

Stimulus	Response	Reference
LPS	• CD14 coimmunoprecipitates with phosphorylated $p56^{lyn}$, $p58^{hck}$, and $59^{c\text{-}fgr}$	10
	• Adenine nucleotide-dependent GTPase activation	5, 18
	• Phospholipase C and phospholipase A2 activation	25, 26
	• Calcium fluxes in platelets are induced by lipid A (This response has been difficult to demonstrate definitively with LPS, probably because LPS can bind a significant amount of Ca^{2+}, which may influence detection).	79, 80
	• Protein kinase C and mitogen-activated protein (MAP) kinase activation	21, 28
	• Phosphorylation of MAD3 ($IF_\kappa B$-like), releasing $NF_\kappa B$	36
	• Activation of OTF-2 in B cells	38
	• Increased JunB transcription	40
ATP	• GTP-dependent phospholipase C, phospholipase A2, or phospholipase D activation	23, 24, 56
	• Calcium release from intracellular stores and influx through pores	57
	• Protein kinase C activation in endothelial cells	20
	• Increased level of c-fos mRNA	63

this LPS-sensitive G protein is postulated to be regulated by a purinoreceptor, hence documented macrophage purinoreceptor effects are also listed in Table 1. Intermediate signaling enzymes activated by either ATP or LPS treatment can cause the stimulation of PKC isoforms (20–26), PKC activation by LPS is probably indirect, as direct activation has been shown only in the presence of very high calcium concentrations (21). The MAP kinase cascade (27) is also activated in LPS-treated cells (28), probably through PKC-mediated phosphorylation of Raf (29). The inhibitory effects of 2-MeS-ATP on LPS-induced signal transduction may be due to its ability to bind purinoreceptors tightly (30), therefore competing with or affecting ATP activation of a purinoreceptor and influencing LPS signal transduction that occurs, at least in part, through a purinoreceptor-linked G protein.

An alternative model (model B) to account for the initial events of LPS-stimulated macrophage activation is shown on the right side of Fig. 1. In this model, the purinoreceptor-liked G protein is not central to LPS signaling. The activation of Lyn, Hck, and c-Fgr by association with CD14 may stimulate PKC and the MAP kinase cascade independently of intermediate phospholipase involvement. The Lyn, Hck, and c-Fgr kinases could activate Raf directly, but it is also possible that Raf activation is through Ras, a small-molecular-weight

G protein that has recently been shown to serve as a membrane anchor for Raf (31). Activation of Ras can occur either through Ras GAP (GTPase-activating protein) regulation or by SH2 interactions with Grb-2, Sos1, and Shc (32,33). Inhibition of LPS signal transduction by 2-MeS-ATP through a purinoreceptor-linked G protein in model B could occur by at least three mechanisms. The effects of this G protein could be directed at the regulatory proteins of Ras and thus affect the MAP kinase cascade. Second, elevated cAMP and PKA activity have been shown to correlate with inhibition of TNF-α transcription (34), so its conceivable that 2-MeS-ATP acts through a purinoreceptor-stimulated adenyl cyclase. Finally, as macrophage purinoreceptors are known to induce calcium fluxes, we cannot eliminate the possibility that 2-MeS-ATP prevents TNF secretion directly.

Because TNF-α is thought to be a central mediator in the sepsis syndrome, the regulation of its production will be discussed. The expression of TNF-α is regulated primarily, but not exclusively, at the transcriptional level. The TNF-α promotor has been identified as a 1.3-kb sequence located between the TNF-β and TNF-α genes (35). This region contains several elements with sequence conservation in the human, mouse, and rabbit genomes, such as an SP1-binding site, an H2TF1/κB site, and two κB/CK-1-related sites, one or two κB-binding sequences (35); other sequence elements may also be involved in species-specific TNF-α expression. NF$_\kappa$B is activated in LPS-treated human THP-1 monocytes and an I$_\kappa$B-like protein, MAD3, is phosphorylated (36), analogous to what has been shown in other cell types where PKC-mediated phosphorylation of I$_\kappa$B allows the release of active NF$_\kappa$B. There is some controversy, however, about the actual role of NF$_\kappa$B in LPS-treated cells. Deletion of the three identified NF$_\kappa$B-binding sites in the human TNF-α promoter ablated NF$_\kappa$B binding in vitro, but did not effect reporter gene expression in LPS-treated murine fibroblasts and monocytes, nor were the isolated NF$_\kappa$B-binding sites sufficient for reporter activity in these cells (37). This result could be due simply to species differences in the transcription factors used for TNF-α initiation, or there could be more than one transcription factor required.

In the murine B lymphoma cell line 70Z/3, LPS treatment activates OTF-2 independent of CD14 expression and of PKC and PKA activities (38). The models in Fig. 1, therefore, suggest that OTF-2 activation might also occur in macrophages via MAP kinases, but this remains to be shown. Leucine zipper heterodimers may also have a regulatory role in LPS signal transduction. The c-Fos/c-Jun heterodimer is induced by PMA stimulation of PKC in macrophages, and the human TNF-α promoter AP-1 site has been reported to be required for TNF reporter construct activity (39). Whether this result mimics LPS treatment is unclear, as the specific PKC isozymes activated by LPS have not been characterized and PMA is known to activate multiple PKC isozymes. Additionally, JunB is activated in LPS-treated murine J774 macrophages via PKA activity

(40), but the influence of JunB on TNF-α expression was not examined in that study. Because elevated cAMP, and therefore PKA activity, has been correlated with an inhibition of TNF-α transcription initiation as mentioned above (34), it is possible that the c-Fos/JunB heterodimer acts as a negative regulatory factor of TNF-α transcription (model B, Fig. 1). This idea is consistent with the finding that JunB expression and JunB heterodimer formation is maximal at times greater than 1 h post-LPS (1μg/mL) stimulation (40) in J774 macrophages, which is the time frame wherein TNF levels in LPS-challenged mice have already peaked and are beginning to fall.

In both models presented, substituted adenine nucleotides may work to protect mice from lethal endotoxemia by influencing LPS signal transduction. This strategy is in contrast to most of the novel therapeutics available, which focus on inhibiting cytokines, neutralizing LPS, or preventing the interaction of LPS with an LPS receptor. Because the field of LPS signal transduction is currently emerging, and because purinoreceptors may modulate LPS action, the remainder of this chapter will review some purinoreceptor biology and the data leading to the model proposed in Fig. 1. We will also compare adenine nucleotide analogs and other LPS signal transduction inhibitors with the more traditional therapeutic modalities directed at the prevention of mortality due to endotoxemia.

II. EXTRACELLULAR ADENINE NUCLEOTIDES AND PURINORECEPTORS

Extracellular adenine nucleotides have been recognized as physiological regulators or hormones since 1929 (reviewed in Ref. 41). Tissues affected by these compounds were thought mainly to be cardiac and nerve. ATP was subsequently identified as a co-transmitter or as a principal neurotransmitter depending on the nerve type (reviewed in Ref. 41). Recently, ATP has been shown to act as a mitogenic growth factor in NIH3T3 cells (42). This effect was shown to be synergistically enhanced by lipids such as lysophosphatidic acid and phosphatidic acid (42), analogous to the synergism we have observed between ATP and LPS in stimulating GTPase activity in vitro.

There are multiple sources for extracellular ATP and its metabolites under normal conditions; e.g., several cell types store ATP in secretory granules for ready release (reviewed in Ref. 43). Depolarizing stimuli can release these granules from nerve terminals, an event that can be quantified in brain slices and synaptosomes. Platelets also store large quantities of ATP in dense granules, such that upon activation by thrombin in vitro, the extracellular concentration of ATP plus ADP reaches approximately 20 μM. The adrenal medulla is another large source of secretory ATP, and the quantities of ATP released far exceed other adrenal gland products during a stress response. ATP is released along with catecholamines from adrenal cells, and incubation of adrenalcortical cells with ATP alone results in the release of cortisol (44), suggesting roles in both the acute and chronic stress responses. The majority of cell types, however, contain only nonsecretory, cytoplasmic ATP which is about 5 mM. Endothelial and smooth muscle cells can release small amounts of ATP from this cytoplasmic pool with no detectable lactate dehydrogenase escape in vitro, suggesting a selecting release of ATP through pores. More significant concentrations of adenine nucleotides are released into the extracellular space during periods of cellular damage. The metabolism of nucleotides in the vasculature is rapid, particularly upon reaching the lung. Several cells and tissues contain ectonucleotidases and nonspecific phosphatases with K_m values for ATP in the high micromolar range. Thus, large amounts of ATP are released from host cells under varying conditions, and the signaling by ATP is limited by extracellular metabolism.

Specific high-affinity purinoreceptors for extracellular ATP, and its phosphohydrolyzed metabolites, have been documented in several cell types and tissues, including pancreatic cells, lung and thyroid epithelial cells, hepatocytes, neurons, cardiovascular tissues, renal tissues, platelets, erythrocytes, and leukocytes (45–47). As the scope of this chapter allows only an abbreviated overview of purinoreceptors with particular emphasis on those found on immune cells, please refer to other excellent reviews for more detailed information (30, 43, 45–47). These receptors have been pharmacologically divided into the P1 class with at least three subclasses (A1, A2, and A3) that bind adenosine > AMP >>> ADP > ATP, and the P2 receptor class with at least five subclasses (P2t, P2u, P2x, P2y, and P2z) that bind ATP > ADP >>> AMP > adenosine. Receptors from all three of the P1 subclasses (48–50), as well as two of the P2 subclasses (P2u and P2y) (51–53) have been cloned and sequenced, with the finding that they all contain significant sequence homology to the family of G protein-linked seven-transmembrane-domain-containing receptors.

Adenosine, the most common P1 receptor ligand, can modulate vasodilation, cardiac contractility, and antiinflammatory effects on leukocytes. [Other P1 receptor effects are reviewed by Stiles (46)]. ATP can stimulate P2 purinoreceptors, and the P2 family can be divided into those that are G-protein dependent and those that activate ion channels. That some P2 receptors activate ion channels is not surprising, as the evolutionary origin of seven-transmembrane-domain receptors is thought to be bacteriorhodopsin, a bacterial pore (54). P2 purinoreceptors associated with channels include the P2x receptor, which is a ligand gated ion channel, and the P2z receptor, which mediates formation of large pores. Pharmacological studies show that the P2x receptor is expressed in the bladder, vas deferens, and several arterial tissues to mediate contraction (43), whereas the P2z receptor can be found on lymphocytes, mast cells, and macrophages affecting DNA synthesis, degranulation, and membrane permeability (43,47).

P2 purinoreceptors that are G-protein dependent include those in the P2y P2t,

P2u, and P2z groups. The P2y class has a wide distribution and can mediate smooth muscle relaxation and/or vasodilation at several sites (47). The P2t receptor is found only on platelets, where ADP binding mediates aggregation while ATP acts an antagonist (47). The P2u receptor is also known as the nucleotide receptor because it binds UTP as well as ATP (45). The P2u class has a wide distribution, including expression in macrophages, neutrophils, and HL60 cells, and it mediates several G protein-linked effects (45). As more purinoreceptors are cloned, their distribution will have to be reexamined by Northern and Western analysis, probably revealing the existence of more than one class on an individual cell. The macrophage, for example, is already known to express A1, A2, P2z, and probably P2u purinoreceptors from individual pharmacological and biochemical studies (55–57). Thus, these observations are consistent with the hypothesis that purinoreceptors are involved in the pathogenesis of endotoxic shock, since they are found on cells in the cardiovascular and immune systems.

Because macrophage activation is fundamental to the endotoxin response and because our previous evidence suggests that LPS interacts in some way with a macrophage purinoreceptor pathway, several purinoreceptor-mediated effects on phagocytic and immune cells are discussed below. Recently, Salmon et al. (55) showed that ligand binding to the A1 class of P1 receptors on either cultured human peripheral blood monocyte-derived macrophages or rheumatoid synovial fluid mononuclear phagocytes caused an induction of the expression of the A2 class of P1 receptors, whereas primary monocytes before in-vitro passage did not express the A2 receptor. Using an antiidiotypic antibody mimicking the A1 receptor ligand and the adenosine analog NECA, which has greater affinity for A2 receptors, Salmon et al. were able to delineate the effects of these two receptors: A1 receptor activation enhanced FcgR1-mediated phagocytosis, while events initiated by the A2 receptor blocked this response (55). Based on differences in affinity for adenosine, they hypothesize that low concentrations of this agonist are proinflammatory, but as the concentration increases in the area of tissue damage, adenosine is then antiinflammatory (55). This contrasts somewhat with the findings of Sullivan et al. (58), where high concentrations of adenosine or some of its derivatives was able to fully reverse the TNF-α-mediated inhibition of directed neutrophil migration to fMLP. Based on a pharmacological analysis, Sullivan et al. (58) suggest that this effect is not mediated through the A1 or A2 receptor classes but possibly via the A3 receptor of the P1 class. Therefore, this apparent discrepancy may be due simply to multiple receptor types with different affinities for adenosine. Another possibility is that TNF-α may prevent migration to fMLP as a signal to promote adherence, phagocytosis, and killing. Reversal of this effect by high concentrations of adenosine could be a way to limit tissue damage by making inflammatory cells less adherent to keep them migrating to other areas of infection. In support of a damage-limiting role for adenosine, Parmely et al. (59) found that adenosine and a related carbocyclic nucleoside derivative reduced the cytotoxicity of culture supernatants from LPS-treated mouse peritoneal macrophages, and the J774 and RAW 264.7 cell lines. This result correlated with a decrease in the steady-state level of TNF-α mRNA in vitro as well as with an increase in survival of mice challenged with a lethal dose of LPS plus D-galactosamine when the mice were also given the carbocyclic derivative (59).

Macrophages, neutrophils, and B cells also express P2 purinoreceptors that bind ATP and effect several intracellular signaling pathways. Early work with J774 macrophages showed that low doses of ATP could elicit calcium mobilization from intracellular stores (via P2u receptors) as well as an influx of extracellular calcium (57). The wave of Ca^{2+} influx was divided into a low threshold response, probably mediated through P2u (the response was elicited by ATP or UTP) receptors, and a high threshold response, probably induced via P2z receptor action (the effect is stimulated only by ATP) (57). Whereas P2u receptors are thought to release calcium via G protein-dependent PI-PLC activity (60), P2z receptor activation can open nonselective pores permeable to ions and small organic molecules ($<$ 950 Da) as well as mediate responses through a GTP-regulated PLD activity that is independent of calcium fluxes (56). The pore-forming activity of P2z receptors is dependent on the physical state of ATP: Tetrabasic ATP (ATP^{-4}) causes rapid pore formation that is reversed by the addition of divalent cations, particularly Mg^{2+}, forming $Mg \cdot ATP^{-2}$ (61). This reversible pore formation can be repeated without damaging the cells (61,62) and can be dissociated from the PLD activity (61). Extracellular calcium was found to be required for a P2u receptor-mediated release of arachadonic acid in dibutyryl cylcic-AMP-differentiated HL60 cells (24). In other systems, arachadonic acid plus calcium activate some isozymes of protein kinase C (22), which can lead to the phosphorylation of Raf and eventual MAP kinase stimulation (29). Although the influence of ATP treatment on transcription of specific genes in macrophages has not been characterized in much detail, ATP stimulation of B cells results in an increase in the steady-state levels of c-fos and c-myc mRNA (63). Because MAP kinases may be phosphorylated in ATP-treated macrophages and because B cells up-regulate gene transcription in response to adenine nucleotides, extracellular ATP is likely to cause induction of specific genes in macrophages as well. Thus, both P1 and P2 purinoreceptors have been found to modulate inflammatory cell function.

III.   THE LPS-STIMULABLE, ADENINE NUCLEOTIDE-DEPENDENT GTPase IN RAW 264.7 MACROPHAGES

The working hypothesis, based on our work and that of others, is that GTP-binding proteins (G proteins) are linked in an important way to LPS signal transduction in macrophages. Evidence from studies using clinical and animal models suggests that a cellular amplification system is needed because minute quantities of endotoxin can elicit toxicity (6,7). In many signal transduction systems, binding of a ligand to a receptor leads to a conformational change in the receptor. This alteration modulates G-protein structure, which allows the G protein to release GDP and bind a molecule of GTP to become active. In fact, both heterotrimeric (e.g., $G\alpha_s$) and small-molecular-weight (e.g., Ras) G proteins bind GTP in their active state and return to the resting state by hydrolyzing the gamma phosphate of GTP via an intrinsic GTPase activity; i.e., GTPase activity is a hallmark of G proteins undergoing activation. In terms of LPS signaling, indirect support for the involvement of G proteins in LPS activation of macrophages has come from studies wherein increased G-protein expression was found to correlate with LPS-induced IL-1 production in U937 cells (64). Moreover, several LPS-induced changes in macrophages (e.g., increased PLC and PLA2 activities, Table 1) are linked to G proteins in other known signal transduction systems (25,26). Therefore, we began to test the hypothesis that a G protein is involved in LPS action using a GTPase assay that measures the release of $^{32}P_i$ into the reaction supernatant as described (18). This approach would be sensitive to G-protein activation regardless of type, which was a necessary concern given that it was unknown which of the dozens of identified (or perhaps undescribed) G proteins may be involved with the endotoxin response.

LPS was found to stimulate GTPase activity in RAW 264.7 macrophage membranes (18). Two types of specificity were sought for this LPS-stimulable GTPase: (a) that it was not due to non-G-protein hydrolysis of GTP, and (b) that it was specific for LPS. Because GTPase activity might come from multiple sources of GTP hydrolysis, including G proteins, nonspecific ATPases, nucleotidases, etc., high levels of ATP (100 μM) and AMPPNP (200 μM) were initially included as inhibitors of non-G-protein enzymes. Under these conditions, LPS was found to cause a two- to threefold increase in macrophage membrane GTPase activity that was evident as early as 1 min into the reaction and that had a low apparent K_m for GTP (18), which is consistent with the timing of LPS signal transduction (65) and with the affinity of G proteins for GTP (see Ref. 18). Several inhibitors of ATPases, including oubain and bafilomycin, were also tested, without any effect on the activation of GTPase activity by LPS (18). Hence, the GTPase activity had many properties consistent with it being attributable to a G protein.

These effects appeared to be LPS-specific because other lipids, such as phosphatidyl serine, phosphatidyl choline, and phosphatidic acid, were unable to cause a similar increase in GTPase activity, nor were they able to block the enhancement by LPS (18). Interestingly, the lipid A substructure, lipid X, which has been shown to protect mice from lethal endotoxemia (66), did not enhance activity by itself, but it was able to block the stimulation by LPS (18). Additional evidence for specificity has been obtained in that the phenol-extracted LPS preparations used are resistant to heat inactivation (3), suggesting that GTPase stimulation is not due to a protein contamination, and that the response can be blocked by polymyxin B (3). Although the standard endotoxin used in our laboratory is a commercially prepared, phenol-extracted LPS from *Escherichia coli* serotype 0111B4, we have also tested several preparations of LPS from different bacteria (generous gifts of Dr. Kuni Takayama), and these endotoxins also activate the macrophage membrane GTPase (Fig. 2). Furthermore, the endotoxin from *Brucella abortus* and *Neisseria meningiditis* are very poor activators, which correlates with their documented endotoxicities (67,68). The dose-response curve to LPS is steep, with a 50% stimulation of GTPase activity at 100 μg/mL and maximal activity at LPS levels greater than or equal to 300 μg/mL (18). These doses of LPS are high, but large doses of ligand are commonly required to stimulate G-protein activity in membranes purified from cells. This effect was apparent in the classic studies by Cassel and Selinger that first de-

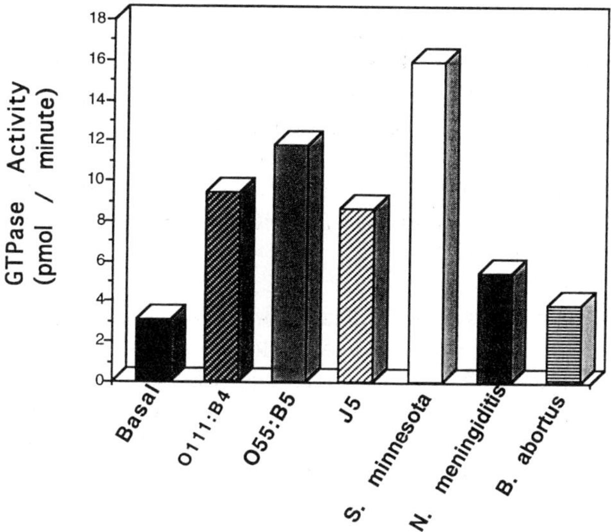

Figure 2 Comparison of GTPase activity induced by different species of LPS. The GTPase activity in RAW 264.7 macrophage membranes was measured as the pmol inorganic phosphate released per minute from (γ-^{32}P) GTP in a 5 min reaction at 30°C. Samples contained 300 μg/mL LPS, 10 μM ATP, 2 μM GTP, 5 mM $MgCl_2$, and 250 mM $(NH_4)_2SO_4$ in 20 mM HEPES pH 7.4. The results are presented as the average activity stimulated by three serotypes of *E. coli* LPS (0111:B4, 055:B5, and J5), *Salmonella minnesota, Neisseria meningiditis,* and *Brucella abortus.* Standard deviations (not shown) were within 5% of the mean.

scribed G-protein linkage to β-adrenergic receptors (69). Using membranes containing β-adrenergic receptors, they found that 1000 times the physiological dose of ligand was required for activation (69), probably due to inefficient receptor–G-protein coupling as a result of disruption of membrane architecture during membrane preparation.

The association between an LPS-stimulable GTPase and a purinoreceptor came from an unexpected observation in experiments performed without ATP and AMPPNP. As mentioned previously, these compounds were included in the GTPase assay to block the activity of nonspecific ATPases that might contribute to apparent GTPase activity. If some of the GTPase activity was due to nonspecific ATPases hydrolyzing GTP, then removal of these inhibitors would be expected to result in an increase in GTP hydrolysis. The exact opposite was observed; i.e., in the absence of adenine nucleotides, LPS was unable to effectively stimulate GTPase activity above baseline levels (5). However, addition of various concentration of ATP or ADP with the LPS resulted in a biphasic dose-dependent activation of GTPase activity, wherein 10 μM ATP or 30 μM ADP was found to be optimal for LPS stimulation (5). At 100 μM ATP or 300 μM ADP, significant declines in LPS stimulation were seen, probably due to the high concentrations of ATP/ADP competing with GTP binding to the G protein (5). Using 10 μM ATP, the increase in LPS stimulation of GTPase activity was three- to sixfold in comparison to the two- to threefold stimulation seen initially with the combination of 100 μM ATP and 100 μM AMPPNP (5). Finally, it was noted that ATP or ADP alone could stimulate the GTPase activity slightly, but that the combination of LPS with ATP or ADP resulted in a synergistic increase in GTPase activity (5).

There are two interpretations of these data. (a) A high-K_m phosphatase or nucleotidase is responsible for GTPase activity that quickly lowers the GTP concentration in the assay below an optimal level required for significant enzyme activity. Stimulation by ATP is due to a nucleotide phosphoryl transferase that replenishes the level of GTP so that more effective levels of GTP (and lower levels of the product inhibitor GDP) are present during the assay, thereby permitting greater apparent GTPase activity. The evidence against this model is that the non- and poorly hydrolyzable adenine nucleotide analogs AMPPNP and ATPγS also synergize with LPS in their stimulation of GTPase activity (5), and that the membrane GTPase has an apparent low K_m for GTP (low micromolar range) (18) whereas phosphatases and/or nucloetidases have higher K_m's (high micro- to millimolar range). (b) A macrophage purinoreceptor–G-protein system is stimulated by LPS and requires the presence of ATP or ADP as the agonist needed for full activity. A well-known analogy to this kind of synergy is the inactivation by cholera toxin of the heterotrimeric G-protein subunit $G\alpha_s$. ADP-ribosylation of this G protein by CT inactivates the GTPase activity, but the modification remains silent until agonist is present to occupy the receptor and turn on the G protein. Without the ability to cleave GTP, modified $G\alpha_s$ is now unable to down-regulate, resulting in continuous stimulation of adenylate cyclase. Whereas LPS probably does not covalently modify the membrane GTPase directly as does CT, our in-vitro results suggest that LPS also does not affect GTPase activity until ATP or ADP is present to act as a signal to stimulate this receptor system. Synergy between extracellular ATP and other lipids for promoting mitogenesis in NIH3T3 cells has been documented (42), suggesting that the interaction of LPS and purinoreceptors may represent a fundamental biological phenomenon.

Dose-response studies with several ATP and adenosine analogs suggest that the LPS-stimulate GTPase is not working through a P1 class of receptor and probably not through P2x, P2t, or P2u. Specifically, adenosine does not stimulate baseline GTPase activity, nor does it synergize with LPS (5). Two P1 receptor antagonists, caffeine and theophylline, do not prevent stimulation by ADP and LPS (5). The analog α-β-CH_2-ATP, which is thought to be selective for P2x receptors, does not stimulate baseline activity, synergize with LPS, or block the effect of ADP and LPS (3). ATP is an antagonist for the P2t receptor, thus eliminating this class from consideration because 10 μM ATP stimulates maximal synergistic GTPase activity, whereas ADP, the preferred ligand for the P2t receptor, requires a concentration of 30 μM for the same effect (5). Finally, UTP stimulates P2u receptors, but it is inactive (like α-β-CH_2-ATP) in the GTPase assay, thus arguing against the involvement of the P2u class in the LPS-stimulable GTPase activity (3). Thus, the purinoreceptor that is associated with the LPS-stimulable GTPase activity has characteristics most like the P2y or P2z classes.

The analog 2-methylthio-ATP had been noted by others to bind very tightly to P2 receptors including P2y (and possibly P2z), yet this ligand only mediates partial stimulation of effects such as G-protein and phospholipase activation (30). A dose response of this analog showed that it alone was capable of a lower biphasic stimulation of GTPase activity, analogous to the behavior of ATP/ADP. Interestingly, 2-MeS-ATP did not cause a synergistic increase in GTPase activity with LPS, as was seen with ATP or ADP (5). Furthermore, 2-MeS-ATP potently inhibited the stimulation of GTPase activity mediated by LPS and ADP (5).

Given this background, correlations between GTPase activity and biological responses to LPS were sought. 2-MeS-ATP treatment lowered LPS-induced TNF-α release from RAW264.7 cells as determined by assaying cytotoxic activity of culture supernatants in the L929 bioassay (19). Extending this to mice, we found that simultaneous administration of LPS and 2-MeS-ATP significantly reduced the amount of serum TNF-α at 1 h and IL-1α at 4 h posttreatment as detected by ELISA; however, IL-6 responses to LPS were not altered (5). Thus, 2-MeS-ATP serves as an immunomodulator, as opposed to a generalized inhibitor of host responses. In performing mortality studies, a single dose (36.6 mg/kg) of 2-MeS-ATP protected 49 of 52 C57B1/6 mice from a dose of *E. coli* O111B4 LPS that killed over 90% of the controls. Subsequent studies have shown that the 2-MeS-ATP can be administered up to 2 h after giving the LPS without compromising the protective effect (3).

Because others have now reported that adenosine derivatives can also be protective against endotoxicity (59,70), we wanted to know whether 2-MeS-ATP or one of its phosphohydrolyzed metabolites was the active species in vitro and in mice. In the LPS-stimulable GTPase assay, 2-MeS-ADP also inhibited GTPase activity induced by ADP and LPS, but 2-MeS-adenosine had no effect (3). If the adenosine derivative was active in vivo, we reasoned that an equimolar dose of 2-MeS-ADP or another metabolite would be equally protective relative to the effects of 2-MeS-ATP. We observed that 2-MeS-ADP protected half of the mice challenged with LPS, 2-MeS-AMP protected none of the LPS-treated animals, and 2-MeS-adenosine again protected only half of the LPS-challenged mice (3,5). These results suggest that both the ATP and the adenosine derivative are active in mice, but that 2-MeS-ATP is most effective, possibly because this compound is able to possibly interact with P2 receptors and remains active through P2 and P1 receptors after hydrolysis to the 2-MeS-ADP or 2-MeS-adenosine derivatives. In this sense, the GTPase assay was predictive only with respect to effects mediated through a putative P2 receptor.

Other adenine nucleotides also have protective efficacy. 2-Choloro-ATP (2-Cl-ATP) potently inhibits the synergistic actions of ADP plus LPS in the GTPase assay (Fig. 3), and it protected 5 of 6 mice from a lethal challenge of endotoxin, whereas the 2-Cl-adenosine derivative interestingly does not do either (no mice were protected, in contrast to the results seen with 2-MeS-adenosine). One drug that has been used clinically in an attempt to lower LPS-stimulated TNF-α levels is pentoxifylline [3,7-dimethyl-1-(5-oxo-hexyl)-xanthine, POF]. Because this drug is a methyl xanthine derivative and is therefore structurally related to adenine nucleotides, we were interested to see if it had any effect on LPS activation of the adenine nucleotide-dependent GTPase activity. POF inhibits the synergistic stimulation of GTPase activity only at high concentrations (Fig. 3), and it does protect mice (71), but only at seizure-threshold doses, again showing correlation, but not causation, between GTPase and biological activity. Finally, ATP was not as effective as 2-MeS-ATP or 2-Cl-ATP in protecting mice from lethal endotoxemia [only 50% of the mice were protected (3)]. Because ATP synergizes with LPS in the GTPase assay and because adenosine derivatives have shown partial protection against endotoxicity, the protection mediated by ATP is probably through metabolism to adenosine. These results suggest that fully protective adenine nucleotides require substitution at the 2-position of the adenine ring, as well as the presence of two or three 5'-phosphates. Because the GTPase assay has been at least partially predictive in vitro of LPS-stimulated effects in vivo,

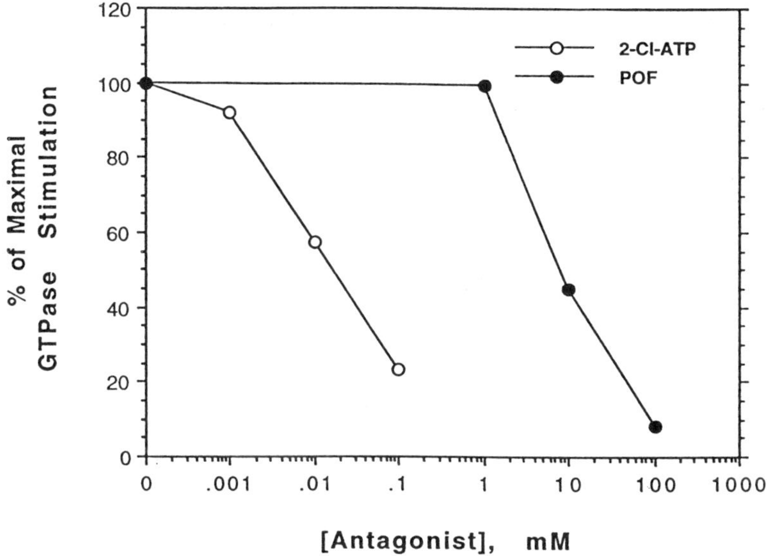

Figure 3 Effect of 2-Cl-ATP and pentoxifylline on GTPASE activity. GTPase
activity was measured as described in Fig. 2, utilizing 300 μg/mL *E. coli* 0111:B4
LPS and 30 μM ADP (open circles) or 10 μM ATP (filled circles). Data are presented
as the percent of maximal LPS/ADP- or LPS/ATP-induced GTPase activity. The range
of results fall within 5% the mean.

we hope to use it to screen other adenine nucleotide derivatives that may be
effective at lower doses in vivo.

In summary, our data strongly suggest that purinoreceptors can influence
LPS action. The LPS-stimulable adenine nucleotide dependent GTPase has been
shown to be stimulated by several LPS preparations from different genera and
species, it has appropriate ligand dose responses for adenine nucleotides, an
apparent low K_m for GTP, and a time course of activity that is consistent with
the effects of LPS signaling on cultured cells (65). Biological correlations between the in-vitro GTPase assay and in-vivo activities of different endotoxins
and of adenine nucleotides suggest, but do not prove, that purinoreceptors may
be active in vivo, and their regulation may facilitate the protection of LPS-
challenged mice. Of interest, inflammation and tissue damage which accompanies most gram-negative bacterial infections, can release large quantities of ATP
from cells (43), thus providing the agonist for the purinoreceptor in the presence
of the co-factor, i.e., LPS, for synergistic activation of the purinoreceptor signal
transduction system in host cells. Because the cellular events necessary for LPS

signaling are yet to be fully identified, we cannot predict whether the actions of macrophage purinoreceptors are central to LPS action as opposed to having a modulatory role on another pathway that can influence LPS action as depicted in Fig. 1. Isolation of the macrophage LPS-stimulable adenine nucleotide GTPase will therefore be a significant step toward understanding the mechanism of the protective effect of 2-MeS-ATP.

IV. COMPARISON OF THERAPEUTIC APPROACHES AND CONCLUSION

Novel therapeutic approaches for gram-negative sepsis can be classified according to four main actions (Table 2): neutralization of endotoxin, competition for endotoxin receptors, inhibition of specific steps in LPS signal transduction, and reduction of inflammatory mediators. Although the therapeutics aimed specifically at mediator release attack the pathophysiological process, directly this approach may be a two-edged sword. For example, therapeutics directed against TNF-α and Il-1α, two cytokines thought to be central to the development of the sepsis syndrome, have already been disappointing. Perhaps removal of too much TNF-α and IL-1α leaves the host immunocompromised. Previous studies have shown that pretreatment of animals with TNF-α or IL-1α can protect them from an otherwise lethal bacterial challenge (72; 73). An advantage shared by therapeutics directed at LPS neutralization, LPS receptor antagonism, and signal transduction inhibition is that they act prior to signal amplification and for this reason could possibly be more potent. One disadvantage of focusing on LPS neutralization or LPS receptor antagonism, however, is that the efficacy of the therapeutics in these categories could be overwhelmed by unusually high concentrations of endotoxin. Another problem with the LPS-neutralization or with LPS-receptor antagonism approaches is that once LPS has been bound to the effector cells, the efficacy of these agents may be compromised. This is certainly the case for many other toxins (e.g., botulinum toxin or pertussis toxin), for which the antitoxin must be given very early or as a vaccine for the therapeutic to be effective. Therapeutics directed at the inhibition of LPS signal transduction, therefore, are unique in that their effects might be relatively independent of the amount of endotoxin and/or inflammatory mediators already present, and they could still be effective even after endotoxin is bound to its receptor or transported into the cell. As more information is learned about the specific steps in LPS signaling, opportunities for the development of new drugs should expand rapidly.

Several therapeutics targeted against LPS signal transduction may already be available: tyrphostins, adenosine derivatives, pentoxifylline, and adenine nucleotides. Inhibition of tyrosine kinases and protection from endotoxic death has recently been shown by the use of tyrphostins (74). These drugs work by mimick-

Table 2 Classification of Novel Gram-Negative Sepsis Therapeutics

Agents that are targeted primarily at:	Reference
LPS neutralization	
• Anti-LPS monoclonal antibodies	81, 82
• Cationic antibacterial proteins including bactericidal/ permeability-increasing protein (BPI)	83, 84
• LBP-BPI chimera	85
• Lysozyme	86
• *Limulus* amebocyte endotoxin-neutralizing proteins	87
• High-density lipoprotein	88
• Polymyxin B	68
• Magainin	89
LPS receptor antagonism	
• Lipid IV A	90
• *Rhodobacter spheroides* lipid A	91
• Lipid X derivatives	92
• Monophosphoryl lipid A and synthetic lipid A derivatives	93
Signal transduction inhibition	
• 2-methylthio-ATP, 2-chloro-ATP	5
• Adenosine derivatives	59, 70
• Pentoxifylline	71
• Tyrphostins	74
Inflammatory mediator prevention	
• Monoclonal antibodies	
Anti-TNF-α	94
Anti-macrophage migration inhibitory factor (MIF)	95
• Soluble TNF-α receptor	96
• TNF-processing inhibitor	97
• Interleukin-1α receptor antagonist	98
• Interleukin-6	99
• Interleukin-10	100
• Tissue factor pathway inhibitor	101
• Platelet-activating factor antagonists	102
• Phosphatidic acid inhibitors	103
• Bradykinin antagonists	104

ing tyrosine, as they are able to irreversibly bind multiple tyrosine kinases at the phosphoanhydride intermediate stage of the phosphoryl transfer reaction (from ATP to tyrosine residues), thus preventing these enzymes from phosphorylating other substrates required in the LPS signaling pathway. A note of caution should be made in that the tyrphostins are not specific for any one particular kinase, and they also have the potential to affect other enzymes requiring a tyrosine phosphoanhydride intermediate, such as topoisomerase, and therefore might be very toxic in humans.

Adenosine derivatives have been shown to have antiinflammatory effects on macrophages and to be somewhat effective in protecting mice from a lethal dose of endotoxin (55,58,59,70). While the effects of adenosine on macrophage P1 receptors may be beneficial, cardiac contractility is depressed and vasodilation is increased when adenosine interacts with cardiac and endothelial P1 receptors. This may be why we and others (70) have not been able to obtain 100% protection with adenosine derivatives in LPS-challenged mice (Firestein et al. show a twofold increase in survival using an adenosine derivative, compared to a ninefold increase with 2-MeS-ATP shown by Proctor et al.).

As mentioned above, pentoxifylline does not seem to work through P2 receptors, but may interact with P1 receptors as well as to inhibit phosphodiesterases directly, resulting in increased intracellular levels of cAMP. This effect has been associated with reduced levels of TNF-α production due to inhibition of transcription initiation, as effects on transcript stability or on the transnational control of TNF have been ruled out (75,76). Because elevated cAMP activates PKA, it is possible that pentoxifylline reduces TNF-α by PKA modulation of an LPS signal transduction pathway or by a PKA-mediated phosphorylation of a transcription factor that serves to block transcript initiation (Fig. 1). However, the high doses of pentoxifylline required for therapeutic responses lead to toxicity, perhaps because this drug is hydrophobic and can pass through the blood–brain barrier to cause seizures.

We have shown that extracellular adenine nucleotides can have a profound effect on endotoxicity, resulting in full protection in mice (5). Our in-vitro results suggest that LPS may interact with a P2 purinoreceptor–G-protein system for cellular signaling. Inhibition could occur at several levels, including the prevention of a signal en route to TNF-α transcription or by a blockade of TNF-α secretion. An intriguing possibility for 2-MeS-ATP arises from its weak agonist stimulation of GTPase activity, its inability to act synergistically with LPS, yet its tight binding to P2 receptors (30); namely, it may lower the levels of important cytokines by preventing macrophage purinoreceptor signaling by more potent agonists such as ATP or ADP. The specific mechanism may involve competitive inhibition versus other adenine nucleotides at a purinoreceptor, or it may interact with a separate class of receptors that can down-regulate signals from a purinoreceptor occupied with ATP. However, demonstrating that 2-MeS-ATP prevents endotoxicity by interacting with a purinoreceptor will require other approaches, e.g., purification of the relevant components, cloning the putative receptor, and creating a genetic knockout cell line. Regardless of the mechanism, toxicity with this type of compound versus other LPS-targeted therapeutics may be less of a problem, as the only side effect noted has been a reversible potentiation of anesthesia. Additional substituted analogs may be found that are specific for macrophage P2 purinoreceptors and that are less rapidly hydrolyzed, hopefully eliminating possible CNS side effects by making them more slowly metabolized (allowing the use of lower doses), and by preventing transmission across the blood–brain barrier.

ATP and UTP have already been used clinically to modulate ion secretion in the lungs of cystic fibrosis patients via putative P2u receptors (77). In experimental models of shock and organ ischemia, ATP has been documented to improve blood flow in the microvasculature, tissue ATP concentrations, cellular functioning, and survival in animals (78), but it is unclear whether this is due to purinoreceptor effects or to a supplementation of the depleted intracellular energy stores found in ischemic tissues. If this is the case, a substituted analog may have a protective effect by reducing the amount of inflammatory cytokines, as well as improving tissue perfusion.

The recent advances in endotoxin research have led to the development of a variety of novel therapeutic approaches which are aimed at reducing the mortality of gram-negative sepsis. A rapidly expanding area of research is the attempt to alter LPS-induced signal transduction in macrophages. The goal is to find specific, nontoxic, small compounds (which might be easily and inexpensively synthesized) that can reduce the release of toxic inflammatory mediators in a way that does not cause immunoparalysis. Adenine nucleotides offer one such possibility. Understanding the mechanism(s) of LPS action and being able to manipulate this system may also have benefits that extend to other clinical situations, such as cerebral malaria or rheumatoid arthritis, where overactive inflammation plays a major role in the disease process.

REFERENCES

1. Hoffman WD, Suffredini AF, Eichacker PQ, Danner RL, Natanson C. Selected treatment strategies for septic shock based on proposed mechanisms of pathogenesis. Ann Intern Med 1994; 120:771–783.
2. Glauser MP, Zanetti G, Baumgartner JD, Cohen J. Septic shock: pathogenesis. Lancet 1991; 338:732–736.
3. Proctor RA, Denlinger LC, Bertics PJ. Lipopolysaccharide and bacterial virulence. In: Minion C, Roth JA, eds. Virulence Mechanisms of Bacterial Pathogens, 2nd ed. American Society for Microbiology. In press.,
4. Bourne HR, Sanders DA, McCormick F. The GTPase superfamily: a conserved switch for diverse cell functions. Nature 1990; 348:125–132.
5. Proctor RA, Denlinger LC, Leventhal PS, et al. Protection of mice from endotoxic death by 2-methylthio-ATP. Proc Natl Acad Sci USA 1994; 91:6017–6020.
6. Casey LC, Balk RA, Bone RC. Plasma cytokine and endotoxin levels correlate with survival in patients with the sepsis syndrome. Ann Intern Med 1993; 119:771–778.
7. Morrison DC, Bucklin S, Leeson M, Fujihara Y. Bacteremia vs endotoxemia in

antibiotic treatment of experimental gram-negative sepsis. Intensive Care Med 1994; 20:20.

8. Ulevitch RJ, Tobias PS. Recognition of endotoxin by cells leading to transmembrane signaling. Curr Opin Immunol 1994; 6:125–130.

9. Hailman E, Lichenstein HS, Wurfel MM, et al. Lipopolysaccharide (LPS)-binding protein accelerates the binding of LPS to CD14. J Exp Med 1994; 179:269–277.

10. Stefanova I, Corcoran ML, Horak EM, Wahl LM, Bolen JB, Horak ID. Lipopolysaccharide induces activation of CD14-associated protein tyrosine kinase p53/561yn. J Biol Chem 1993; 268:20725–20728.

11. Lynn WA, Liu Y, Golenbock DT. Neither CD14 nor serum is absolutely necessary for activation of mononuclear phagocytes by bacterial lipopolysaccharide. Infect Immun 1993; 61:4452–4461.

12. Goyert S. Development of animal models to study mechanisms of endotoxic shock and possible therapeutics. IBC's Fourth Annual Conference on The Shift in R&D Strategies for the Prevention & Treatment of Endotoxemia & Sepsis, Philadelphia, PA, June 13–15, 1994.

13. Risco C, Carrascosa JL, Bosch MA. Uptake and subcellular distribution of *Escherichia coli* lipopolysaccharide by isolated rat type II pneumocytes. J Histochem Cytochem 1991; 39:607–615.

14. Haziot A, Chen S, Ferrero E, Low MG, Silber R, Goyert SM. The monocyte differentiation antigen, CD14, is anchored to the cell membrane by a phosphatidylinositol linkage. J Immunol 1988; 141:547–552.

15. Sargiacomo M, Sudol M, Tang Z, Lisanti MP. Signal transducing molecules and glycosyl-phosphatidylinositol-linked proteins form a caveolin-rich insoluble complex in MDCK cells. J Cell Biol 1993; 122:789–807.

16. Tsai MH, Hall A, Stacey DW. Inhibition by phospholipids of the interaction between R-ras, Rho, and their GTPase-activating proteins. Mol Cell Biol 1989; 9:5260–5264.

17. Wedegaertner PB, Chu DH, Wilson PT, Levis MJ, Bourne HR. Palmitoylation is required for signaling functions and membrane attachment of $G_q\alpha$ and Gsα. J Biol Chem 1993; 268:25001–25008.

18. Tanke T, van de Loo JW, Rhim H, Leventhal PS, Proctor RA, Bertics PJ. Bacterial lipopolysaccharide-stimulated GTPase activity in RAW264.7 macrophage membranes. Biochem J 1991; 277:379–385.

19. Bertics PJ, van de Loo JW, Denlinger L, et al. The purine analog, 2-methylthio-ATP (2-MeS-ATP), protects mice from endotoxin death. In: Levin J, Alving CR, Munford RS, Stutz PL, eds. Bacterial Endotoxins: Recognition and Effector Mechanisms. 1993: 233–241.

20. Purkiss JR, Boarder MR, Stimulation of phosphatidate synthesis in endothelial cells in response to P2-receptor activation. Evidence for phospholipase C and phospholipase D involvement, phosphatidate and diacylglycerol interconversion and the role of protein kinase C. Biochem J 1992; 287:31–36.

21. Wightman PD, Raetz CRH. The activation of protein kinase C by biologically active lipid moieties of lipopolysaccharide. J Biol Chem 1984; 259:10048–10052.

22. Schaechter JD, Benowitz LI, Activation of protein kinase C by arachidonic acid

selectively enhances the phosphorylation of GAP-43 in nerve terminal membranes. J Neurosci 1993; 13:4361–4371.

23. Cockcroft S, Stutchfield J, ATP stimulates secretion in human neutrophils and HL60 cells via a pertussis toxin-sensitive guanine nucleotide-binding protein coupled to phospholipase C. Elsevier Sci Pub B V 1989; 245:25–29.

24. Xing M, Thevenod F, Mattera R. Dual regulation of arachidonic acid release by P_{2U} purinergic receptors in dibutyryl cyclic AMP-differentiated HL60 cells. J Biol Chem 1992; 267:6602–6610.

25. Prpic V., Weiel JE, Somers SD, et al. The effects of bacterial entotoxin on the hydrolysis of phosphatidyl inositol-4,5-biophosphate in murine pentoneal macrophages. J Immunol 1987: 139:526–533.

26. Hatch GM, Vance DE, Wilton DC, Rat liver mitochondrial phospholipase A2 is an endotoxin-stimulated membrane-associated enzyme of Kupffer cells which is released during liver perfusion. Biochem J 1993; 293:143–150.

27. Pelech SL, Sanghera JS. MAP kinases: charting the regulatory pathways. Science 1992; 257:1355–1356.

28. Weinstein SL, Gold MR, DeFranco AL, Bacterial lipopolysaccharide stimulates protein tyrosine phosphorylation in macrophages. Proc Natl Acad Sci USA 1991; 88:4148–4152.

29. Gardner AM, Vaillancourt RR, Johnson GL, Activation of mitogen-activated protein kinase/extracellular signal-regulated kinase by G protein and tyrosine kinase oncoproteins. J Biol Chem 1993; 268:17896–17901.

30. O'Connor SE, Dainty IA, Leff P, Further subclassification of ATP receptors based on agonist studies. Trends Pharmacol Sci 1991; 12:137–141.

31. Stokoe D, Macdonald SG, Cadwallader K, Symons M, Hancock JF. Activation of Raf as a result of recruitment to the plasma membrane. Science 1994; 264:1463–1467.

32. Rozakis-Adcock M, McGlade J, Mbamalu G, et al. Association of the Shc and Grb2/Sem5 SH2-containing proteins is implicated in activation of the Ras pathway by tyrosine kinases. Nature 1992; 360:689–692.

33. Boguski MS, McCormick F. Proteins regulating Ras and its relatives. Nature 1993; 366:643–654.

34. Tannenbaum CS, Hamilton TA, Lipopolysaccharide-induced gene expression in murine peritoneal macrophages is selectively suppressed by agents that elevate intracellular cAMP. J Immunol 1989; 142:1274–1280.

35. Shakhov AN, Kuprash DV, Azizov MM, Jongeneel CV, Nedospasov SA, Structural analysis of the rabbit TNF locus, containing the genes encoding TNF-β (lymphotoxin) and TNF-α (tumor necrosis factor). Gene 1990; 95:215–221.

36. Cordle SR, Donald R, Read M, Hawiger J. Lipopolysaccharide induces phosphorylation of MAD3 and activation of c-Rel and related NF-kappa B proteins in human monocytic THP-1 cells. J Biol Chem 1993; 268:11803–11810.

37. Goldfield AE, Doyle C, Maniatis T. Human tumor necrosis factor α gene regulation by virus and lipopolysaccharide. Proc Natl Acad Sci USA 1990; 87:9769–9773.

38. Rooney JW, Emery DW, Sibley CH, 1.3E2, a variant of the B lymphoma 70Z/3, defective in activation of $NF_{\kappa}B$ and OTF-2. Immunogenetics 1990; 31:73–78.

39. Rhoades KL, Golub SH, Economou JS, The regulation of the human tumor necrosis factor α promoter region in macrophage, T cell, and B cell lines. J Biol Chem 1992; 267:22102–22107.

40. Fujihara M, Masashi J, Muroi Y, Ito N, Suzuki T, Mechanism of lipopolysaccharide-triggered junB activation in a mouse macrophage-like cell line (J774). J Biol Chem 1993; 268:14898–14905.

41. Burnstock G, Kennedy C, Is there a basis for distinguishing two types of P^2-purinoceptor? Gen Pharmacol 1985; 16:433–440.

42. Wang D-J, Huang N-N, Heller EJ, Heppel L. A. A novel synergistic stimulation of Swiss 3T3 cells by extracellular ATP and mitogens with opposite effects of cAMP levels. J Biol Chem 1994; 269:16648–16655.

43. Gordon JL, Extracellular ATP: effects, sources and fate. Biochem J 1986; 233:309–319.

44. Hoey ED, Nicol M, Williams BC, Walker SW, Primary cultures of bovine inner zone adrenocortical cells secrete cortisol in response to adenosine triphosphate, adenosine diphosphate, and uridine triphosphate via a nucleotide receptor which may be coupled to two signal generation systems. Endocrinology 1994; 134:1553–1560.

45. Dubyak GR, Signal transduction by P_2-purinergic receptors for extracellular ATP. Am J Respir Cell Mol Biol 1991; 4:295–300.

46. Stiles GL, Adenosine receptors. J Biol Chem 1992; 267:6451–6454.

47. El-Moatassim C, Dornand J, Mani J-C. Extracellular ATP and cell signalling. Biochim Biophys Acta 1992; 1134:31–45.

48 Olah ME, Ren H, Ostrowski J, Jacobson KA, Stiles GL. Cloning, expression, and characterization of the unique bovine A_1 adenosine receptor. J Biol Chem 1992; 267:10764–10770.

49. Stehle JH, Rivkees SA, Lee JJ, Weaver DR, Deeds JD, Reppert SM. Molecular cloning and expression of the cDNA for a novel A_2-adenosine receptor subtype. Mol Endocrinol 1992; 6:384–393.

50. Zhou Q-Y, Li C, Olah ME, Johnson RA, Stiles GL, Civelli O. Molecular cloning and characterization of an adenosine receptor: the A3 adenosine receptor. Proc Natl Acad Sci USA 1992; 89:7432–7436.

51. Lustig KD, Shiau AK, Brake AJ, Julius D. Expression cloning of an ATP receptor from mouse neuroblastoma cells. Proc Natl Acad Sci USA 1993; 90:5113–5117.

52. Erb L, Lustig KD, Sullivan DM, Turner JT, Weisman GA. Functional expression and photoaffinity labeling of a cloned P_{2U} purinergic receptor. Proc Natl Acad Sci USA 1993; 90:10449–10453.

53. Webb TE, Simon J, Krishek BJ, et al. Cloning and functional expression of a brain G-protein-coupled ATP receptor. FEBS Lett 1993; 324:219–225.

54. Dixon RAF, Kobilka BK, Strader DJ, et al. Cloning of the gene and cDNA for mammalian β-adrenergic receptor and homology with rhodopsin. Nature 1986; 321:75–79.

55. Salmon JE, Brogle N, Brownlie C, et al., Human mononuclear phagocytes express adenosine A^1 receptors. J Immunol 1993; 151:2775–2785.

56. El-Moatassim C, Dubyak GR. A novel pathway for the activation of phospholipase D by P_{2z} purinergic receptors in BAC1.2F5 macrophages. J Biol Chem 267:23664–23673.

57. Greenberg S, Di Virgilio F, Steinberg TH, Silverstein SC. Extracellular nucleotides mediate Ca^{2+} fluxes in J774 macrophages by two distinct mechanisms. J Biol Chem 1988; 263:10337–10343.

58. Sullivan GW, Linden J, Hewlett EL, Carper HT, Hylton JB, Mandell GL. Adenosine and related compounds counteract tumor necrosis factor-α inhibition of neutrophil migration: implication of a novel cyclic amp-independent action on the cell surface. J Immunol 1990; 145:1537–1544.

59. Parmely MJ, Zhou W-W, Edwards CK III, Borcherding DR, Silverstein R, and Morrison DC. Adenosine and a related carbocyclic nucleoside analogue selectively inhibit tumor necrosis factor-α production and protect mice against endotoxin challenge. J Immunol 1993; 151:389–396.

60. Lazarowski ER, Harden TK. Identification of a uridine nucleotide-selective G-protein-linked receptor that activates phospholipase C. J Biol Chem 1994; 269:11830–11836.

61. El-Moatassim C, Dubyak GR. Dissociation of the pore-forming and phospholipase D activities stimulated via P_{2z} purinergic receptors in BAC1.2F5 macrophages. J Biol Chem 1993; 268:15571–15578.

62. Steinberg TH, Silverstein SC. Extracellular ATP^{4-} promotes cation fluxes in the J774 mouse macrophage cell line. J Biol Chem 1987; 262:3118–3122.

63. Padeh S, Cohen A, Roifman CM. ATP-induced activation of human B lymphocytes via P_2-purinoreceptors. J Immunol 1991; 146:1626–1632.

64. Daniel-IssaKani S, Spiegel AM, Strulovici B. Lipopolysaccharide response is linked to the GTP binding protein, Gi2, in the promonocytoc cell line U937. J Biol Chem 1989; 264:20240–20247.

65. Gallay P, Jongeneel CV, Barras C, et al. Short time exposure to lipopolysaccharide is sufficient to activate human monocytes. J Immunol 1993; 150:5086–5093.

66. Proctor RA, Will JA, Burhop KE, Raetz CRH. Protection of mice against lethal endotoxemia by a lipid A precursor. Infect Immun 1986; 52:905–907.

67. Goldstein J, Hoffman T, Frasch C, et al. Lipopolysaccharide (LPS) from *Brucella abortus* is less toxic than that from *Escherichia coli*, suggesting the possible use of *B. abortus* or LPS from *B. abortus* as a carrier in vaccines. Infect Immun 1992; 60:1385–1389.

68. Baldwin G, Alpert G, Caputo GL, et al. Effect of polymyxin B on experimental shock from meningococcal and *Escherichia coli* endotoxins. J Infect Dis 1991; 164:542–549.

69. Cassel D, Selinger Z. Catecholamine-stimulated GTPase activity in turkey erythrocyte membranes. Biochim Biophys Acta 1976; 452:538–551.

70. Firestein GS, Boyle D, Bullough DA, et al. Protective effect of an adenosine kinase inhibitor in septic shock. J Immunol 1994; 152:5853–5859.

71. Schade UF. Pentoxifylline increases survival in murine endotoxin shock and decreases formation of tumor necrosis factor. Circ Shock 1990; 31:171–181.

72. Bortolussi R, Rajaraman K, Serushago B. Role of tumor necrosis factor-alpha and interferon-gamma in newborn host defense against *Listeria monocytogenes* infection. Pediatr Res 1992; 32:460–464.

73. Vogels MT, Cantoni L, Carelli M, Sironi, M Ghezzi, P van der Meer JW. Role of acute-phase proteins in interleukin-1-induced nonspecific resistance to bacterial infections in mice. Antimicrob Agents Chemother 1993; 37:2527–2533.

74. Novogrodsky A, Vanichkin A, Patya M, Gazit A, Osherov N, Levitzki A. Prevention of lipopolysaccharide-induced lethal toxicity by tyrosine kinase inhibitors. Science 1994; 264:1319–1322.

75. Doherty GM, Jensen JC, Alexander HR, Buresh CM, Norton JA. Pentoxifylline suppression of tumor necrosis factor gene transcription. Surgery 1991; 110:192–198.

76. Han J, Thompson P, Beutler B. Dexamethasone and pentoxifylline inhibit endotoxin-induced cachectin/tumor necrosis factor synthesis at separate points in the signaling pathway. J Exp Med 1990; 172:391–394.

77. Knowles MR, Clarke LL, Boucher RC. Activation by extracellular nucleotides of chloride secretion in the airway epithelia of patients with cystic fibrosis. N Engl J Med 1991; 325:533–538.

78. Chaudry IH. Use of ATP following shock and ischemia. In: Dubyak GR, Fedan JS, eds. Biological Actions of Extracellular ATP. New York: New York Academy of Sciences, 1990:130–140.

79. Romano M, Molino M, Cerletti C. Endotoxic lipid A induces intracellular Ca^{2+} increase in human platelets. Biochem J 1991; 278:75–80.

80. Ferris FG. Metallic ion interactions with the outer membrane of gram-negative bacteria. In: Beveridge TJ, Doyle RJ, eds., Metal Ions and Bacteria. New York: Wiley, 1989:295–323.

81. McCloskey RV, Straube RC, Sanders C, Smith SM, Smith CR, CHESS Trial Study Group. Treatment of septic shock with human monoclonal antibody HA-1A. A randomized, double-blind, placebo-controlled trial. Ann Intern Med 1994; 121:1–5.

82. Warren HS, Danner RL, Munford, RS. Anti-endotoxin monoclonal antibodies. N Engl J Med 1992; 326:1153–1156.

83. Kohn F. R., Ammons W. S., Horwitz A., et al. Protective effect of a recombinant amino-terminal fragment of bactericidal/permeability-increasing protein in experimental endotoxemia. J Infect Dis 1993; 168:1307–1310.

84. Hirata M, Shimomura Y, Yoshida M, et al. Characterization of a rabbit cationic protein (CAP18) with lipopolysaccharide-inhibitory activity. Infect Immun 1994; 62:1421–1426.

85. Marra M. Bactericidal/permeability increasing protein (BPI) and lipopolysaccharide binding protein (LBP) fusion chimeras. IBC's Fourth Annual Conference on The Shift in R&D Strategies for the Prevention & Treatment of Endotoxemia & Sepsis, Philadelphia, PA, June 13–15, 1994.

86. Takada K, Ohno N, Yadomae T. Binding of lysozyme to lipopolysaccharide suppresses tumor necrosis factor production *in vivo*. Infect Immun 1994; 62:1171–1175.

-87. Fletcher MA, McKenna TM, Quance JL, Wainwright NR, Williams TJ. Lipopolysaccharide detoxification by endotoxin neutralizing protein. J Surg Res 1993; 55:147–154.

-88. Levine DM, Parker TS, Donnelly TM, Walsh A, Rubin AL. In vivo protection against endotoxin by plasma high density lipoprotein. Proc Natl Acad Sci USA 1993; 90:12040–12044.

-89. Williams, TJ. Magainin compounds act systemically to kill bacteria and/or neutralize endotoxin. IBC's Fourth Annual Conference on The Shift in R&D Strategies for the Prevention & Treatment of Endotoxemia & Sepsis, Philadelphia, PA, June 13–15, 1994.

-90. Kovach NL, Yee E, Munford RS, Raetz CRH, Harlan JM. Lipid IV^A inhibits sythesis and release of tumor necrosis factor induced by lipopolysaccharide in human whole blood ex vivo. J Exp Med 1990; 172:77–84.

91. Qureshi N, Takayama K, Kurtz R. Diphosphoryl lipid A obtained from the nontoxic lipopolysaccharide of *Rhodopseudomonas sphaeroides* is an endotoxin antagonist in mice. Infect Immun 1991; 59:441–444.

92. Danner RL, Eichacker PQ, Doerfler ME, et al. Therapeutic trial of lipid X in a canine model of septic shock. J Infect Dis 1993; 167:378–384.

93. Rossignol DP. Interactions of LPS and lipid A-like LPS antagonists with endotoxin binding proteins. IBC's Fourth Annual Conference on The Shift in R&D Strategies for the Prevention & Treatment of Endotoxemia & Sepsis, Philadelphia, PA, June 13–15, 1994.

94. Saravolatz LD, Wherry JC, Spooner C, et al. Clinical safety, tolerability, and pharmacokinetics of murine monoclonal antibody to human tumor necrosis factor-α. J Infect Dis 1994; 169:214–217.

95. Bernhagen J, Calandra T, Mitchell RA, et al. MIF is a pituitary-derived cytokine that potentiates lethal endotoxaemia. Nature 1993; 365:756–759.

96. Lesslauer W, Tabuchi H, Gentz R, et al. Recombinant soluble tumor necrosis receptor proteins protect mice from lipopolysaccharide-induced lethality. Eur J Immunol 1991; 21:2883–2886.

97. Mohler KM, Sleath PR, Fitzner JN, et al. Protection against a lethal dose of endotoxin by an inhibitor of tumour necrosis factor processing. Nature 1994; 370:218–220.

98. Mancilla J, Garcia P, Dinarello CA. The interleukin-1 receptor antagonist can either reduce or enhance the lethality of *Klebsiella pneumoniae* sepsis in newborn rats. Infect Immun 1993; 61:926–932.

99. Barton BE, Jackson JV. Protective role of interleukin 6 in the lipopolysaccharide-galactosamine septic shock model. Infect Immun 1993; 61:1496–1499.

100. Howard M, Muchamuel T, Andrade S, Menon S. Interleukin 10 protects mice from lethal endotoxemia. J Exp Med 1993; 177:1205–1208.

101. Galluppi G. R. Prevention of death due to septic shock by tissue factor pathway inhibitor in a primate model of E. coli infection. IBC's Fourth Annual Conference on The Shift in R&D Strategies for the Prevention & Treatment of Endotoxemia & Sepsis, Philadelphia, PA, June 13–15, 1994.

102. Torley LW, Pickett WC, Carroll ML, et al. Studies of the effect of a platelet-activating factor antagonist, CL 184,005, in animal models of gram-negative bacterial sepsis. Antimicrob Agents Chemother 1992; 36:1971–1977.

103. Rice GC, Brown PA, Nelson RJ, Bianco JA, Singer JW, Bursten S. Protection from endotoxic shock in mice by pharmacologic inhibition of phosphatidic acid. Proc Natl Acad Sci USA 1994; 91:3857–3861.

104. Rodell TC. The role of bradykinin antagonists in the treatment of sepsis. IBC's Fourth Annual Conference on The Shift in R&D Strategies for the Prevention & Treatment of Endotoxemia & Sepsis, Philadelphia, PA, June 13–15, 1994.

14

Carbocyclic Nucleosides as Potential Therapeutic Agents for the Treatment of Septic Shock

Michael J. Parmely, Elda H. S. Hausmann, and David C. Morrison
University of Kansas Medical Center
Kansas City, Kansas

I. INTRODUCTION

Septic shock is a pathophysiological condition that results from a systemic response to serious bacterial infection. The low success rate associated with our current strategies for the prevention of this disease or the management of patients in shock underscores our lack of detailed information on the essential pathogenic mechanisms that contribute to disease progression. Although there exists an extensive literature describing the range of host immune and inflammatory responses to gram-negative bacteria, information is lacking that would identify which of the many described pathophysiological processes are actually necessary for the development of this life-threatening condition. This chapter reviews recent studies that suggest the potential efficacy of a novel synthetic structural analog of adenosine in the treatment of septic shock. Perhaps equally important, we describe how one can use such a reagent in an experimental context to identify the inflammatory responses that make essential contributions to the pathogenesis of endotoxic septic shock.

II. APPLICATION OF ADENYL CARBOCYCLIC NUCLEOSIDES TO SEPTIC SHOCK

Carbocyclic nucleosides have received considerable attention over the years as potential antiviral agents. A number of novel synthetic nucleosides have been designed with the intent of inhibiting specific viral polymerases or enzymes catalyzing steps in the metabolism of viral nucleic acids. Examples include 3'-azidothymidine (AZT), acyclovir, and the ribovirin phosphates that have multiple effects on viral transcriptases or other enzymes involved in nucleoside or nucleic acid biosynthesis. More recently, nucleoside inhibitors of viral replication have been characterized that act on *cellular* enzymes. Notable among these is a group of naturally occurring and synthetic adenyl carbocyclic nucleosides, for which a strong correlation exists between antiviral activity and inhibitory activity for the enzyme *S*-adenosyl homocysteine (SAH) hydrolase. This enzyme catalyzes the degradation of SAH to adenosine and homocysteine, thus preventing feedback inhibition of biological transmethylation reactions by SAH (1). Relative to potential antiviral effects, the inhibition of SAH hydrolase activity by these compounds would be expected to reduce 5'-cap methylation of viral mRNAs, which is essential for transcript stability, RNA processing, and the efficient translation of viral mRNAs (2). The naturally occurring fungal metabolites aristeromycin and neplanocin A (Fig. 1) have long been recognized as potent and specific inhibitors of SAH hydrolase (3,4). However, their inherent toxicities have limited their therapeutic value and encouraged the synthesis of additional analogs with less severe biological side effects. One such compound, dihydroxycyclopentenyladenine or DHCeA (Fig. 1), is an analog of neplanocin A showing comparatively low toxicity and high inhibitory activity for SAH hydrolase. A number of structurally related, low-toxicity analogs have also been produced that have potent biological effects, although their mechanisms of action have not been fully characterized (5). One such compound is MDL201,112 or 9-[(1S,3R)-*cis*-cyclopentan-3-ol]adenine (abbreviated cPA)(Fig. 1). This compound was synthesized by David Borcherding at the Marion Merrell Dow Research Institute (Cincinnati, OH). Like aristeromycin, cPA shares with adenosine the adenine base and contains a substituted 9,1-linked cyclopentane ring instead of the usual sugar group.

One of the first reported successful applications of synthetic adenyl carbocyclic nucleosides to the treatment of experimental inflammatory diseases was the use of cPA in a mouse model of endotoxin lethality (6). The animal model employed was first described by Galanos et al. (7), who showed that mice treated with the hepatotoxin D-galactosamine (D-galNH$_2$) were highly sensitive to the lethal effects of bacterial endotoxic LPS. Indeed, the 50% lethal dose (LD$_{50}$) for smooth forms of LPS is typically reduced in mice treated with D-galNH$_2$ by as much as four orders of magnitude. This treatment also results in a reproducible acute shock response to LPS challenge, and deaths in CF1 mice occur within 12 h.

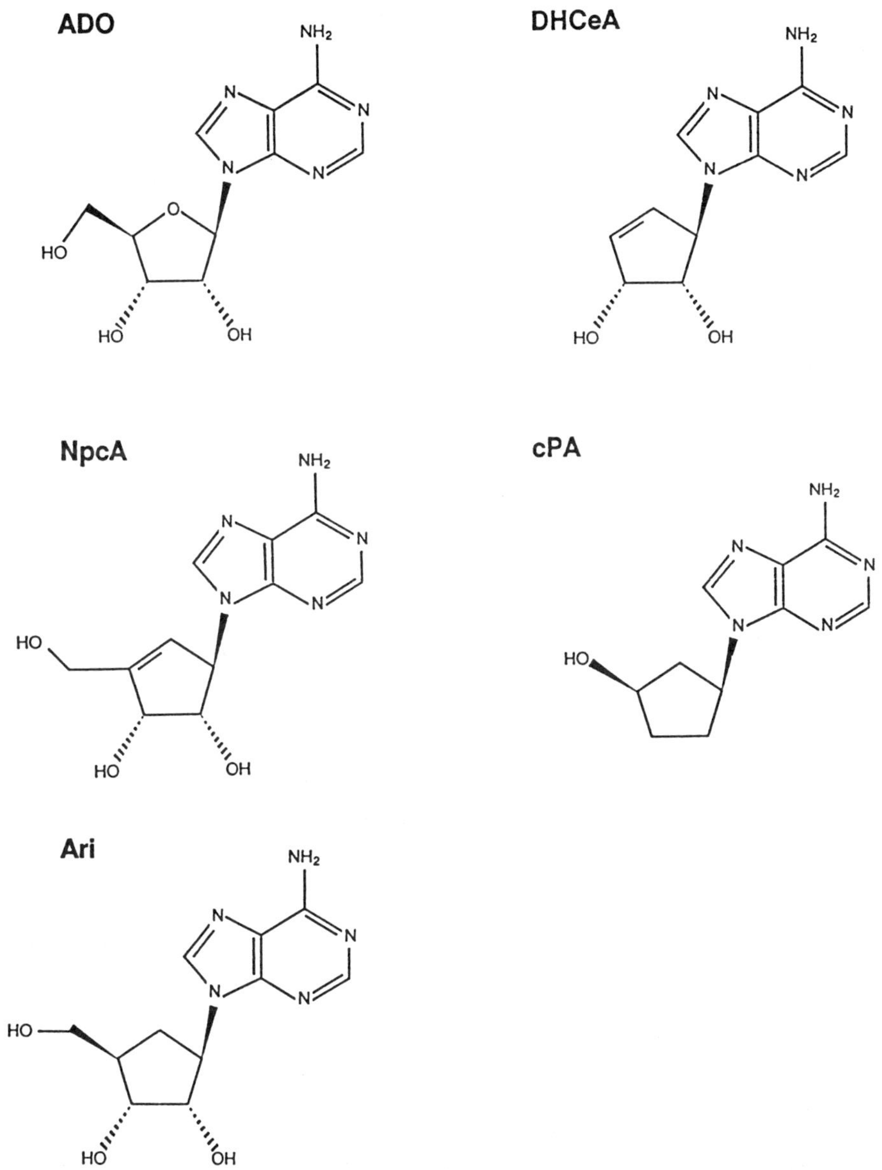

Figure 1 Structures of adenosine (ADO), neplanocin A (NpcA), aristeromycin (Ari), DHCeA, and cPA (MDL201, 112).

In one group of experiments (6), mice challenged with 20–50 ng LPS + D-galNH$_2$ showed 81% mortality (40 deaths of 49 mice). In contrast, a single intraperitoneal injection of cPA (100 mg cPA/kg body weight) 1 h prior to challenge reduced mortality to 6% (3 deaths in 49 mice). Mice were also protected if the compound was given at the time of endotoxin + D-galNH$_2$ challenge, indicating that cPA did not protect animals by inducing endotoxin tolerance due to contaminating LPS in the drug preparation. Likewise, because the compound did not prevent lethality caused by challenge with recombinant TNF-α + D-galNH$_2$, potential interactions between cPA and D-galNH$_2$ that might render the animals more resistant to LPS-induced lethality did not appear to explain the beneficial effects of cPA. Importantly, treatment of mice with cPA caused a significant reduction in serum TNF-α in response to LPS challenge, indicating that a correlation existed between the prevention of lethal shock and an inhibition of the production of this important pro-inflammatory cytokine.

III. MECHANISMS OF ACTION OF cPA ON MOUSE MACROPHAGES ACTIVATED BY LPS IN VITRO

LPS-activated macrophages appear to play a central role in the pathogenesis of endotoxin shock by virtue of the types and quantities of pro-inflammatory mediators they produce. These include the cytokines IL-1β, IL-6, and TNF-α, a number of lipid and arachidonic acid metabolites, and the free radicals superoxide (O_2^-) and nitric oxide (NO). The most compelling evidence for a role of macrophages in this regard includes the elegant studies of Michalek et al. (8) and Galanos and his colleagues (9) showing that the ability to induce endotoxin lethality in mice can be adoptively transferred to naive mice either by bone marrow cells or LPS-activated macrophages. Pretreatment of the recipients with anti-TNF-α antibodies prevented lethality in these experimental systems (10), demonstrating the essential role that TNF-α plays in this particular model. Similar results with neutralizing antibodies have been forthcoming in a number of other animal models of endotoxin shock (6,11–13), indicating that TNF-α is an important, if not essential, component in the pathogenesis of endotoxin lethality in a number of animal species.

Because macrophages and their secretory products appear to play a central role in shock pathogenesis, we recently have focused our attention on characterizing the effects of cPA on mouse macrophage activation in vitro, with particular interest in the pro-inflammatory mediators produced by this cell type. Using a variety of techniques, we have established that cPA is a potent and selective inhibitor of macrophage gene expression both in mouse peritoneal macrophages and in the macrophagelike cell lines RAW 264.7 and J774.1. Typical findings are shown in Fig. 2, which illustrates the effects of cPA and adenosine on TNF-α production by thiogylcollate-elicited mouse peritoneal macrophages following

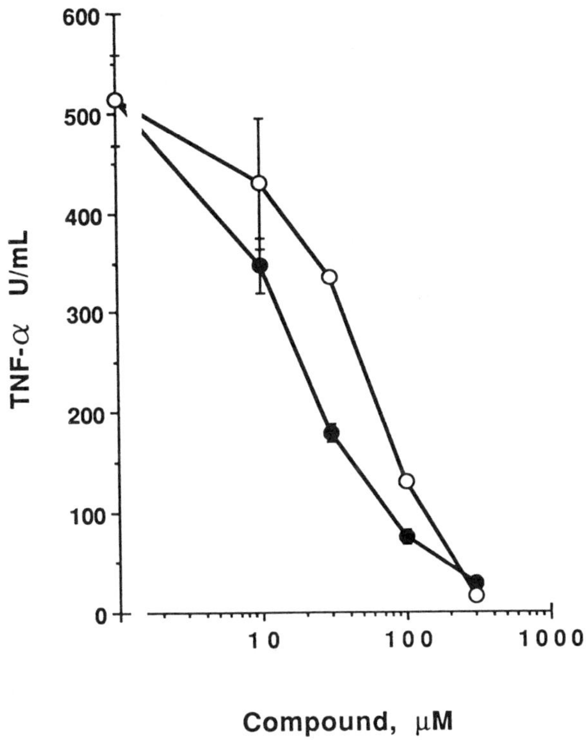

Figure 2   Effects of cPA and adenosine on TNF-α production by C3HeB/FeJ thioglycollate-elicited peritoneal macrophages activated with LPS plus IFN-γ. Culture supernatant fluids were recovered 9 h after activation with 1 ng LPS/mL plus 3 U IFN-γ/mL and assayed for TNF-α by the L929 cell bioassay (14). The indicated concentrations of either adenosine (○) or cPA (●) were added at the same time as were LPS and IFN-γ.

activation with LPS plus interferon-γ (IFN-γ). In this experiment cPA acted in a dose-dependent fashion, showing an IC_{50} of approximately 20 μ M. A number of additional findings help define the specificity of cPA in terms of its effects on mouse macrophages. At concentrations less than 100 μ M, cPA did not inhibit LPS-induced IL-1 or IL-6 production as measured by bioassay or ELISA, respectively. While cPA inhibited TNF-α mRNA expression in RAW 264.7 cells activated by LPS plus IFN-γ, it slightly enhanced expression of IL-1β mRNA by the same cells (6). Because the inhibitory effect of cPA on steady-state TNF-α mRNA expression could not be attributed to a change in mRNA stability in RAW 264.7 cells, we have tentatively concluded that cPA may have a direct effect on *TNF*-α gene transcription. However, it should be noted that to date no direct evidence exists indicating that cPA or related compounds have any effect on the transcription of macrophage cytokine genes. As shown in Fig. 2, adenosine also inhibited the production of TNF-α in vitro as assessed by bioassay. Although mouse macrophages bear receptors for adenosine, several findings indicate that cPA does not act through these classical adenosine receptors. First, competitive binding assays have failed to detect the binding of cPA to A1 or A2 receptors (6). Second, the mechanism by which adenosine inhibits TNF-α production by macrophages is not the same as that described above for cPA. For example, adenosine has no effect on the expression of TNF-α mRNA by activated RAW 264.7 cells, J774.1 cells (6) or mouse peritoneal macrophages (Parmely et al., unpublished observations).

The effects of cPA on TNF-α production are not limited to LPS-stimulated macrophages. The results reported in Table 1 indicate that cPA inhibited TNF-α production by mouse macrophages, whether the cells were activated by LPS, LPS plus IFN-γ, heat-killed *Listeria monocytogenes* organisms, or opsonized zymosan. Together with the observation that IL-1 and IL-6 production were relatively unaffected by cPA, these findings strongly suggest that the compound acts at a site proximal to the expression of the *TNF*-α gene rather than by

Table 1 Effects of cPA on TNF-α and NO Production by Mouse Macrophages Activated by a Variety of Different Stimuli

Activating agent[a]	100 μ cPA	TNF-α[b]		Nitrite[c]	
		U/mL	Percent inhibition	μ	Percent inhibition
None	−	<10		<0.5	
LPS	−	666		14.0	
	+	120	82	9.3	34
LPS + IFN-γ	−	3001		56.6	
	+	285	91	52.0	8
HKLM	−	2057		3.9	
	+	287	86	8.0	0
Zymosan	−	1375		16.4	
	+	124	91	14.7	10
IFN-γ + TNF-α	−	N.D.[d]		24.5	
	+	N.D.		26.1	0

[a]100 ng LPS/mL; 1 ng LPS/mL + 10 U IFN-γg/mL; 50 heat-killed *Listeria monocytogenes* per macrophage; 50 μ g zymosan/mL.
[b]TNF-α was measured by bioassay (14) on culture supernatants collected 9 h after addition of the activating agents.
[c]Nitrite was measured with the Griess reagent (15) on 30-h culture supernatants.
[d]N.D. = not determined.

inhibiting a much earlier signal transduction event triggered by LPS receptor–ligand interactions. The data in Table 1 also demonstrate that NO production in response to these cell-activating agents was generally not inhibited by cPA. The implications of this specificity to septic shock pathogenesis will be discussed in more detail in Section V.

Overall, the data reviewed to this point indicate that cPA is a potent and selective inhibitor of TNF-α production by LPS-activated mouse macrophages in vitro and may act, at least in part, by inhibiting *TNF-α* gene transcription. This observation is consistent with the ability of the compound to prevent endotoxin lethality in mice in vivo and supports the general conclusion that macrophages play a central role in the pathogenesis of endotoxin shock by virtue of their ability to produce large amounts of the pro-inflammatory cytokine TNF-α. The exact role of macrophages and/or TNF-α in disease progression is not completely understood, although a number of possibilities exist, including the induction of altered neutrophil migration, adhesion and activation, platelet aggregation, and changes in vascular tone. Recently, considerable attention has focused on the free radical NO as a potentially important component in shock pathogenesis, and we have utilized cPA to test two hypotheses related to NO and endotoxin shock: (a) that TNF-α-induced NO plays an essential role in endotoxin shock in mice and (b) that *macrophage-derived* NO production is essential to disease progression in this species.

IV. NITRIC OXIDE PRODUCTION AS A POTENTIAL THERAPEUTIC TARGET IN SEPTIC SHOCK

Considerable clinical and experimental evidence exists supporting the conclusion that the potent vasodilator NO mediates many of the pathological changes resulting in abnormal blood flow that are seen in septic and endotoxin shock. Urinary and plasma nitrates are elevated in patients with the disease (16,17), as they are in animals challenged with LPS (18,19). Endotoxin challenge of human beings and laboratory animals induces a state of hypotension similar to that seen in septic shock (20), and this hypotension has been successfully treated in a limited number of patients (21) or prevented in experimental animals (22,23) by the administration of L-arginine analogs that block intracellular NO synthase (NOS) activity. Accompanying these cardiovascular abnormalities is an elevated expression of NOS activity in several tissues that reflects the action of the constitutive, calcium-dependent as well as the calcium-independent, inducible isoforms of this enzyme (24). Several reports indicate that dexamethasone, which inhibits the expression of inducible NOS (iNOS), but not that of the constitutive NOS isoforms (25,26), can also block the hypotension induced by endotoxin in rats (23,27). This suggests that much of the deleterious effects of NO in shock result from LPS-induced iNOS expression. Thus, there is a growing body of evidence that supports the hypothesis that LPS-induced NO production is an important, if not essential, step in the development of the cardiovascular shock response to endotoxin challenge, if not septic shock itself.

There is also considerable evidence linking TNF-α to the induction of NO, both in vitro and in LPS-challenged animals. Injection of TNF-α can mimic many of the effects of LPS, including the induction of hypotension in human beings (28) and laboratory animals (12,22,29,30). Anti-TNF-α antibodies can protect animals against LPS lethality (6,11,12) and block many (but not all) of the symptoms of endotoxin shock. Thus, there is experimental support for the conclusion that endotoxin shock is mediated, in part, by NO induced by TNF-α produced by LPS-activated cells. This has led to the speculation that the macrophage is central in this cascade of events, both as a source of TNF-α and as an important producer of NO. Likewise, it is tempting to assume that TNF-α-induced NO production is a necessary step in the pathogenesis of *septic* shock. In fact, very little evidence exists for either of these last two conclusions.

In an effort to determine the validity of the hypothesis that NO serves a harmful role in endotoxin shock, several investigators have administered NOS inhibitors to laboratory animals prior to endotoxin challenge. Certain L-arginine analogs, such as N^G-monomethyl-L-arginine (NMMA), can inhibit NOS activity, acting on both the inducible and constitutive enzyme isoforms. Although these compounds have shown protective effects in experimental models of endotoxemia (27,31,32), overly aggressive treatment of endotoxin shock with NOS inhibitors can lead to an exacerbation of the hypotensive effects of LPS, intense vasoconstriction, end organ damage, and rapid death (27,31–33). The positive effects of supportive NO therapy (i.e., either inhaled NO gas or injected NO donors) (27,34) have suggested that the indiscriminate inhibition of both inducible and constitutive isoforms of NOS may be particularly damaging, and that the ultimate outcome in endotoxin shock may be determined by the overall degree of inhibition of NO biosynthesis. Because a number of cell types express both isoforms of NOS (24), it has not been a simple matter to identify either the potentially beneficial or harmful NO-producing cells that participate in this condition. Thus, at the present time, no firm data exist that clearly identify a given cell type as the principal source of vasoactive, pathogenic NO in shock.

V. EFFECTS OF cPA ON NO PRODUCTION BY LPS-ACTIVATED MACROPHAGES

The availability of cPA and knowledge of its effects on mouse macrophages has afforded us the opportunity to ask two questions related to the role of NO production in endotoxin shock. First, we wished to know to what extent autocrine/paracrine TNF-α contributes to LPS-induced NO production by mouse macrophages in vitro. Studies with neutralizing anti-TNF-α antibodies have suggested that mouse macrophage NO production induced by IFN-γ plus muramyl dipeptide is TNF-α-dependent (35), but insufficient data exist to conclude with certainty whether, and to what extent, a similar cascade mediates LPS-induced NO production. The second objective of our studies was to determine the relative contribution of *macrophage-derived* NO to the pathogenesis of endotoxin shock in mice. Although this latter goal was somewhat more elusive, we reasoned that any information obtained would be valuable in terms of establishing the likely therapeutic benefit of inhibiting macrophage NO production as a means of treating septic shock.

Whereas cPA has proven to be an effective inhibitor of TNF-α production in mouse macrophages activated with LPS as well as a number of other stimuli (Table 1), NO production by the same cells was only marginally affected by cPA. Perhaps the greatest effect of cPA on NO biosynthesis in mouse peritoneal macrophages was observed when the cells were activated with LPS alone, in which case 100 μM cPA caused only a 30–35% inhibition of the response. This compared to >90% inhibition of NO production by 350 μM NMMA and 80–90% inhibition by cPA of TNF-α production by the same cells (Table 1 and Ref. 36). When peritoneal macrophages were co-activated with 1 ng LPS per mL and 0.1–10 U IFN-γ /mL, cPA had no statistically significant effect on NO production, while it inhibited TNF-α production by more than 90% (Table 1 and Ref. 36). These differences between TNF-α and NO production by cPA-treated cells could not be attributed to changes in the kinetics of the responses, as NO production was unaffected by cPA over the entire 24 h of culture. In contrast, TNF-α production was inhibited by the compound at all time points tested.

The induction of TNF-α by heat-killed *Listeria monocytogenes* or opsonized zymosan was also inhibited by cPA, whereas NO responses were not significantly reduced in either case. These data suggest that the activation of mouse macrophages for NO production by a number of different agents is not dependent on TNF-α as a co-activating agent, as suggested by an earlier report (35) for responses to IFN-γ plus muramyl dipeptide. As a final test of the hypothesis that cPA regulates NO biosynthesis, we have also determined whether cPA inhibits NO induced directly by TNF-α. By itself, TNF-α does not activate mouse peritoneal macrophages for NO production, but Ding et al. (37) have shown that IFN-γ and TNF-α can synergize for the induction of NO. As shown in Table 1, cPA had no significant effect on the production of the reactive nitrogen intermediate induced by IFN-γ plus TNF-α, indicating that cPA-treated macrophages produce normal NO levels despite being significantly inhibited in terms of their ability to synthesize TNF-α.

With regard to our initial questions, the following conclusions appear justified: (a) The induction of NO biosynthesis by LPS-activated mouse peritoneal macrophages is not highly dependent on co-stimulation of the cells with autocrine/

paracrine TNF-α, and the minor activating role TNF-α may play in this LPS-induced response is easily replaced by other co-activating stimuli, including IFN-γ; (b) nitric oxide production by tissue macrophages is not essential to the pathogenesis of endotoxin lethality in mice. This second conclusion is derived from the findings that cPA protected mice against LPS-induced lethality but had no significant effect on NO production by mouse macrophages in vitro. The anatomical distribution of macrophages is also inconsistent with their playing a dominant role in the acute effects on vessel walls, despite the diffusibility of NO. Moreover, the general failure of human monocytes and macrophages to respond to LPS by producing large amounts of NO suggests that cells of other histogenic types are the principal sources of the damaging levels of vasoactive NO seen in endotoxin, and perhaps septic, shock. Our current efforts are aimed at determining the specificity of cPA in vivo, as further support for our conclusions would be derived from finding that cPA had no effect on LPS-induced macrophage NOS activity in the intact mouse.

VI. THERAPEUTIC APPROACHES

Although experimental endotoxin lethality models of septic shock have been extremely valuable in defining host responses to this important component of the bacterial cell wall, in the strictest sense the clinical challenge is in managing *septic*, rather than *endotoxin*, shock. It is clear that these are not completely equivalent disease processes. For example, whereas NMMA can lessen the severity of lethal shock in mice challenged with endotoxin, Evans et al. (38) reported that NMMA failed to improve survival of mice challenged either by the intravenous or the intraperitoneal routes with lethal doses of *Escherichia coli*. Eskandari et al. (39) were similarly unable to prevent lethality in mice receiving live bacterial challenge by treating with anti-TNF-α antibodies, despite earlier successful efforts by other investigators with baboons and mice (40,41). It is also clear that the effective treatment of patients in septic shock, or at risk to develop this condition, may require combined therapies involving agents that target different aspects of the disease. The rational selection of multiple therapies will require a more complete understanding of the interactions between known pathogenic processes. While our findings suggest that macrophage-derived NO may not play a critical role in the cardiovascular changes seen in the shock syndrome, prevention of TNF-α production by this cell type can still be an important therapeutic component in the prevention and/or treatment of this disease. Inhibiting TNF-α production would be expected to reduce the levels of vasoactive NO produced by endothelial cells and/or smooth muscle cells of the vessel walls. However, a recent report indicates that this too may be a more complicated process. Yoshizumi et al. (42) have reported that very low concentrations of TNF-α (IC_{50} = 0.1 ng/mL) can inhibit constitutive endothelial cell NOS mRNA expression in vitro. This finding suggests that the pathogenesis of endotoxin shock may include inhibition of basal constitutive NO production in addition to the induction of iNOS activity. Thus, the effectiveness of any therapeutic approach involving TNF-α will require systematic studies that carefully define the target cell population, the nature of its response to TNF-α, and its precise contribution to shock pathogenesis.

ACKNOWLEDGMENTS

The authors wish to thank Terry Bolin, Carl Edwards, and David Borcherding of Marion Merrell Dow Research Institute for providing cPA for these studies. This research was supported, in part, by NIH grant 1-PO1-CA54474.

REFERENCES

1. Wolfe MS, Borchardt RT. S-adenosyl-L-homocysteine hydrolase as a target for antiviral chaemotherapy. J Med Chem 1991; 34:1521–1530.
2. Furuichi Y, Shatkin AJ. Capping and methylation of mRNA. In: Higgins SJ, Hames BD, eds. RNA Processing: A Practical Approach. Oxford: Oxford Univ Press, 1994: 35–67.
3. Cools M, DeClercq E. Correlation between the antiviral activity of acyclic and carbocyclic adenosine analogues in murine L929 cells and their inhibitory effect on L929 cell S-adenosylhomocysteine hydrolase. Biochem Pharm 1989; 38:1061–1067.
4. Borchardt RT. S-Adenosyl-L-methionine-dependent macromolecular methyltransferases: potential targets for the design of chemotherapeutic agents. J Med Chem 1980; 23:347–357.
5. Borcherding DR, Edwards CK. J Med Chem 1995; in press.
6. Parmely MJ, Zhou W-W, Edwards CK, Borcherding DR, Silverstein R, Morrison DC. Adenosine and a related carbocyclic nucleoside analogue selectively inhibit tumor necrosis factor-α production and protect mice against endotoxin challenge. J Immunol 1993; 151:389–396.
7. Galanos C, Freundenberg MA, Reutter W. Galactosamine-induced sensitization of to the lethal effects of endotoxin. Proc Natl Acad Sci USA 1979; 76:5939–5943.
8. Michalek SM, Moore RN, McGhee JR, Rosentstreich DC, Mergenhagen SE. The primary role of lymphoreticular cells in the mediation of host responses to bacterial endotoxin. J Infect Dis 1980; 141:55–63.
9. Freudenberg MA, Keppler D, Galanos C. Requirement for lipopolysaccharide-responsive macrophages in galactosamine-induced sensitization to endotoxin. Infect Immun 1986; 51:891–895.
10. Galanos C, Freudenberg MA, Katschinski T, Salomao R. Mossman H, Kumazawa Y. Tumor necrosis factor and host response to endotoxin. In: Morrison DC, Ryan JL, eds. Bacterial Endotoxic Lipopolysaccharides. Boca Raton, FL: CRC Press, 1992: 75–104.

11. Beutler B, Milsark IW, Cerami A. Passive immunization against cachectin/tumor necrosis factor protects mice from lethal effect of endotoxin. Science 1985; 229:869–871.

12. Mathison JC, Wolfson E, Ulevitch RJ. Participation of tumour necrosis factor in the mediation of gram negative bacterial lipopolysaccharide-induced injury in rabbits. J Clin Invest 1988; 81:1925–1937.

13. Silva AT, Bayston KF, Cohen J. Prophylactic and therapeutic effects of a monoclonal antibody to tumor necrosis factor-α in experimental gram-negative shock. J Infect Dis 1990; 162:421–427.

14. Parmely MJ, Gale A, Clabaugh M, Horvat R, Zhou W-W. Proteolytic inactivation of cytokines by *Pseudomonas aeruginosa*. Infect Immun 1990; 58:3009–3015.

15. Green LC, Wagner DA, Giogowski J, Skipper PL, Wishnock JS, Tannenbaum SR. Analysis of nitrate, nitrite and [^{15}N] nitrite in biological fluids. Anal Biochem 1982; 126:5241–5244.

16. Evans T, Carpenter A, Kinderman H, Cohen J. Evidence of increased nitric oxide production in patients with the sepsis syndrome. Circ Shock 1993; 41:77–81.

17. Ochoa JB, Udekwu AO, Billiar TR, et al. Nitrogen oxide levels in patients after trauma and during sepsis. Ann Surg 1991; 214:621–626.

18. Granger DL, Hibbs JB Jr, Broadnax LM. Urinary nitrate excretion in relation to murine macrophage activation. J Immunol 1991; 146:1294–1302.

19. Shultz PJ, Raiji L. Endogenously synthesized nitric oxide prevents endotoxin-induced glomerular thrombosis. J Clin Invest 1992: 90:1718–1725.

20. Suffrendini AF, Fromm RE, Parker MM, et al. The cardiovascular response of normal humans to the administration of endotoxin. N Engl J Med 1989; 321:280–287.

21. Petros A, Bennett D, Vallance P. Effect of nitric oxide synthase inhibitors on hypotension in patients with septic shock. Lancet 1991; 338:1557–1558.

22. Kilbourn RG, Gross SS, Jubran A, et al. N^G-methyl-L-arginine inhibits tumor necrosis factor-induced hypotension: implications for the involvement of nitric oxide. Proc Natl Acad Sci USA 1990; 87:3629–3632.

23. Szabo C, Mitchell JA, Thiermermann C, Vane JR. Nitric oxide-mediated hyporeactivity to noradrenaline precedes the induction of nitric oxide synthase in endotoxin shock. Br J Pharmacol 1993; 108:786–792.

24. Knowles RG, Moncada S. Nitric oxide synthases in mammals. Biochem J 1994; 298:249–258.

25. Knowles RG, Salter M, Brooks SL, Moncada S. Anti-inflammatory glucocorticoids inhibit the induction by endotoxin of nitric oxide synthase in the lung, liver and aorta of the rat. Biochem Biophys Res Commun 1990; 172:1042–1048.

26. Radomski MW, Palmer RMJ, Moncada S. Glucocorticoids inhibit the expression of an inducible, but not the constitutive, nitric oxide synthase in vascular endothelial cells. Proc Natl Acad Sci USA 1990; 87:10043–10047.

27. Wright CE, Rees DD, Moncada S. Protective and pathological roles of nitric oxide in endotoxin shock. Cardiovasc Res 1992; 26:48–57.

28. Kilbourn RG, Griffith OW. Overproduction of nitric oxide in cytokine-mediated and septic shock. J Natl Cancer Inst 1992; 84:827–831.

29. Billiau A, Vandekerckhove F. Cytokines and their interactions with other inflammatory mediators in the pathogenesis of sepsis and septic shock. Eur J Clin Invest 1991; 21:559–573.
30. Tracey KJ, Beutler B, Lowry SF, et al. Shock and tissue injury induced by recombinant human cachectin. Science 1986; 234:470–474.
31. Nava E, Plamer RMJ, Moncada S. The role of nitric oxide in endotoxic shock: effects of N^G-monomethyl-L-arginine. J Cardio Pharm 1992; 20: 132–134.
32. Moncada S, Higgs A. The L-arginine-nitric oxide pathway. N Engl J Med 1993; 329:2002–2012.
33. Minnard EA, Shou J, Naama H, et al. Inhibition of nitric oxide synthesis is detrimental during endotoxemia. Arch Surg 1994; 129:142–148.
34. Weitzberg E, Rudehill A, Lundberg JM. Nitric oxide inhalation attenuates pulmonary hypertension and improves gas exchange in endotoxin shock. Eur J Pharm 1993; 233:85–94.
35. Drapier J-C, Wietzerbin J, Hibbs JB Jr. Interferon-γ and tumor necrosis factor induce the L-arginine-dependent cytotoxic effector mechanism in murine macrophages. Eur J Immunol 1988; 18:1587–1592.
36. Parmely MJ, Hao S-Y, Morrison DC, Pace JL. Role of macrophage-derived nitric oxide in endotoxin lethality in mice. J Endotoxin Res 1995; 2:45–52.
37. Ding A, Nathan CF, Graycar J, Derynck R, Stuehr DH, Srimal S. Macrophage deactivating factor and transforming growth factors-β 1, -β 2 and -β 3 inhibit induction of macrophage nitrogen oxide synthesis by IFN-γ. J Immunol 1990; 145:940–945.
38. Evans T, Carpenter A, Silva A, Cohen J. Inhibition of nitric oxide synthetase in experimental gram-negative sepsis. J Infect Dis 1994; 169:343–349.
39. Eskandari MK, Bolgos G, Miller C, et al. Anti-tumor necrosis factor antibody therapy fails to prevent lethality after cecal ligation and puncture or endotoxemia. J Immunol 1992; 148: 2724–2730.
40. Tracey KJ, Fong Y, Hesse DG, et al. Anti-cachectin/TNF monoclonal antibodies prevent septic shock during lethal bacteraemia. Nature 1987; 330:662–664.
41. Hinshaw LB, Tekamp-Olsen P, Chang ACK, et al. Survival of primates in LD_{100} septic shock following therapy with antibody to tumor necrosis factor (TNFα). Circ Shock 1990; 30:279–292.
42. Yoshizumi M, Perrella MA, Burnett JC Jr, Lee M-E. Tumor necrosis factor down-regulates endothelial nitric oxide synthase mRNA by shortening its half-life. Circ Res 1993; 173:205–209.

15

Sepsis and Pentoxifylline Therapy: From Newborn to Adult

Michael P. Sherman
University of Kansas Medical Center
Kansas City, Kansas

William E. Truog
University of Missouri—Kansas City School of Medicine
and Children's Mercy Hospital
Kansas City, Missouri

I. INTRODUCTION

The "sepsis syndrome" is manifest clinically by an escalating immune response to microbial toxins (1–3). In its severest form, inflammatory mediators of host defense cause shock, multiple organ failure, and high mortality (4,5). The lung is a particularly vulnerable target during this explosive effort at host protection, and an acute form of pulmonary injury called the adult respiratory distress syndrome (ARDS) often coexists during sepsis. The adult respiratory distress syndrome is characterized by high-permeability pulmonary edema, refractory hypoxemia, and respiratory failure (6). Tumor necrosis factor-α (TNF-α), which has been shown to be pivotal in tissue damage, multiple organ failure, shock, and death, is elevated in blood and alveolar fluid during the course of ARDS (7,8). Alveolar macrophages recovered from patients with ARDS have increased expression of the TNF-α gene (9), suggesting that these phagocytes manifest enhanced TNF-α secretion during the course of this condition. The activation of polymorphonuclear leukocytes (PMN) and pulmonary endothelial cells during the host's response to microbial components (10) is also mediated, in part, by TNF-α. Accordingly, the proposed pathogenesis of ARDS associated with endotoxemia includes production of TNF-α which initiates adherence of polymorphonuclear leukocytes (PMN) to pulmonary endothelium, and these phagocytes, in turn, release oxidants and lysosomal components which cause endothelial

267

damage (11–13). Even in the absence of neutrophils, endothelium can be damaged by TNF-α (14), but neutrophils are reported to enhance the injury (15). Thus, TNF-α appears to be a central effector responsible for the loss of alveolar–capillary barrier function, increased permeability pulmonary edema, and pulmonary vascular occlusion seen in ARDS (16).

Lack of a definitive treatment for either the sepsis syndrome (17) or ARDS (6,18) has resulted in the search for a ''magic therapeutic bullet.'' Immediate interest in pentoxifylline (PTXF) as a major advance in treating sepsis came when Raffin and colleagues reported that this agent attenuated acute lung injury in septic guinea pigs and reduced TNF-α-mediated cytotoxicity of endothelium when PMN were present (19,20). Other reports have corroborated and extended these findings (21–25). The observation that PTXF might mitigate ARDS was exciting because PTXF reduces monocyte TNF-α production, diminishes leukocyte adherence and aggregation, decreases neutrophil superoxide anion release and degranulation, lessens PMN responsiveness to TNF-α and interleukin-1, and lowers PMN priming by platelet-activity factor (26–29 and reviewed in Refs. 30 and 31). During the immune response to endotoxin, these effects of PTXF would be expected to reduce pulmonary endothelial damage mediated by TNF-α and neutrophils. Additional effects of PTXF that would also favor recovery from either the sepsis syndrome and/or ARDS are increased red blood cell deformability, reduced platelet and erythrocyte aggregation, diminished platelet adhesion, stimulation of fibrinolysis and anticoagulant properties, and inhibition of vasoconstriction (31–34). Each of these effects of PTXF would reduce pulmonary vascular occlusion, alleviate ventilation–perfusion mismatching, and enhance systemic oxygen delivery in ARDS induced by endotoxemia.

The preceding effects of PTXF have been largely studied in adult animal models of sepsis and/or ARDS. In these models, either gram-negative bacteria themselves or endotoxin isolated from these microorganisms have been utilized to initiate immune activation. Thus, the beneficial effects of PTXF on the sepsis syndrome and ARDS cannot be easily extrapolated to animals at younger ages or to gram-positive bacterial pathogens. For this reason, the authors have utilized infantile animal models of sepsis or pneumonia to study whether PTXF has therapeutic benefits in group B streptococcal (GBS) infections during infancy. Unlike the sepsis syndrome of adults, wherein gram-negative organisms predominate, group B streptococci (GBS) are the major pathogens responsible for neonatal pneumonia and bacteremia shortly after birth (35–37). Interestingly, the clinical features of neonatal GBS infections have many of the same characteristics seen in adults with sepsis and/or ARDS. These findings include (a) intense pulmonary inflammation with vascular occlusion involving PMN and platelets, (b) loss of capillary integrity manifest by pleural effusions, (c) profound hypoxemia, (d) shock, and (e) a high mortality.

The goals of this review are not to cover every physiological effect or novel therapeutic use of PTXF which have been reported recently (30,31). Rather, three specific topics will be discussed which are not included in recent reviews of pentoxifylline therapy. First, the use of PTXF therapy in experimental, neonatal GBS sepsis and pneumonia will be described. Our studies have utilized infantile piglets to offer new insights into the mechanisms whereby PTXF affects pulmonary hemodynamics and oxygen exchange during GBS sepsis, and this model established the relationships between TNF-α production and release of endogenous vasoactive effectors in the pulmonary circulation (38–40). Since GBS pneumonia and bacteremia have their most devastating effects in premature human newborns, a premature-rabbit model of pulmonary infection caused by GBS was developed. These animals were infected with GBS aerosols, and the studies showed that PTXF was effective in reducing TNF-α production in pulmonary alveoli during infection. Although the content of TNF-α was diminished, the lung's phagocytic defenses against GBS were not hindered (41). Second, our observations using neonatal animals infected with group B streptococci will be contrasted to PTXF treatment of adult models of sepsis and ARDS which are initiated by endotoxin or gram-negative bacteria. Finally, future directions for defining pentoxifylline's mechanisms of action during sepsis and ARDS will be outlined, and the importance of proper design to delineate the effectiveness of pentoxifylline in clinical trials of septic newborns and adults will be discussed.

II. INFANT MODELS OF GROUP B STREPTOCOCCAL (GBS) INFECTION

A. Infantile Piglets and GBS Bacteremia

The 2-week-old piglet is an ideal model for studying the hemodynamic, metabolic, and inflammatory consequences of GBS bacteremia on the cardiopulmonary system (38–40). Anesthetized and paralyzed animals are ventilated via a tracheostomy, and catheters are placed in the external jugular vein, aorta and left pulmonary artery (5 Fr Swan-Ganz thermodilution). The animals receive sigh breaths every 20 min to minimize atelectasis. Animals are maintained under a radiant heat source with core temperature monitoring.

To study the hemodynamic, metabolic, and inflammatory effects of GBS bacteremia, a bacterial suspension is infused at a rate of 1.25×10^9 colony-forming units (CFU) per kilogram body weight per hour via the jugular catheter. Prior to GBS infusion, each animal receives 10 mL of 0.9% sterile saline/kg B.W. to ensure a standardized euvolemic state. The GBS suspension is tested for endotoxin contamination and has < 0.03 endotoxin units/mL (<150 pg/mL) based on the Limulus amoebocyte lysate assay. The following parameters are monitored prior to and at 1, 2, and 4 h after beginning the GBS infusion: systemic arterial pressure, pulmonary artery and wedge pressures, cardiac output, arterial and mixed venous blood gas tensions, thromboxane B_2 (TxB_2), 6-keto-prostaglandin $F_{1\alpha}$, and tumor necrosis factor-α. Eicosanoids in aortic blood are drawn into a cold inhibitor solution containing indomethacin and sodium EDTA. A competitive radioimmunoassay is used to measure eicosanoid concentrations in plasma (42). A sandwich ELISA using rabbit anti-TNF-α and horseradish peroxidase-conjugated mouse monoclonal antibody (Genentech, Inc., San Francisco, CA) and the L-929 cell lytic bioassay are used to determine TNF levels in serum.

Pentoxifylline-treated animals received a bolus injection of the drug at 20 mg/kg B.W. given intravenously followed by a 20-mg/kg/h continuous infusion rate. In separate studies, animals also received a bolus injection of indomethacin (3 mg/kg) i.v. along with the PTXF. The GBS infusion was begun one-half hour after treatment. Control animals received either saline alone or PTXF alone.

B. Premature Rabbits and GBS Pneumonia

Although human newborns die from the hemodynamic and cardiopulmonary consequences of GBS infections, mortality is strongly linked to premature birth and the presence of congenital pneumonia. Immunologically nascent host defenses of the premature infant, particularly those present in the lung at birth, contribute to the high mortality (43). For this reason, a premature-animal model of GBS infection of the lung was developed (41). Briefly, at 28 days of completed gestation, preterm rabbit pups are delivered by hysterotomy. Thirty-one days of gestation is term in the rabbit, and 28 days of gestation in the premature rabbit is equivalent to 32 weeks of gestation in human infants. At 1 h of age, the animals are infected with GBS using an aerosol exposure chamber that produces uniform lung infection. Following aerosol exposure, the animals to be studied at later time intervals received 25 mg/kg B.W. of PXTF given by intraperitoneal injection. Pentoxifylline was administered again i.p. at 6 and 12 h after infection (12.5 mg/kg/dose). Immediately after aerosol infection, and at 4 and 24 h thereafter, numbers of viable GBS are measured in the aseptically removed left lung by standard pour-plate techniques. The remaining right lung is lavaged, and the numbers of leukocytes present at different intervals after infection are ascertained by counting cells recovered after centrifugation of the lavaged specimens. Wright-Giemsa-stained cytocentrifuge preparations are examined microscopically to determine the types of cells present and the numbers of GBS associated with alveolar macrophages versus neutrophils. The first two passages of cell-free lavage effluent are concentrated to dryness and, after rehydration, are used to measure the amount of TNF and lysozyme present in epithelial lining fluid (ELF). The L-929 cell lytic bioassay and the *Micrococcus lysodeikticus* lysoplate method were utilized to determine TNF and lysozyme content of ELF, respectively. The TNF content of ELF evaluates whether PTXF inhibited its production by macrophages and other pulmonary cells, while lysozyme serves as a marker of lysosomal degranulation and its blockade by PTXF. Although these animals weigh between 30 and 45 g, bacteremia can be assessed by obtaining blood via aseptic cardiac puncture. In addition to blood cultures, pentoxifylline levels could be analyzed in the serum of the recovered blood. We contrasted the concentrations of PTXF in blood with the amount present in epithelial lining fluid. Pentoxifylline and metabolite I in blood and ELF were measured by gas chromatography (44).

III. THE EFFECT OF PENTOXIFYLLINE ON THE BIOLOGICAL RESPONSES OF INFANTS TO GBS BACTEREMIA AND PNEUMONIA

A. Attenuation of TNF-α Production and Improvement in Pulmonary Hemodynamics and Hypoxemia During GBS Bacteremia in Piglets Receiving Pentoxifylline

It was postulated that the inhibitor of TNF production, pentoxifylline, would attenuate GBS-induced TNF production and ameliorate the late hemodynamic effects of GBS bacteremia (38). PTXF would act by reducing a TNF-mediated increase in thromboxane A_2 (TxA_2), a pulmonary vasoconstrictor, and by lowering a TNF-induced increase in prostacyclin (PGI_2), a systemic vasodilator. In piglets infused with 1.25×10^9 CFU/kg/h of GBS, Figure 1 shows that serum TNF levels (pg/mL, ELISA assay) increased significantly by 4 h ($1{,}047 \pm 41$) compared to animals given GBS + PTXF concurrently (208 ± 39, mean $\pm$ SEM, $p < 0.02$). Piglets given saline or PTXF i.v. had no detectable TNF after 4 h. Despite this fivefold reduction in the blood's TNF content, PTXF therapy was associated with a more modest reduction in pulmonary vascular resistance (Fig. 2) and less dramatic improvement in oxygenation after 4 h of GBS bacteremia ($PaO_2 = 59 \pm 3$ mm Hg for GBS alone versus 72 ± 2 mm Hg for GBS + PTXF, $p < 0.05$). The finding that PTXF therapy had less substantial benefit on pulmonary gas exchange was explained by similar serum levels of TxB_2 after 4 h of bacteremia (GBS alone $= 139 \pm 33$ pg/0.1 mL versus GBS + PTXF $= 176 \pm 45$). As indicated above, pulmonary hypertension during GBS bacteremia is associated with increased TxA_2 and has been evaluated during in-vivo infection by measuring its stable metabolite, TxB_2. Furthermore, PTXF therapy did not attenuate the systemic hypotension and reduced cardiac output seen in piglets receiving a continuous infusion of GBS. PTXF actually enhanced the production of 6-keto-$PGF_{1\alpha}$, the stable metabolite of PGI_2, in piglets subjected to 4 h of GBS bacteremia (GBS + PTXF $= 306 \pm 75$ pg/0.1 mL versus GBS alone $= 85 \pm 18$, $p < 0.05$). This observation suggests that GBS stimulates

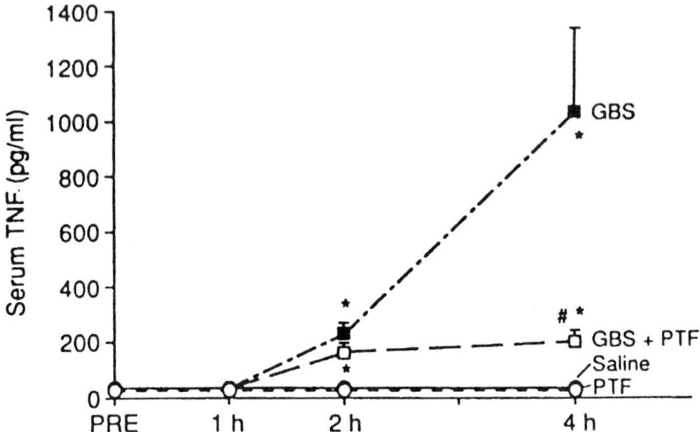

Figure 1 The effect of pentoxifylline (PTF) on tumor necrosis factor (TNF) production induced by group B streptococci (GBS). The four experimental groups are identified in the figure. Data presented as mean $\pm$ SEM. The asterisk indicates $p <$ 0.05 compared to the intragroup PRE value. The # signifies $p < 0.05$ for GBS + PTF compared to GBS at the same time point.

release of TxA^2 and PGI^2 independently of TNF production, or that residual GBS-induced TNF activity was sufficient to contribute to elevations of these arachidonic acid metabolites. Higher doses of PTXF might have further reduced TNF production in this piglet model of GBS sepsis, but done so at the risk of a more pronounced reduction in systemic resistance. For this reason, a second study was undertaken in which piglets were pretreated with a combination of PTXF and indomethacin, an inhibitor of arachidonic acid metabolism, prior to the initiation of GBS bacteremia (39). Indomethacin, which had no effect on GBS-induced TNF production, prevented increases in TxB_2 and 6-keto-$PGF_{1\alpha}$ after 4 h of GBS bacteremia when utilized in combination with PTXF (each being <10 pg/0.1 mL). Cardiac output was also higher in piglets receiving both agents (0.66 $\pm$ 0.05 L/min) when compared to animals receiving either GBS alone (0.50 $\pm$ 0.04) or GBS + indomethacin (0.38 $\pm$ 0.06, $p < 0.05$). We conclude that the beneficial effects of PTXF and indomethacin in GBS bacteremia suggest that there is no "magic bullet therapy" and that adjunctive therapy for GBS sepsis will require more than one agent if there is to be clinical success.

B. Reduced Intraalveolar TNF-α and Improved Intrapulmonary Inactivation of GBS in Premature Rabbits Treated with Pentoxifylline

It was postulated that PTXF therapy would reduce intraalveolar TNF content after intrapulmonary GBS infection of premature rabbits, but it was unknown

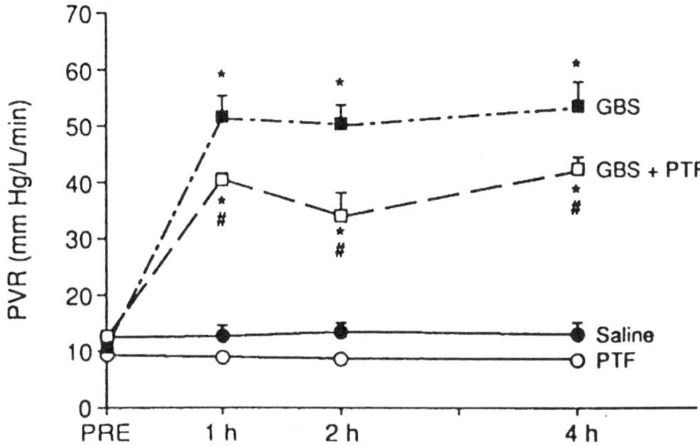

Figure 2 The effect of pentoxifylline (PTF) on increases in pulmonary vascular resistance (PVR) induced by group B streptococci (GBS). The four experimental groups are identified in the figure. Data presented as mean ± SEM. The asterisk indicates $p < 0.05$ compared to the intragroup PRE value. The # signifies $p < 0.05$ for GBS + PTF compared to GBS at the same point.

whether this effect would benefit or hinder phagocytic host defenses against GBS. In this preterm-animal model, pulmonary alveolar macrophages are present in low numbers at the time of birth. This circumstance is also observed in premature human neonates at the time of parturition. Thus, recruitment of functioning PMN is essential to intrapulmonary host defense when congenital bacterial pneumonia is present. Previous in-vitro reports indicate that PTXF treatment of PMN reduces their mobility, superoxide production, and degranulation. Each of these components of PMN function is thought to be important in killing intraalveolar GBS, and concern was raised whether PTXF's effects on neutrophils might impair host defense.

Twenty-four hours after GBS aerosol infection, the L-929 lytic assay showed that TNF in bronchoalveolar lavage fluid was significantly lower in PTXF-treated rabbit pups (828 ± 82 U/mL) compared to untreated, GBS-infected animals (12,840 ± 5520 U/mL, mean ± SEM, $p < 0.005$). The difference remained if corrected for the numbers of macrophages present in the lavage effluent (13 ± 5 versus 91 ± 40 U/macrophage, $p < 0.03$). Importantly, this reduction in TNF content at the alveolar surface did not impair phagocytic function. Twenty-four hours after infection, the numbers of GBS in the lungs of PTXF-treated animals was more than fourfold below that seen in untreated pups (Fig. 3, top). Calculated intrapulmonary clearance of GBS, which is based on comparing the numbers of GBS in the lungs at 24 h versus bacterial counts measured in a separate group of animals immediately after aerosol infection, verified the benefit of PTXF therapy (Fig. 3, bottom). As expected, there were small numbers of PAM, and essentially no PMN, in the lavage effluent of both PTX and saline groups immediately after infection (Fig. 4). Nevertheless, total cell counts rose rapidly after aerosol infection, and at 24 h after infection, PMN were the predominate type of phagocyte present in lavage specimens. At no time point were significant differences noted in either PMN or macrophage counts between the PTXF- and placebo-treated animals. Furthermore, microscopic analysis of the phagocytes recovered from lavage specimens revealed that similar phagocytic rates and profiles were seen in macrophages and neutrophils regardless of whether animals received PTXF therapy (Table 1). Thus, we have concluded that PTXF did not impair PMN or macrophage mobility or phagocytosis as has been suggested by previous in-vitro studies. The assumption that PTXF therapy would impair degranulation of neutrophils, however, did seem to be evident. Lysozyme activity in the bronchoalveolar lavage fluid of PTXF-treated animals was 7.2 ± 4.4 µg/mL compared to 19.8 ± 4.4 µg/mL in newborn rabbits receiving placebo therapy ($p < 0.02$). Since newborn alveolar macrophage have very low concentrations of lysozyme, the lysozyme activity in bronchoalveolar lavage fluid was corrected for PMN content in the specimen and the differences remained (PTXF = 11.6 ± 9.2 versus placebo = 21.3 ± 7.5, $p < 0.03$). We speculated that the retention of microbicidal effectors in the lysosomes of PMN may have enhanced their antibacterial activity once they reached the alveoli. This would explain the reduced numbers of GBS in the lungs of PXTF-treated animals. Nevertheless, the mechanisms responsible for improved GBS killing in the lungs of premature animals treated with PTXF remain incompletely defined. Finally, the incidence of bacteremia at 24 h after aerosol infection was very high in both PTXF- (16 of 17) and placebo-treated (19 of 20) pups, while mortality at 24 h was comparable in the two groups (PTXF = 6/25 and placebo = 4/25). Our findings support pentoxifylline as an adjunctive therapy for GBS pneumonia and bacteremia in newborns, but we propose that this agent is not the entire answer to this devastating disease. Perhaps the most important aspect of the PTXF studies using premature animals is that TNF production can be reduced locally without impairing host defense. Lower TNF production in tissues may be associated with less organ injury and a better overall outcome. Clinical trials using PTXF as an adjunctive treatment need to address this presumption.

IV. COMPARISON OF PENTOXIFYLLINE EFFECTIVENESS IN TREATING THE SEPSIS SYNDROME IN NEWBORNS VERSUS ADULTS

There are limited animal and human studies which have examined the benefits of PTXF on cardiopulmonary stability during endotoxemia. Demling and colleagues pretreated adult sheep with a 20-mg/kg bolus of PTXF followed by a constant

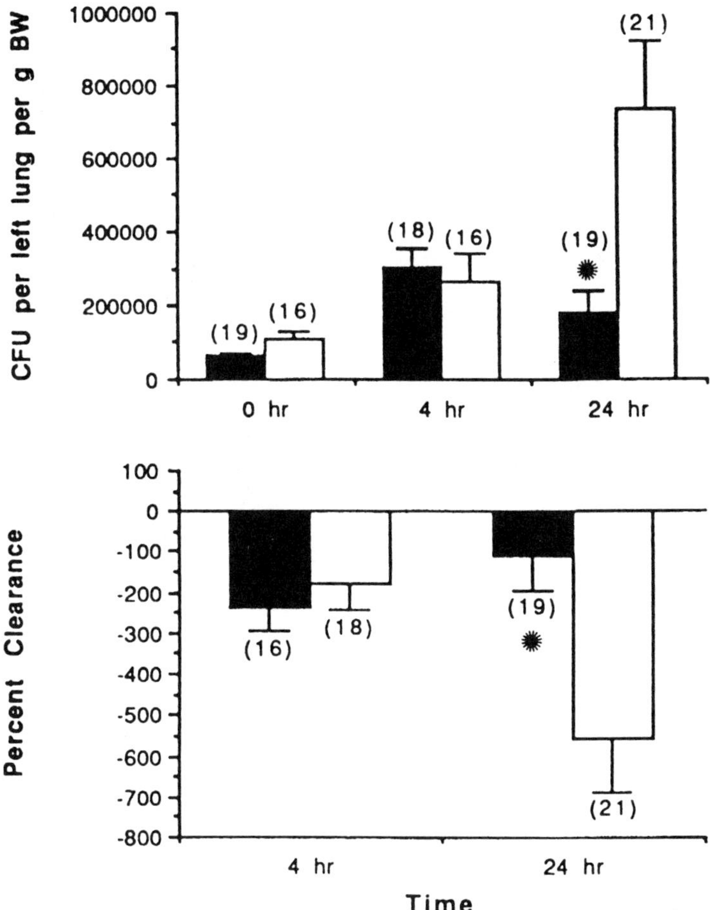

Figure 3 Top: Effect of pentoxifylline on the numbers in group B streptococci in lung at the three time intervals (0, 4, and 24 h) after aerosol infection of premature rabbits. Pentoxifylline-treated animals are indicated by the solid bars, while placebo (saline)-treated animals are depicted by the open bars. Error bars represent SEM; values in parentheses are the number of animals studied. The asterisk signifies $p < 0.03$ for pentoxifylline- versus placebo-treated animals. Abbreviations: CFU = colony-forming units; BW = birth weight. Bottom: Intrapulmonary clearance of group B streptococci at 4 and 24 h after aerosol infection. Mean clearance of inhaled group B streptococci is shown for the pentoxifylline-treated animals (solid bars) and for the placebo (saline)-treated animals (open bars). A negative clearance, which was always present in treated and control animals, indicates net bacterial proliferation from 0 h. Error bars represent SEM; values in parentheses indicate the number of animals studied. The asterisk signifies $p < 0.01$ for pentoxifylline versus placebo.

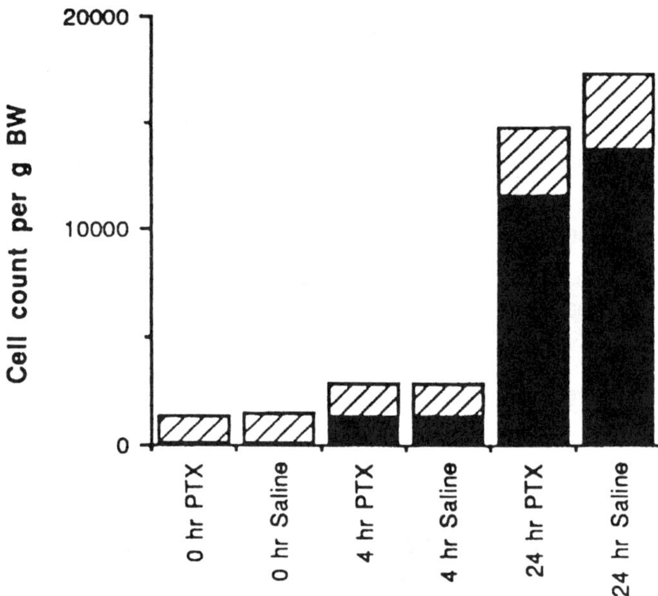

Figure 4   Intrapulmonary phagocyte kinetics observed by lavaging the right lung at three intervals (0, 4, and 24 h) after aerosol infection. Mean neutrophil counts (solid bars) and alveolar macrophage counts (hatched bars) in the bronchoalveolar lavage fluid were equated to gram body weight. Abbreviations: BW = body weight; PTX = pentoxifylline.

infusion rate of 6 mg/kg/h to evaluate the hemodynamic state of these animals following the intravenous administration of 5 µg/kg of endotoxin (45). PTXF pretreatment did not attenuate the initial pulmonary hypertension observed in sheep given an endotoxin infusion, but it did improve the late hyperdynamic state observed after endotoxin administration. These findings contrast with studies by Sigurdsson and Youssef, where pretreatment of sheep with PTXF improved mean arterial pressure and gas exchange four hours after *Escherichia coli* endotoxin was infused, although increased pulmonary artery pressure and reduced cardiac output were unaffected (46). These investigators emphasized that pretreatment with PTXF was absolutely essential to reduce platelet sequestration in the pulmonary vasculature. At a lower dose (3 mg/kg/h i.v.), PTXF attenuated the systemic hypotension, reduced cardiac output, and elevated pulmonary wedge pressure observed in Yucatan minipigs made septic with an i.p. injection of *E. coli* (47). These three studies illustrate the mitigating effects of PTXF on the hemodynamic responses of adult animals who have endotoxemia; they also stress that species differences, the nature of the inciting agent, and the manner of the drug's adminis-

Table 1 Phagocytic Profiles of Neutrophils and Pulmonary Alveolar Macrophages Obtained from Bronchoalveolar Lavage Fluid at 24 h After Aerosol Infection

		Ingestion rate (%)	Phagocytic index
Treatment group			
Pentoxifylline (16)[a]	Neutrophils	34.4 ± 4.2[b]	2.9 ± 0.5
	Macrophages	59.2 ± 4.2	16.4 ± 2.6
Control group			
Saline (19)	Neutrophils	34.8 ± 3.8	4.2 ± 0.7
	Macrophages	56.3 ± 4.0	18.1 ± 2.3

[a]Number of animals.
[b]Mean ± SEM.

tration may influence the study's results. Furthermore, these studies suggest that endotoxemia in adult animals may respond less favorably to PTXF therapy compared to the cardiopulmonary improvement observed in neonatal animals given PTXF during GBS infection. From newborn and adult studies, it is apparent that pretreatment enhances PTXF's effectiveness, an observation which has substantial clinical importance.

Healthy human subjects have been given oral ibuprofen or pentoxifylline before endotoxin administration, and these individuals showed no improvement in their cardiac output or oxygen delivery versus subjects receiving endotoxin alone (48). Over a 6-h period, patients with ARDS also showed no improvement in their hemodynamic status or gas exchange while receiving a 1-mg/kg bolus of PTXF followed by an infusion of 1.5 mg/kg/h (49). PTXF (5 mg/kg/h for 6 h) did improve the oxygenation of a newborn infant with pneumonia and pulmonary hypertension caused by *E. coli* (50). These isolated reports, however, will not substitute for controlled, randomized clinical trials, which are needed to demonstrate the efficacy of PTXF in the treatment of the sepsis syndrome.

Neonatal and adult responses to PTXF therapy extended beyond its effects on hemodynamics and gas exchange. In-vitro studies of adult alveolar macrophages reported that their stimulated migration would be inhibited by PTXF (51). This proved not to be the case during in-vivo GBS pneumonia of newborn rabbits; in our studies, interstitial or intravascular macrophages were recruited to the alveoli after aerosol infection, wherein they were actively phagocytic. Furthermore, in premature rabbits receiving PTXF, intrapulmonary neutrophils appeared to function more optimally in GBS infection, a finding consistent with in-vitro studies of human neonatal PMN (52,53). Thus, one cannot conclude that PTXF's effects on adult phagocytes are comparable to those observed in newborn PMN, monocytes, and tissue macrophages. The beneficial effects of PTXF on newborn PMN may be dose-dependent, as pointed out by Krause et al. (53). Given the wide range of pentoxifylline's actions in newborns and adults, investigators must decide where research using this drug should be headed in the future.

V. FUTURE DIRECTIONS

This review started by defining the relationships between the sepsis syndrome and ARDS. The similarities between GBS sepsis in neonates and an ARDS-like clinical presentation were also outlined. Interestingly, the benefits of PTXF in these clinical states may be related to the drug's action in modulating the lung's response to injury. In the future, PTXF may assist in the lung's repair after injury via the following actions. Pentoxifylline may reverse the inhibition of surfactant synthesis induced by TNF-α (54), and PTXF may assist in the remodeling of the lung's vasculature (55).

Pentoxifylline's effects may extend beyond the inhibition of TNF production. Recently, PTXF was shown to inhibit HIV replication by blocking nuclear factor kappa B (NF-κB) activation and nuclear binding (56). Since expression of inducible nitric oxide synthase requires NF-κB activation, we tested whether PTXF could inhibit the nitric oxide synthase activity of rat alveolar macrophages exposed to endotoxin. These activated macrophages had a 50% reduction in nitric oxide production when incubated with 5 mM PTXF (M. P. Sherman and D. C. Morrison, unpublished observations). Since excessive nitric oxide production may mediate hypotension during endotoxemia, PTXF may be responsible for reversing shock via this mechanism. Clearly, the actions of PTXF during endotoxemia may be more complex than were previously appreciated, and new mechanisms for its effects must be explored.

Finally, despite a wealth of reports about pentoxifylline's activity in septic animals, there is little information regarding its effectiveness in the clinical bacterial infections. One reason for a lack of clinical trials may be that PTXF is not licensed for intravenous use in the United States. Randomized trials studying newborns and adults are needed to establish or reject PTXF as an adjunctive therapy for the sepsis syndrome. This research may require special permission from the FDA to obtain and use intravenous preparations which are available in Europe. The design of these trials will be crucial. The aforementioned animal studies repeatedly indicated that PTXF must be given before or near the onset of endotoxemia. It may have been early administration which was responsible for pentoxifylline's success in preventing toxicity associated with bone marrow transplantation (57). Studies on the effectiveness of pentoxifylline to alleviate morbidity and mortality in the sepsis syndrome may also be best undertaken by targeting potential victims early in their hospital course. These subjects might include patients who have experienced extensive burns, significant trauma, cardiopulmonary bypass, or extreme prematurity. Only well-designed studies will answer whether pentoxifylline is a pretender to the throne or a drug with a lofty place in medical history.

REFERENCES

1. Bone RC. The pathogenesis of sepsis. Ann Intern Med 1991; 115:457–469.
2. Nathan C, Sporn M. Cytokines in context. J Cell Biol 1991; 113:981–986.
3. Dinarello CA, Wolff SM. The role of interleukin-1 in disease. N Engl J Med 1993; 328:106–113.
4. The Veterans Administration Systemic Sepsis Cooperative Study. Effect of high-dose glucocorticoid therapy on mortality in patients with clinical signs of systemic sepsis. N Engl J Med 1987; 317:659–665.
5. Danner RL, Elin RJ, Hosseini JM, Wesley RA, Reilly JM, Parrillo JE. Endotoxemia in septic shock. Chest 1991; 99:165–175.
6. Repine JE. Scientific perspectives on adult respiratory distress. Lancet 1992; 339:466–469.
7. Tracey KL, Lowry SF, Cerami A. Cachectin/TNF-α in septic shock and septic adult respiratory distress syndrome. Am Rev Respir Dis 1988; 138: 1377–1379.
8. Suter PM, Suter S, Girardin E, Roux-Lombard P, Grau GE, Dayer JM. High bronchoalveolar levels of tumor necrosis factor and its inhibitors, interleukin-1, interferon and elastase, in patients with adult respiratory distress syndrome after trauma, shock, and sepsis. Am Rev Respir Dis 1992; 145:1016–1022.
9. Tran Van Nhieu J, Misset B, Lebargy F, Carlet J, Bernaudin J-F. Expression of tumor necrosis factor-α gene in alveolar macrophages from patients with the adult respiratory distress syndrome. Am Rev Respir Dis 1993; 147:1585–1589.
10. Meyrick B, Brigham KL. Acute effects of *E. coli* endotoxin on the pulmonary microcirculation of anesthetized sheep. Lab Invest 1983; 48:458–470.
11. Gamble JR, Smith WB, Vadas MA. TNF modulation of endothelial and neutrophil adhesion. In: Beutler B, ed. Tumor Necrosis Factors: The Molecules and Their Emerging Role in Medicine. New York: Raven Press, 1992:65–86.
12. Zimmerman GA, Renzetti AD, Hill HR. Functional and metabolic activity of granulocytes from patients with ARDS. Am Rev Respir Dis 1983; 127:290–300.
13. Haslett C, Worthen GS, Giclas PC, Morrison DC, Henson JE, Henson PM. The pulmonary vascular sequestration of neutrophils in endotoxemia is initiated by an effect of endotoxin on the neutrophil in the rabbit. Am Rev Respir Dis 1987; 136:9–18.
14. Horvath CJ, Ferro TH, Jesmok G, Malik AB. Recombinant tumour necrosis factor increases pulmonary vascular permeability independent of neutrophils. Proc Natl Acad Sci USA 1988; 85:9219–9223.
15. Zheng H, Crowley JJ, Chan JC, et al. Attenuation of tumor necrosis factor induced endothelial cytotoxicity and neutrophil chemiluminescence. Am Rev Respir Dis 1990; 142:1073–1078.
16. Bachofen M, Weibel ER. Structural alterations of lung parenchyma in adult respiratory distress syndrome. Clin Chest Med 1982; 3:35–56.

17. Natason C, Hoffman WD, Suffredini AF, Eichacker PQ, Danner RL. Selected treatment strategies for septic shock based on proposed mechanisms of pathogenesis. Ann Intern Med 1994; 120:771–783.

18. Lewis JF, Jobe AH. Surfactant and the adult respiratory distress syndrome. Am Rev Respir Dis 1993; 147:218–233.

19. Ishizaka A, Wu Z, Stephens KE, et al. Attenuation of acute lung injury in septic guinea pigs by pentoxifylline. Am Rev Respir Dis 1988; 138:376–382.

20. Lilly CM, Sandhu JS, Ishizaka A, et al. Pentoxifylline inhibits prevents tumor necrosis factor-induced lung injury. Am Rev Respir Dis 1989; 139:1361–1368.

21. Welsh CH, Lien D, Worthen GS, Weil JV. Pentoxifylline decreases endotoxin-induced pulmonary neutrophil sequestration and extravascular protein accumulation in the dog. Am Rev Respir Dis 1988; 138:1106–1114.

22. Lilly CM, O'Hanley PT, Raffin TA. The effects of aminophyline and pentoxifylline on multiple organ damage after *Escherichia coli* sepsis. Am Rev Respir Dis 1989; 140:974–980.

23. Seenar MD, Hannam VL, Kaapa P, Raj JU, O'Brodovich HM. Effect of pentoxifylline on hemodynamics, alveolar fluid reabsorption, and pulmonary edema in a model of acute lung injury. Am Rev Respir Dis 1990; 142:1083–1087.

24. McDonald RJ. Pentoxifylline reduces injury to isolated lungs perfused with human neutrophils. Am Rev Respir Dis 1991; 144:1347–1350.

25. Sato K, Stelzner TJ, O'Brien RF, Weil JV, Welsh CH. Pentoxifylline lessens the endotoxin-induced increase in albumin clearance across pulmonary artery endothelial monolayers with and without neutrophils. Am J Respir Cell Mol Biol 1991; 4:219–227.

26. Bessler H, Gilgal R, Djaldetti M, Zahavi I. Effect of pentoxifylline on the phagocytic activity, cAMP levels, and superoxide anion production by monocytes and polymorphonuclear cells. J Leukoc Biol 1986; 40:747–754.

27. Sullivan GW, Carper HT, Novick WJ Jr, Mandell GL. Inhibition of the inflammatory action of interleukin-1 and tumor necrosis factor (alpha) on neutrophil function by pentoxifylline. Infect Immun 1988; 56:1722–1729.

28. Strieter RM, Remick DG, Ward PA, et al. Cellular and molecular regulation of tumor necrosis factor-alpha production by pentoxifylline. Biochem Biophys Res Commun 1988; 155:1230–1236.

29. Currie MS, Rao KMK, Padmanabhan J, Jones A, Crawford J, Cohen HJ. Stimulus-specific effects of pentoxifylline on neutrophil CR3 expression, degranulation, and superoxide production. J Leukoc Biol 1990; 47:244–250.

30. Zabel P, Schade FU, Schlaak M. Inhibition of endogenous TNF formation by pentoxifylline. Immunobiol 1993; 147:147–163.

31. Samlaska CP, Winfield EA. Pentoxifylline. J Am Acad Dermatol 1994; 30:603–621.

32. Ohdama S, Takano S, Ohashi K, Miyaka S, Aoki N. Pentoxifylline prevents tumor necrosis factor-induced suppression of endothelial cell surface thrombomodulin. Thromb Res 1991; 62:745–755.

33. Ollivier V, Tarnisiene C, Vu T, Hakim J, de Prost D. Pentoxifylline inhibits

expression of tissue factor mRNA in endotoxin-activated human monocytes. FEBS Lett 1993; 322:231–234.

34. Levi M, ten Cate M, Bauer KA, et al. Inhibition of endotoxin-induced activation and fibrinolysis by pentoxifylline or a monoclonal anti-tissue factor antibody in chimpanzees. J Clin Invest 1994; 93:114–120.

35. Sherman M, Goetzman B, Ahlfors C, Wennberg R. Tracheal aspiration and its clinical correlates in the diagnosis of congenital pneumonia. Pediatrics 1980; 65:258–263.

36. Sherman MP, Chance KH, Goetzman BW. Gram's stains of tracheal secretions predict neonatal bacteremia. Am J Dis Child 1984; 138:848–850.

37. Webber S, Wilkinson AR, Lindsell D, Hope PL, Dobson SRM, Issacs D. Neonatal pneumonia. Arch Dis Child 1990; 65:207–211.

38. Gibson RL, Redding GJ, Henderson WR, Truog WE. Group B *Streptococcus* induces tumor necrosis factor in neonatal piglets. Effect of the tumor necrosis factor inhibitor pentoxifylline on hemodynamics and gas exchange. Am Rev Respir Dis 1991; 143:598–604.

39. Gibson RL, Truog WE, Henderson WR Jr Redding GJ. Group B streptocoocal sepsis in piglets: effect of combined pentoxifylline and indomethacin pretreatment. Pediatr Res 1992; 31:222–227.

40. Truog WE, Gibson RL Jr, Henderson WR Jr, Redding GJ, Standaert TA. Effect of pentoxifylline on cytokine- and eicosanoid-induced acute pulmonary hypertension in piglets. Pediatr Res 31; 31:163–169.

41. Mah MP, Aeberhard EE, Gilliam MB, Sherman MP. Effects of pentoxifylline on *in vivo* leukocyte function and clearance of group B streptococci from preterm rabbit lungs. Crit Care Med 1993; 21:712–720.

42. Truog WE, Gibson RL, Juul SE, Henderson WR, Redding GJ. Neonatal group B streptococcal sepsis: effects of late treatment with dazmegrel. Pediatr Res 1988; 23:352–356.

43. Sherman MP, Ganz T. Host defense in pulmonary alveoli. Annu Rev Physiol 1992; 54:331–350.

44. Burrows JL. Determination of oxpentifylline and three metabolites in plasma by automated capillary gas chromatography. J Chromatogr 1987; 423:139–146.

45. Youn YK, Knox J, Lalonde C, Demling R. Pentoxifylline does not prevent endotoxin induced lung and liver lipid peroxidation in the adult sheep. Circ Shock 1993; 39:39–49.

46. Sigurdsson GH, Youssef H. Effects of pentoxifylline on hemodynamics, gas exchange and multiple organ platelet sequestration in experimental septic shock. Acta Anaesthesiol Scand 1993; 37:396–403.

47. Law WR, Nadkarni VM, Fletcher MA, et al. Pentoxifylline treatment of sepsis in conscious Yucatan minipigs. Circ Shock 1992; 37:291–300.

48. Martich GD, Parker MM, Cunnion RE, Suffredini AF. Effects of ibuprofen and pentoxifylline on the cardiovascular response of humans to endotoxin. J Appl Physiol 1992; 73:925–931.

49. Montravers P, Fagon J-Y, Gilbert C, Blanchet F, Novara A, Chastre J. Pilot study

of cardiovascular risk from pentoxifylline in adult respiratory distress syndrome. Chest 1993; 103:1017–1022.

50. Lauterbach R. Pentoxifylline treatment of persistent pulmonary hypertension of newborn. Eur J Pediatr 1993; 152:460.

51. Williams JH Jr, Heshmati S, Tamadon S, Guerra J. Inhibition of alveolar macrophages by pentoxifylline. Crit Care Med 1991; 19:1073–1078.

52. Krause PJ, Kristie J, Wang W-P, et al. Pentoxifylline enhancement of defective neutrophil function and host defense in neonatal mice. Am J Pathol 1987; 129:217–222.

53. Krause PJ, Maderazo EG, Contrino J, et al. Modulation of neutrophil function by pentoxifylline. Pediatr Res 1991; 29:123–127.

54. Balibrea-Cantero JL, Arias-Diaz J, Garcia C, et al. Effect of pentoxifylline on the inhibition of surfactant synthesis induced by TNF-α in human type II pneumocytes. Am J Respir Crit Care Med 1994; 149:669–706.

55. Kullman A, Vaillant P, Muller V, Martinet Y, Martinet N. *In vitro* effects of pentoxifylline on smooth muscle migration and blood monocyte production of chemotactic activity for smooth muscle cells: potential therapeutic benefit in adult respiratory distress syndrome. Am J Respir Cell Mol Biol 1993; 8:83–88.

56. Biswas DK, Dezube BJ, Ahlers CM, Pardee AB. Pentoxifylline inhibits HIV-1 LTR-driven gene expression by blocking NF-κB action. J Acquir Immune Defic Syndr 1993; 6:778–786.

57. Bianco JA, Appelbaum FR, Nemuniatis J, et al. Phase I-II trial of pentoxifylline for the prevention of transplant-related toxicities following bone marrow transplantation. Blood 1991; 78:1205–1211.

16

The Potential Role of PAF Antagonists in the Therapy of Sepsis

Daniel H. Albert, James B. Summers, and Hollis D. Kleinert
Abbott Laboratories
Abbott Park, Illinois

I. PLATELET-ACTIVATING FACTOR

A. Basics

1. Structure

Platelet activating factor (PAF, 1-O-alkyl-2-(R)-acetyl-sn-glyceryl-3-phospho-choline) is an endogenous phospholipid which serves as an immunologic mediator. The alkyl ether group is usually 16 or 18 carbons in length but varies with cell type and species.

2. Biosynthesis of PAF

The synthesis of PAF proceeds primarily through a remodeling pathway in which a long-chain fatty acid is first removed from the C_2 position of the ether-linked analogs of phosphatidyl choline to produce biologically inactive *lyso*-PAF. This species is then acetylated in the presence of acetyl coenzyme A to produce PAF(1). Although a de-novo synthetic pathway has also been described (2), the remodeling pathway is believed to be primarily responsible for PAF synthesis in the inflammatory response.

3. Location of PAF, Receptorology, and Functional Properties

PAF is synthesized by a variety of cells, including inflammatory cells and noninflammatory cells such as eosinophils, macrophages, monocytes, mast cells, platelets, Kupffer cells, endothelial cells, fibroblasts, kidney cells, and gastric mucosal cells.

PAF binds primarily to a single class of high-affinity GTP-coupled receptors (1), located on platelets, eosinophils, neutrophils, and macrophages, and in brain, kidney, liver, eye, uterus, small intestine, and lung tissue. These receptors are located on the cell surface and intracellularly. The phospholipid nature of PAF allows for cell penetration and participation in intracellular biochemical events, as well as cell membrane activities. The term PAF does not do justice to the versatile nature of this molecule. As described below, PAF is involved in modulating not only platelet activation, but also a variety of organ systems. This substance has the capacity to function as autocoid, paracoid, or truly humoral in manner, depending on whether it remains within the cell of origin, is secreted outside the cell of origin to act on an adjacent cell, or travels through the body to a distant site following synthesis and secretion at a primary site, respectively.

4. In-Vivo Fate

PAF has an in-vivo half-life of only a few minutes, due to the action of extracellular and intracellular PAF acetylhydrolase, which converts PAF to *lyso*-PAF (3). *lyso*-PAF can in turn be reacylated by a transacylase.

5. Quantification of PAF

Several methods to assay PAF have been reported, including rabbit bioassays after chromatographic separation of the lipid extract, radioimmunoassays, gas chromatography in conjunction with mass spectrometry, and radioreceptor-binding assays (4). The quantitation of PAF, however, is challenging and not routinely performed either in animal or clinical studies. The difficulty in quantitating PAF lies both in the elaborate extraction procedures required to isolate it and in its rapid metabolism.

B. PAF and the Pathophysiology of Sepsis

The association of PAF with sepsis is multifold. First, the administration of PAF mimics the sepsis state. Table 1 delineates the functions implicating PAF in sepsis (4). These hemodynamic and inflammatory effects result in organ injury, dysfunction, and possibly failure, with ensuing death. Second, PAF levels have been reported to be elevated following endotoxin administration to rats (5) and in the blood of sepsis patients (6). Third, as described in the section below, PAF antagonists attenuate the untoward sequelae of sepsis and septic shock.

Table 1 Pharmacological Actions of PAF: Mimicry of Shock Pathophysiology

Blood	Respiratory system
Platelet activation	Increased airway resistance
Leukocyte activation	Compliance reduction
Hyperfibrinolysis	Congestion
Cardiovascular system	Production of leukotrienes
Arrhythmias	Bronchial hyperreactivity
Negative inotropism	Edema
Coronary constriction	Liver
Extravasation	Vascular constriction
Hemoconcentration	Glycogenolysis
Systemic hypotension	Inositol turnover
Pulmonary hypertension	Gastrointestinal tract
Skin	Ischemic necrosis
Erythema	Ileum contraction
Edema	Gastric ulceration
Leukocyte infiltration	Kidney
Metabolism	Diminution of blood flux
Hyperglycogenesis	Diminution of filtration
Hyperglycemia	Diminution of Na excretion
Hypoinsulinemia	
Hypertriglyceridemia	

Source: From Ref. 4, with permission.

II. ACTIVITY OF PAF ANTAGONISTS IN ANIMAL MODELS OF SEPTIC SHOCK

A. Rodent Models of Septic Shock

Lipopolysaccharide (LPS, endotoxin) from gram-negative organisms evokes in rodents many of the hallmarks of septic shock. Responses to LPS injection or infusion include: systemic hypotension, increased vascular permeability and organ damage, disseminated intravascular coagulation (DIC), and high mortality. As described below, each of these responses can be ameliorated, albeit to different degrees, by administration of PAF antagonists.

1. Hypotension

Infusion or intraperitoneal injection of LPS (10–30 mg/kg) into rats induces a transient fall in mean arterial pressure followed by a partial recovery and then a sustained period of hypotension which reaches a maximum of about 60% baseline 30 min after challenge (Fig. 2). Virtually all PAF antagonists tested in the rat have displayed at least some efficacy for blocking this hypotension. In general, the dosage necessary for blocking the hypotensive response is related

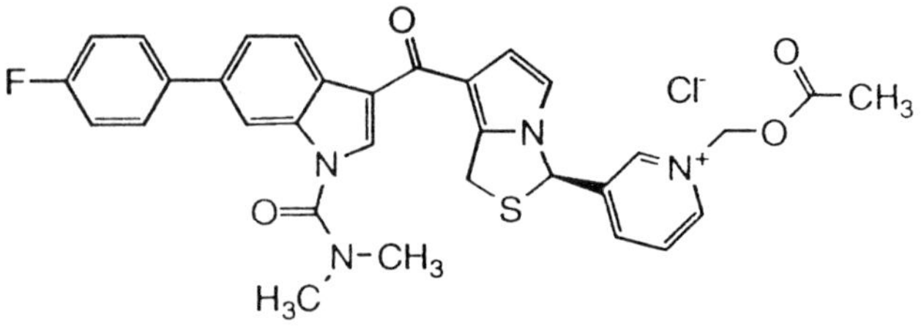

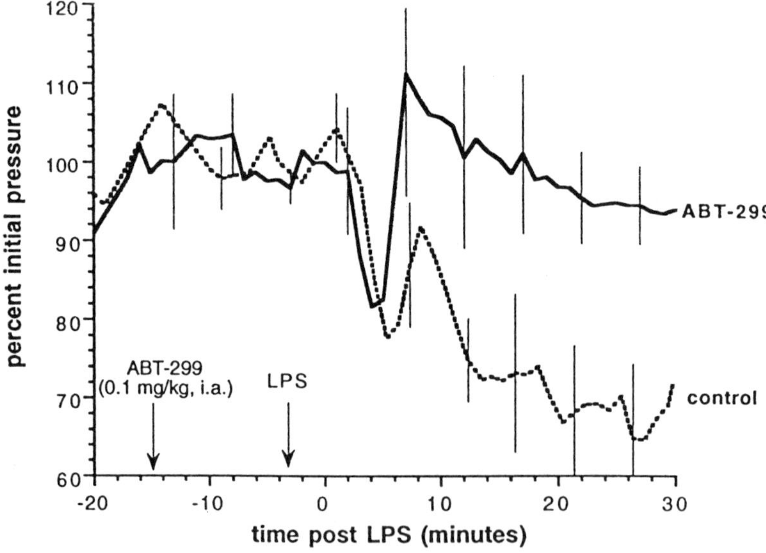

Figure 1 Structure of the platelet-activating factor receptor antagonist, ABT-299.

to the potency of the antagonists against a PAF challenge. Early antagonists with in-vivo potencies in the mg/kg range (CV-3988, Kadsurenone, WEB 2086, BN52021) are less effective, whereas the newer, more potent (0.01–0.1 mg/ kg) antagonists (ABT-299, CL 184,005) completely prevent hypotension when administered prior to LPS (5,7–10). This is illustrated for ABT-299 (Fig. 1), an example of an indole-containing pyrdinium pyrrolothiazole that exhibits potent PAF antagonist activity in vitro (human platelets, $K_i = 0.3$ nM) (11).

PAF antagonists are also capable of reversing established LPS-induced hypotension. As shown in Fig. 3, when ABT-299 (0.1 mg/kg, intraarterially) was

Figure 2 Inhibition of LPS-induced hypotension following pretreatment (15 min) with ABT-299 (0.1 mg/kg, intraarterially) in rat. Data are expressed as the mean of the group ($n = 4$) ± standard deviation.

given as late as 60 min after LPS, the ongoing hypotension was reversed and the mean arterial pressure restored to baseline. Other impressive examples are CL 184,005 and TCV-309, which reversed the response at an intravenous (i.v.) dose of 10 μg/kg (10,12).

The effectiveness of PAF antagonists in preventing and reversing LPS-induced hypotension clearly implicates PAF as an important mediator in this aspect of sepsis. Other vasoactive mediators are also induced during sepsis and may have a role in producing the hypotensive response. Cyclooxygenase and 5-lipoxygenase blockade modifies LPS-induced hypotension (13), although not to the same extent as can be achieved with a PAF antagonist. Cytokines such as interleukin-1β (IL-1β) and tumor necrosis factor alpha (TNF-α) are also elevated in sepsis and induce a shocklike syndrome when administered to animals (14). PAF, IL-1β, and TNF-α stimulate the release of each other via positive-feedback cycles (15–17) and may share a common pathway in inducing hypotension via nitric oxide (18).

2. Vascular Permeability and Organ Damage

Administration of LPS to rats leads to hemoconcentration and vascular leakage that is evident in the large airways (19), gastrointestinal tract (5), and pancreas (20). Several PAF antagonists have been shown to be effective in preventing various aspects of LPS-induced vascular damage when administered intraperito-

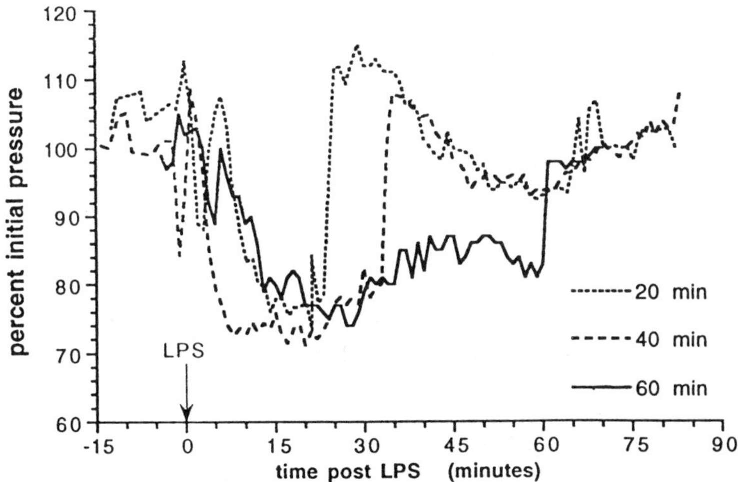

Figure 3 Reversal of LPS-induced hypotension by posttreatment with ABT-299 in rat. ABT-299 (0.1 mg/kg, intraarterially) was administered 20 min, 40 min, or 60 min following LPS challenenge. Standard deviations, omitted for clarity, are within 20% of the mean.

neally (i.p.). For example, BN 50739 (10 mg/kg, i.p.) is effective in blocking LPS-induced hemoconcentration, and CV 3988 (10 mg/kg, i.p.), SRI 63–441 (50 mg/kg, i.p.), and WEB 2086 (10 mg/kg, i.p.) have been shown to inhibit by greater than 50% LPS-induced vascular leakage in the lung (7,21).

PAF antagonists are also effective in preventing LPS-induced increases in vascular permeability in the GI tract. An LPS bolus (25 mg/kg) in the rat produces marked hyperemia and overt lumenal bleeding in the small bowel within 30 min. Early studies demonstrated that CV 3988 (10 mg/kg, i.v.), BN-52021 (10 mg/kg, i.v.), and Ro 19–3704 (1 mg/kg, i.v.) significantly reduced this LPS-induced plasma leakage in rat stomach and small intestine (5). More recently it has been reported that CL 184,005 (0.5 mg/kg, i.p.) blocks LPS-induced vascular leakage into the intestine (10). In a similar study pretreatment with ABT-299 (0.01 mg/kg, i.v.) 30 min prior to LPS challenge provided virtually complete protection against intestinal bleeding assessed by the hemoglobin content of the lumen (0.03 mg/g tissue versus 2.29 mg/g, $p < 0.001$).

The effectiveness of PAF antagonists in preventing LPS-induced vascular permeability and organ damage in the lung and GI tract supports the concept that PAF is a major contributor to organ damage associated with sepsis and related pulmonary and gastrointestinal diseases such as adult respiratory distress syndrome (ARDS) (19) and necrotizing endocolitis (22).

3. Disseminated Intravascular Coagulation

Disseminated intravascular coagulation (DIC) is characterized by systemic activation of the coagulation and fibrinolytic systems. This disorder most frequently occurs after infectious complications such as sepsis. Endotoxin, considered a pivotal mediator of the pathogenesis of DIC, is frequently present in detectable levels in septic patents and can provoke coagulation activation directly and/or through cytokine induction. Coagulation activation in turn results in the formation of microvascular thrombi that are involved in the pathogenesis of multiple organ failure associated with sepsis (23).

In experimental animals, injection or infusion of LPS provokes systemic responses that mimic many of the clinical symptoms of DIC. In the rat, the responses related to coagulation activation include thrombocytopenia, prolongation of prothrombin and partial thromboplastin times, decreased plasma fibrinogen, and elevated levels of fibrinogen/fibrin degradation products (24).

CV-3988, a structural analog of PAF, was the first PAF antagonist to be evaluated in a rat DIC model. Pretreatment and continued infusion of CV-3988 (total dose 10 mg/kg, i.v.) significantly inhibited each of the DIC symptoms mentioned above. These results prompted the hypothesis that PAF was involved in DIC caused by endotoxin (25). Since then, several additional PAF antagonists representing different chemical classes have produced beneficial effects in rat models of DIC. Some of the antagonists tested include: TCV-309, a PAF analog (26); SM-10661, a thiazolidine (27); L-659,989, a tetrahydrofuran (28); and WEB-2170, a hetrazepine (28). ABT-299 also is effective in the rodent DIC model. As shown in Fig. 4, when co-infused with LPS following an intravenous bolus of the antagonist, ABT-299 provides highly significant protection (85–95%, $p < 0.001$) for each of the parameters monitored.

4. Mortality

Septic shock is characterized by a high risk of mortality (40–60%) resulting from hemodynamic collapse, DIC, and multiple organ failure. These lethal effects of endotoxin are also observed experimentally in rat or mouse. An intravenous injection of LPS (5–25 mg/kg) causes 40–100% mortality within 24 h (29).

The first report of a PAF antagonist in a septic shock model included the finding that CV-3988 increased survival (29). A number of chemically diverse PAF antagonists have since been shown to improve survival in rodent shock models. In general, the potency for improving survival corresponds to potency

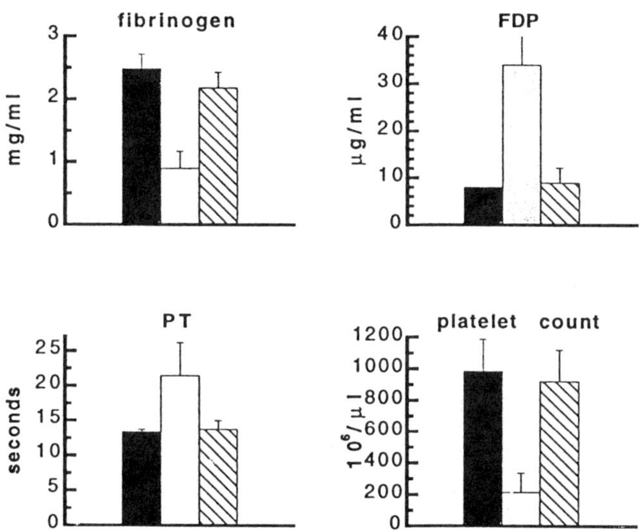

Figure 4 Inhibition of LPS-induced changes in coagulation parameters in rat. ABT-299 (1 mg/kg) or vehicle was administered as an intravenous bolus followed by co-infusion of LPS (0.25 mg/kg/h) and ABT-299 (1 mg/kg/h) for 4 h. At the end of the infusion, blood samples were taken for analysis of fibrinogen, fibrinogen/fibrin degradation products (FDP), prothrombin time (PT), and platelet count. Normal control, solid; LPS, open; LPS + ABT-299, diagonal. Data are expressed as the mean ± standard deviation.

in blocking other sepsis and PAF-challenge responses. The protective effect of PAF antagonists is exemplified by ABT-299. Pretreatment with ABT-299 (0.1 mg/kg) by the intravenous route resulted in a marked improvement in survival (90% survival, $p < 0.05$) of rats given a lethal challenge (50–60% mortality) of LPS. When given by the oral route, ABT-299 was also effective in increasing the survival rate (80% survival, $p < 0.05$).

The protective effect of PAF antagonists demonstrates the potential importance of PAF in the lethal cascade provoked by endotoxin. However, as was noted above, other mediators are also clearly involved. The importance of TNF, IL-1, and IL-6 in shock has been recognized, in part because of the effectiveness of anti-TNF, anti-IL-6, and IL-1 receptor antagonist therapies in experimental shock models (30–32). That both anti-PAF and anti-cytokine therapies are effective suggests complex interactions between these mediators during septic shock. Such interactions are evident in the ability of PAF to prime for TNF-induced tissue damage (33) and for PAF, TNF, and IL-1 to stimulate the release of each other (15–17).

5. Gram-Positive Shock

Cell surface components derived from gram-positive organisms have been shown in vitro to have pro-inflammatory activity. For example, lipoteichoic acid (LTA) isolated from several enterococcal species stimulates cytokine production from human monocytes in a fashion similar to LPS (34). Although studied in less detail, the in-vivo responses induced by LTA are also similar to those of LPS. Administration of LTA to rats produces a hypotensive episode accompanied by extensive intestinal bleeding and damage which are analogous to that produced by LPS. Both the hypotension and increased intestinal permeability are prevented by pretreatment with the PAF antagonist ABT-299 (Figs. 5 and 6). These results raise the possibility that, at least in principle, PAF antagonists may have a utility beyond the treatment of shock caused by gram-negative organisms.

B. PAF Antagonists in Large-Animal Models of Sepsis

In addition to rodent endotoxemia models described above, several groups have utilized larger animal species, including sheep, pig, and primates, to evaluate the potential role of PAF antagonists in sepsis. Unlike rats and mice, these species are much more sensitive to endotoxin, and in that regard more closely mimic the human condition. These species also provide a more convenient and relevant setting to assess the effects on the cardiovascular and pulmonary symptoms of sepsis.

Several groups have reported the effect of early PAF antagonists in LPS-induced lung injury in the sheep. SRI 64-441, BN-52021, and WEB-2086 were shown to attenuate pulmonary hypertension and block increased lung lymph flow

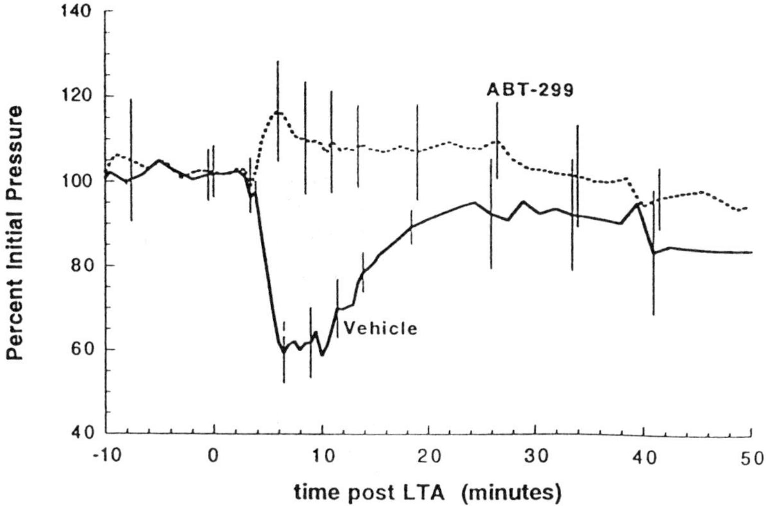

Figure 5 Inhibition of LTA-induced hypotension following pretreatment (15 min) with ABT-299 (0.1 mg/kg, intraarterially) or vehicle in rat. Data are expressed as the mean of the group ($n = 4$) $\pm$ standard deviation.

that result from infusions of endotoxin (35–37). SRI 64-441 was also shown to inhibit the early phases of hypoxemia, reduce leukopenia, and improve the lung compliance in the sheep. All three agents reduced the levels of cyclooxygenase products, particularly TXB_2, which may in part account for some of the effects of the antagonists. None of the compounds had any effect on the systemic hemodynamic changes induced by LPS in the sheep.

In pigs, WEB-2086 and SRI 63-675 were shown to reduce LPS-induced pulmonary hypertension, attenuate leukopenia, and improve airway pressure when administered prior to and during endotoxin challenge (38,39). SRI 63-675, but not WEB-2086, was also reported to inhibit the early systemic hypotension and increase cardiac index associated with endotoxemia. As was seen in the sheep, cyclooxygenase products are elevated in the pig following LPS challenge, and SRI 63-675 inhibited this increase in prostaglandin and thromboxane levels.

In addition, SRI 63-675 has been evaluated in a bacteremia model of sepsis in the pig (40). The antagonist blocked the early pulmonary hypertension, inhibited the early and late hypoxemia, and prevented the late-phase increase in lung edema and albumin flux following infusion of *Pseudomonas aeruginosa*. Unlike with LPS challenge, SRI 63-675 had no significant effect on systemic hypotension and cardiac output changes following bacterial infusion.

The hetrazepine PAF antagonist Ro 24–4736 has been evaluated in a bacter-

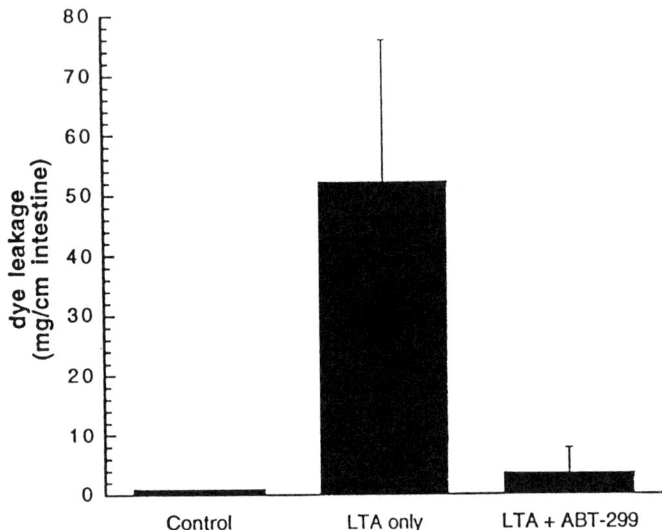

Figure 6 Inhibition of LTA-induced gastrointestinal permeability following pretreatment with ABT-299 (0.1 mg/kg, intraarterially) in rat. Data are expressed as the mean ± standard deviation ($n = 6$).

emia model in baboons (41). No improvement in overall survival was noted when the animals were given the antagonists 2 h prior to a lethal infusion of live *Escherichia coli*, although the baboons receiving Ro 24–4736 had significantly longer survival times. No effect on systemic hypotension was observed, but less fluid resuscitation was required in the treated baboons. There was also a significant improvement in early hypoxemia and circulating lactate levels. Circulating concentrations of the cytokines IL-1β and IL-6, but not TNF, were attenuated in the PAF antagonist-treated group.

Taken together, the data obtained in several large-animal models of septic shock are consistent with a role for PAF antagonists in the management of LPS-induced lung injury. Improvements in pulmonary hypertension, oxygenation, vascular leak, and lung function are commonly observed. Less convincing is the ability of PAF antagonists to block the systemic cardiovascular effects associated with these models. This is in contrast to rodent models, where antagonists are highly effective. Definitive evidence for the role of PAF antagonism in modulating systemic hemodynamic effects may depend on the evaluation of more potent PAF antagonists such as ABT-299. However, ultimately the role of PAF in septic shock will be determined only through carefully designed clinical studies with potent antagonists.

III. CLINICAL APPLICATION

A. Asthma

Empirical evidence has linked PAF to pathophysiological changes (42,43) and to the generation of secondary mediators such as cyclooxygenase products (35) in asthma. Unfortunately, early PAF antagonists with limited potency, such as WEB 2086, were ineffective in asthma patients (43). Nonetheless, these and other studies involving PAF antagonists in humans have provided information useful in the design of sepsis trials.

B. Sepsis

More than 400,000 cases of sepsis are diagnosed each year in the United States. Between 20 and 60% of these patients will fall victim to multiorgan failure and mortality. Despite improved antimicrobial therapy and advanced supportive care, the percentage of mortal events remains unaltered. Further, the number of patients presenting with sepsis is climbing. Clearly, effective, adjunctive therapy for sepsis is in demand.

To describe the task of planning the clinical development program for PAF antagonists for the indication of sepsis as challenging is an understatement. Past clinical disappointments of other mediator blockers, such as anti-endotoxin antibodies, an interleukin-1 receptor antagonist, soluble TNF receptor, and anti-TNF antibodies bears testimony to this statement.

Clinical studies with potent PAF antagonists in sepsis, such as BB-882 and ABT-299, are currently ongoing. The results of studies with BB-882 have not been published to date. Clinical studies are poised to begin with ABT-299.

1. Issues in Clinical Studies

a. Safety Considerations—Phase I. It would be of interest to determine the safety of drugs for sepsis in normal subjects with subsequent confirmation in sepsis patients. One might expect that the pharmacokinetic profile of the xenobiotic would differ in the two populations due to the abnormalities in metabolism in sepsis patients, as well as the degree of liver and/or renal failure in the latter population.

b. Efficacy Protocol Planning. The lack of understanding of the pathophysiology of sepsis syndrome lessens our ability to design the ideal protocol to test immunomodulators as efficacious adjunctive therapy. Which patients should be included in the studies, when should we initiate therapy, for how long should the therapy be administered, how much inhibition of the target should be induced, and which parameters will best predict short- and long-term benefit to the patient? Each of these questions raises a host of related questions and considerations in designing a series of experiments in an attempt to render interpretative results. In designing a clinical program for new sepsis drugs, it may be worthwhile to consider the experience of predecessors in this field.

2. Previous Clinical Experiences with PAF Antagonists

Following is a summary of previous clinical experiences with various PAF antagonists with respect to mechanism of action, safety, and efficacy.

   a. Mechanism of Action in Man
   i. Ex Vivo.   Both ex-vivo and in-vivo determinations of PAF antagonist activity have been conducted in Phase I clinical studies in normal, healthy volunteers or atopic subjects. Platelet aggregation can be induced ex vivo by a variety of stimuli, including epinephrine, ADP, collagen, and PAF. PAF-induced platelet aggregation can be used to assess the level of anti-PAF activity present in the plasma of subjects administered PAF antagonists. For example, PAF (5 × 10^{-8}M)-induced platelet aggregation was inhibited in a dose-related manner in response to single rising doses of the PAF antagonist WEB 2086 given either intravenously (0.5–50 mg) or by inhalation administration (0.05–1.0 mg) (44).

   ii. In Vivo, PAF-Induced Cutaneous Responses.   Intradermal administration of an antigen induces a biphasic inflammatory response portrayed first by the appearance of a wheal-and-flare skin reaction, which is evident within 1 of the insult, followed by infiltration of inflammatory cells, edema, and fibrin deposition during the late phase (45,46). It is believed that the release of histamine is responsible for the early phase of the response (47). However, the mediators of the late phase have not been clearly defined, and PAF may play a role. To this end, the cutaneous response to intradermal injections of 200 ng of PAF given 2 h after treatment with the ginkgolide mixture PAF antagonist BN 52063 was shown to be inhibited in 10 atopic subjects in a double-blind, placebo-controlled study, whereas the response to a histamine challenge was unaffected (48). The acute wheal response was reduced by 50% but not significantly so, and the inhibition of the flare response was unremarkable. However, the volume of the late-onset phase of inflammatory swelling occurring 8 h after the PAF challenge was significantly reduced, suggesting that PAF is a mediator of the immune response. This concept was confirmed in normal subjects pretreated with WEB 2086, in whom the wheal volume and flare responses to 200 ng of PAF intradermally were significantly attenuated, but the response to histamine was unaffected (49).

   b. Endotoxin Challenge.   Attempts to mimic LPS endotoxemia have also been conducted in Phase I trials. Endotoxin challenge with 20 U/kg of National Reference Bacterial Endotoxin given over 5 min elevated circulating pro-inflammatory cytokines TNF-α and IL-6 and the endogenous TNF-α antagonist, sTNFR-I, in 5 normal males compared to a demographically similar placebo control group in a double-blind study (50). This was accompanied by acute increases in circulating titers of cortisol, epinephrine, and glucagon. The symptoms of endotoxemia, such as rigors, myalgias, headache, nausea, and vomiting, were significantly reduced, as was peak cortisol and epinephrine levels if the subjects were pretreated with only 10 mg of the PAF antagonist Ro 24–4736 rather than placebo. Ex vivo, PAF-induced platelet aggregation was completely attenuated for 3 weeks after PAF antagonist treatment. Disappointingly, changes in vital signs elicited by endotoxin, including fever, tachycardia, and falls in blood pressure, as well as the normal hypermetabolic response to LPS, were unaltered by Ro 24–4736. Further, PAF antagonism did not affect elevated cytokines. These findings suggest that PAF does play a role in the consequences of endotoxemia, but that role may be independent of cytokine mechanisms under these conditions in humans. No safety concerns were observed.

    c. Efficacy. In a randomized, placebo-controlled, double-blind clinical trial in 119 patients with documented gram-negative severe sepsis, the PAF antagonist BN 52021 reduced mortality by 42%. This difference compared to placebo was not noted in the absence of documented gram-negative sepsis (51). The relationship of this finding with antagonism of PAF-induced effects remains unclear in view of the modest potency of this compound and the variety of other properties attributed to it. Theoretically, PAF antagonists should be effective in inhibiting the systemic inflammatory response syndrome (SIRS), regardless of the etiology (see Section II.A.5).

    The question of whether PAF antagonism will be effective in gram-positive endotoxemia and other states of induced SIRS, such as pancreatitis, remains to be determined.

IV. PROSPECTUS

The likelihood of adequate efficacy from a single agent as adjunctive treatment of sepsis is low due to the intricate nature of the pathophysiology. Rather, a cocktail of drugs/biologics with various mechanisms of action may provide the greatest promise of success. Nevertheless, a positive trend in end-organ function, morbidity, and mortality resultant of any individual agent will be encouraging and a start to the process of selecting the components of the final therapeutic product. Whether potent PAF antagonists will play a pivotal role in the therapeutics of sepsis syndrome awaits the results of imminent clinical evaluation.

REFERENCES

1. Anderson BO, Bensard DD, Harken AH. The role of platelet activating factor and its antagonists in shock, sepsis and multiple organ failure. Surgery 1991; 172:415–424.
2. Woodard DS, Lee T-L, Snyder F. The final step in the *de novo* biosynthesis of platelet-activating factor. J Biol Chem 1987; 262:2520–2527.

3. Blank ML, Lee TC, Fitzgerald V, Snyder F. A specific hydrolase for 1-alkyl-2-acetyl-*sn*-glycero-3-phosphochloine hypotensive platelet activating lipid. J Biol Chem 1981; 256:175–178.

4. Sanchez Crespo M, Fernandez-Gallardo S. Pharmacological modulation of PAF: a therapeutic approach to endotoxin shock. J Lipid Mediators 1991; 4:127–144.

5. Wallace JL, Steel G, Whittle BJ, Lagente V, Vargaftig B. Evidence for platelet-activating factor as a mediator of endotoxin-induced gastrointestinal damage in the rat. Effects of three platelet-activating factor antagonists. Gastroenterology 1987; 93:765–773.

6. Zeng N. Determination of plasma level of platelet activating factor in cirrhotic patients and its relation to endotoxemia. Chung Hua I Hsueh Tsa Chih 1992; 72:141–143.

7. Chang SW, Feddersen CO, Henson PM, Voelkel NF. Platelet-activating factor mediates hemodynamic changes and lung injury in endotoxin-treated rats. J Clin Invest 1987; 79:1498–1509.

8. Doebber TW, Wu MS, Robbins JC, Choy BM, Chang MN, Shen TY. Platelet activating factor (PAF) involvement in endotoxin-induced hypotension in rats. Studies with PAF-receptor antagonist kadsurenone. Biochem Biophys Res Commun 1985; 127:799–808.

9. Qi M, Jones SB. Contribution of platelet activating factor to hemodynamic and sympathetic responses to bacterial endotoxin in conscious rats. Circ Shock 1990; 32:153–163.

10. Torley LW, Pickett WC, Carroll ML, et al. Studies of the effect of a platelet-activating factor antagonist, CL 184,005, in animal models of gram-negative bacterial sepsis. Antimicrob Agents Chemother 1992; 36:1971–1977.

11. Summers JB, Albert DH, Davidsen SK, et al. ABT-299, A potent antagonist of platelet activating factor. In: Adv. Prost. Leuko. Res. New York Raven, Press 1995; pp 475–477.

12. Terashita Z, Kawamura M, Takatani M, Tsushima S, Imura Y, Nishikawa K. Beneficial effects of TCV-309, a novel potent and selective platelet activating factor antagonist in endotoxin and anaphylactic shock in rodents. J Pharmacol Exp Ther 1992; 260: 748–755.

13. Etienne A, Hecquet F, Soulard C, Spinnewyn B, Clostre F, Braquet P. In vivo inhibition of plasma protein leakage and *Salmonella enteritidis*-induced mortality in the rat by a specific paf-acether antagonist: BN 52021. Agents Actions 1986; 17:368–370.

14. de Boer JP, Wolbink GJ, Thijs LG, Baars JW, Wagstaff J, Hack CE. Interplay of complement and cytokines in the pathogenesis of septic shock. Immunopharmacology 1992; 24:135–148.

15. Camussi G, Bussolino F, Salvidio G, Baglioni C. Tumor necrosis factor/cachectin stimulates peritoneal macrophages, polymorphoculear neutrophils, and vascular endothelial cells to synthesize and release platelet-activating factor. J Exp Med 1987; 166:1390–1404.

16. Bussolino F, Breviario F, Tetta C, Massimo A, Mantovani A, Dejana E. Interleukin-

1 stimulates platelet-activating factor production in cultured human endothelial cells. J Clin Invest 1986; 77:2027–2033.

17. Valone FH, Epstein LB. Biphasic platelet-activating factor synthesis by human monocytes stimulated with IL-1-beta, tumor necrosis factor, or IFN-gamma. J Immunol 1988; 141:3945–3950.

18. Szabo C, Wu CC, Mitchell JA, Gross SS, Thiemermann C, Vane JR. Platelet-activating factor contributes to the induction of nitric oxide synthase by bacterial lipopolysaccharide. Circ Res 1993; 73:991–999.

19. Chang SW. Endotoxin-induced lung vascular injury: role of platelet activating factor, tumor necrosis factor and neutrophils. Clin Res 1992; 40:528–536.

20. Sirois MG, Jancar S, Braquet P, Plante GE, Sirois P. PAF increases vascular permeability in selected tissues: effect of BN-52021 and L-655,240. Prostaglandins 1988; 36:631–644.

21. Chang SW, Fernyak S, Voelkel NF. Beneficial effect of a platelet-activating factor antagonist, WEB 2086, on endotoxin-induced lung injury. Am J Physiol 1990; 258:H153–H158.

22. Hsueh W, Gonzalez-Crussi F, Arroyave JL. Platelet-activating factor: an endogenous mediator for bowel necrosis in endotoxemia. FASEB J 1987; 1:403–405.

23. Levi M, ten Cate H, van der Poll T, van Deventer SJ. Pathogenesis of disseminated intravascular coagulation in sepsis. JAMA 1993; 270:975–979.

24. Yoshikawa T, Furukawa Y, Murakami M, Takemura S, Kondo M. Experimental model of disseminated intravascular coagulation induced by sustained infusion of endotoxin. Res Exp Med 1981; 179:223–228.

25. Imura Y, Terashita Z, Nishikawa K. Possible role of platelet activating factor (PAF) in disseminated intravascular coagulation (DIC), evidenced by use of a PAF antagonist, CV-3988. Life Sci 1986; 39:111–117.

26. Kawamura M, Terashita Z, Imura Y, Shino A, Nishikawa K. Inhibitory effect of TCV-309, a novel platelet activating factor (PAF) antagonist, on endotoxin-induced disseminated intravascular coagulation in rats: possible role of PAF in tissue factor generation. Thromb Res 1993; 70:281–293.

27. Imanishi N, Komuro Y, Morooka S. Effect of a selective PAF antagonist SM-10661 (($\pm$)-cis-3,5-dimethyl-2-(3-pyridyl)thiazolidin-4-one HCl) on experimental disseminated intravascular coagulation (DIC). Lipids 1991; 26:1391–1395.

28. Tang HM, Teshima DY, Lum B. Effects of the PAF antagonists bepafant and L-659,989 in endotoxic and septic shock. Drug Dev Res 1993; 29:216–221.

29. Terashita Z-I, Imura Y, Nishikawa K. Inhibition by CV-2988 of the binding of [^{3}H]-platelet activating factor (PAF) to the platelet. Biochem Pharmacol 1985; 34:1491–1495.

30. Beutler B, Milsark IW, Cerami A. Passive immunization against cachectin/tumor necrosis factor (TNF) protects mice from lethal effect of endotoxin. Science 1985; 229:869–871.

31. Starnes HF, Pearce M, Yim J, Abrams J, Tewari A, Zou J. Anti-IL-6 monoclonal antibodies protect against lethal *Escherichia coli* infection and lethal tumor necrosis factor-alpha challenge in mice [retraction of Starnes HF Jr, Pearce MK, Tewari A,

Yim JH, Zou JC, Abrams JS. In: J Immunol 1990 Dec 15; 145(12):4185–4191].
J Immunol 1992; 148:1968.

32. Wakabayashi G, Gelfand JA, Burke JF, Thompson RC, Dinarello CA. A specific receptor antagonist for interleukin 1 prevents *Escherichia coli*-induced shock in rabbits. FASEB J 1991; 5: 338–343.

33. Sun XM, Hsueh W, Torre-Amione G. Effects of in vivo "priming" on endotoxin-induced hypotension and tissue injury. The role of PAF and tumor necrosis factor. Am J Pathol 1990; 136:949–956.

34. Bhakdi S, Klonisch T, Nuber P, Fischer W. Stimulation of monokine production by lipoteichoic acids. Infect Immun 1991; 59: 4614–4620.

35. Christman BW, Lefferts PL, Blair IA, Snapper JR. Effect of platelet-activating factor receptor antagonism on endotoxin-induced lung dysfunction in awake sheep. Am Rev Respir Dis 1990; 142:1272–1278.

36. Redl H, Vogl C, Schiesser A, et al. Effect of the PAF antagonist BN 52021 in ovine endotoxin shock. J Lipid Mediat 1990; 2:S195–201.

37. Sessler CN, Glauser FL, Davis D, Fowler AA 3d. Effects of platelet-activating factor antagonist SRI 63–441 on endotoxemia in sheep. J Appl Physiol 1988; 65:2624–2631.

38. Dobrowsky RT, Voyksner RD, Olson NC. Effect of SRI 63–675 on hemodynamics and blood PAF levels during porcine endotoxemia. Am J Physiol 1991; 260:H1455–H1465.

39. Olson NC, Joyce PB, Fleisher LN. Role of platelet-activating factor and eicosanoids during endotoxin-induced lung injury in pigs. Am J Physiol 1990; 258:H1674–H1686.

40. Byrne K, Sessler CN, Carey PD, et al. Platelet-activating factor in porcine *Pseudomonas* acute lung injury. J Surg Res 1991; 50:111–118.

41. Thompson WA, Van Zee KJ, Rogy M, Felsen D, Lowry SF, Moldawer LL. Platelet-activating factor antagonist (Ro24–4736) attenuates the metabolic respons to gram-negative sepsis in primates. Surg Forum 1992; 48:84–87.

42. Smith LJ. The role of platelet activating factor in asthma. Am Rev Respir Dis 1991; 143:S100–S102.

43. Freitag A, Watson RM, Matsos G, Eastwood C, O'Byrne PM. Effect of a PAF antagonist WEB-2086, on allergen induced asthmatic response. Thorax 1993; 48:594–598.

44. Adamus WS, Heuer H, Meade CJ. PAF induced platelet aggregation *ex vivo* as a method for monitoring pharmacological activity in healthy volunteers. Meth Find Exp Clin Pharmacol 1989; 11:415–420.

45. Umemoto L, Poothullil J, Dolovich J, Hargreave FE. Factors which influence late cutaneous allergic responses. J Allergy Clin. Immunol 1976; 58:60–68.

46. Solley GO, Gleich GJ, Jordan RE, Shcroeter AL. Late phase of the immediate wheal-and-flare skin reaction: its dependence on IgE antibodies. J Clin Invest 1976; 58:408–420.

47. Phillips MJ, Meyrick Thomas RH, Moodley I, Davies RJ. A comparison of the in vivo effects of ketotifen, clemastine, chlorpheniramine and sodium cromoglycate

on histamine-and allergen-induced weals in human skin. Br J Clin Pharmacol 1983; 15:277–286.

48. Roberts NM, Page CP, Chung KF, Barnes PJ. Effect of a PAF antagonist, BN52063, on antigen-induced, acute, and late-onset cutaneous responses in atopic subjects. J Allergy Clin Immunol 1988; 82:236–241.

49. Hayes JP, Ridge SM, Griffith S, Barnes PJ, Chung KF. Inhibition of cutaneous and platelet responses to platelet-activating factor by oral WEB 2086 in man. J Allergy Clin Immunol 1991; 88:83–88.

50. Thompson WA, Coyle S, Van Zee K, et al. The metabolic effects of PAF antagonism in endotoxemic man. Arch Surg 1994; 129:72–79.

51. Tenaillon A, Dhainaut JF, Letulzo UY, et al. Efficacy of PAF antagonists BN-52021 in reducing mortality of patients with severe gram negative sepsis. Am Rev Respir Dis 1993; 147:A97.

17

Interleukin-10 as a Protective Cytokine Produced During Sepsis

Arnaud Marchant, Jean-Louis Vincent, and Michel Goldman
Hôpital Erasme
Brussels, Belgium

I. INTRODUCTION

Macrophage activation by microbial products is thought to play a central role in the pathogenesis of septic shock. The injection of gram-negative lipopolysaccharide (LPS, endotoxin) to animals has been used extensively as a model for septic shock. Most of the toxicity of LPS is related to the release of pro-inflammatory cytokines such as tumor necrosis factor (TNF) and interleukin-1 (IL-1) by activated macrophages (1). Indeed, passive immunization against TNF or administration of the IL-1 receptor antagonist (IL-1ra) protect animals from lethality associated with endotoxin shock (2–6). These data led to the development of several clinical trials using either anti-TNF monoclonal antibodies (mAb) or IL-1ra for the treatment of patients with sepsis syndrome and septic shock. Although further studies are still needed to establish the interest of these approaches, it is already suggested that pharmacotherapeutic ''cocktails'' may be necessary to reduce the toxicity of the multiple macrophage products that are thought to be responsible for the development of septic shock (1). A valuable alternative to these ''cocktails'' could be the use of molecules that prevent macrophage activation by bacterial products. Glucocorticoids, IL-4, and IL-10 are potent macrophage deactivators, suppressing TNF and IL-1 release by these cells (7–11). In this review, we first summarize data indicating that IL-10 protects mice from lethality associated with endotoxin shock. We then show that IL-10 is produced during murine endotoxemia and that this endogenous IL-10 controls LPS toxicity.

Finally, we discuss the potential role of IL-10 produced during human septicemia and septic shock.

II. INTERLEUKIN-10 AS A MACROPHAGE-DEACTIVATING CYTOKINE

Interleukin-10 (IL-10) was first described as a cytokine produced by mouse "type 2" helper T-cell clones (Th2), which inhibits cytokine production by "type 1" helper T-cell clones (Th1) (12). Th1 cells are specialized in producing interferon-γ (IFN-γ) and IL-2 and therefore play an important role in cell-mediated immunity. Th2 cells secrete IL-4, IL-5, IL-6, and IL-10 and are particularly efficient in helping antibody responses. The cytokine synthesis-inhibitory activity of IL-10 appears to be mostly related to its ability to decrease the costimulatory signals given by antigen-presenting cells to Th1 lymphocytes (13).

One of the major biological properties of IL-10 is to deactivate monocytes and macrophages. In vitro, IL-10 is a very potent inhibitor of cytokine production (including TNF, IL-1, IL-6, IL-8, and IL-12) by LPS-activated monocytes and macrophages (9–11,14) and suppress the tissue factor-dependent procoagulant activity induced by LPS on human monocytes (15). IL-10 also inhibits free-radical release and nitric oxide-dependent microbicidal activity of macrophages against various pathogens (10,16). We observed, in a human whole-blood model, that IL-10 also inhibits LPS-induced IFN-γ release (17). NK cells are thought to be a major source for IFN-γ during experimental endotoxemia, most probably as a consequence of their activation by monocyte/macrophage-derived TNF and IL-12 (18–20). The inhibition of LPS-induced IFN-γ synthesis by IL-10 is therefore probably dependent on its ability to suppress TNF and IL-12 production by monocytes and macrophages (14,19,20).

Interestingly, together with the inhibition of the inflammatory response, it appears that IL-10 does not interfere with the in-vitro production of several antiinflammatory mediators. Indeed, IL-10 does not influence the release of monocyte-derived TGF-β (11), and induces the production of IL-1ra (14).

III. INTERLEUKIN-10 PROTECTS MICE FROM ENDOTOXIN SHOCK

A. Recombinant Interleukin-10 Inhibits TNF and IFN-γ Synthesis and Protects Mice from LPS-Induced Mortality

The macrophage-deactivating properties of IL-10 led us to investigate whether this cytokine is able to modulate the production of TNF and IFN-γ in vivo and to reduce the lethality associated with endotoxemia in mice.

Cytokine release was induced by i.p. injection of 100 μg of LPS (*Escherichia coli* O55:B5). Mice were injected with 1000 U of recombinant IL-10 (rIL-10) 30 min before LPS challenge. A second injection of 1000 U rIL-10 was performed 4 h after LPS when IFN-γ production was studied. Peak TNF and IFN-γ serum levels were measured by ELISA at 90 min and 6 h, respectively. We observed that rIL-10 treatment reduced by 70–90% the release of both TNF and IFN-γ in this model (17,21). Together with this inhibition of pro-inflammatory cytokines release, we also observed a reduction of LPS toxicity. Indeed, pretreatment with 1000 U of rIL-10 totally prevented LPS-induced mortality (21). As both TNF and IFN-γ have been incriminated in the toxicity of LPS (2–5,22–24), the inhibition of the release of both cytokines is probably involved in the protective effect of rIL-10. Similar data were reported by Howard et al. (25). Interestingly, these authors have shown that rIL-10 injection could be delayed until 1 h after LPS and still protect against LPS toxicity.

Together with TNF and IFN-γ, IL-6 is also released in vivo following LPS administration. Although the role of IL-6 in the pathogenesis of endotoxin shock remains controversial (26), several reports suggest that it could have a protective effect against LPS toxicity by blocking TNF synthesis both in vitro and in vivo (27,28). Therefore, it was of interest to examine the effect of rIL-10 pretreatment on IL-6 production during murine endotoxemia. As shown in Fig. 1, we observed that rIL-10 does not influence the LPS-induced production of IL-6 in mice, while TNF release was strongly suppressed in the same experimental conditions (21). These data suggest: (a) that IL-10 could differentially regulate TNF and IL-6 production by macrophages in vivo, in contrast with data obtained in vitro (11); or (b) that other cell types than macrophages are a major source of IL-6 in vivo and are resistant to IL-10. Recent experiments showing that LPS-induced IL-6 production by endothelial cells is not affected or may even be up-regulated by rIL-10 support the second hypothesis (29; and our own observations). This sustained production of a mediator with potential antiinflammatory activity could play a role in the protective effect of rIL-10 against LPS toxicity.

Taken together, these data suggest that rIL-10 could be useful in the treatment of inflammatory disorders associated with macrophage activation. Further studies of the effects of rIL-10 in animal models of bacterial infection are now needed to evaluate its potential interest for patients with sepsis. Interestingly, recent data indicated that rIL-10 is also able to control T-cell activation and to protect mice from lethal shock induced by gram-positive-derived superantigens (30). On the other hand, the inhibitory activity of IL-10 on macrophage microbicidal activity observed in mice infected with *Mycobacterium avium* or *Listeria monocytogenesis* suggests that rIL-10 administration could be deleterious when the host is infected by intracellular pathogens (31–33).

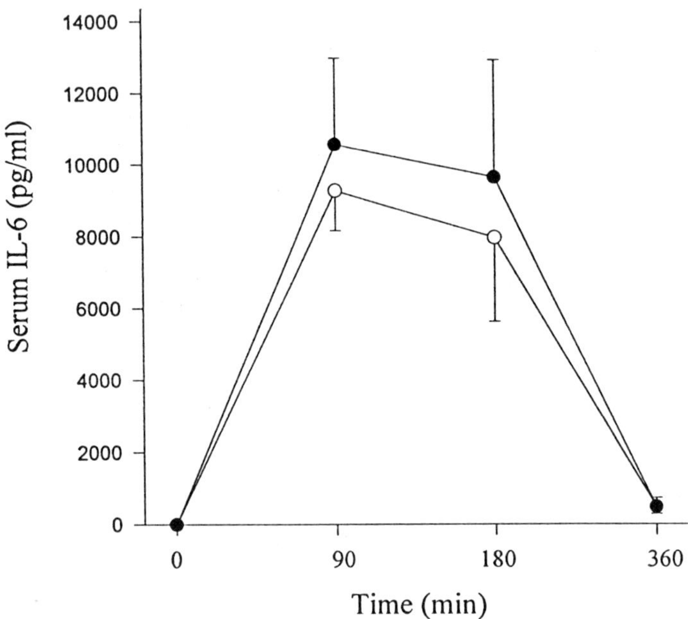

Figure 1   rIL-10 does not influence LPS-induced IL-6 release in vivo. Mice (5 per group) were injected with 100 µg of LPS with (filled circles) or without (open circles) pretreatment with 1000 U of rIL-10 given 30 min before LPS. Bioactive IL-6 serum levels determined with the 7TD1 cell line are represented as mean ± SEM.

B. Production and Role of Endogenous Interleukin-10 During Endotoxin Shock in Mice

Following activation by LPS, monocytes and macrophages produce IL-10 in vitro (11). Although IL-10 is produced later than TNF, IL-1, IL-6, or IL-8 in this setting, monocyte coincubation with LPS and neutralizing anti-IL-10 mAb enhanced the production of these monokines, indicating that IL-10 functions as an autoregulatory mechanism controlling monocyte activation by LPS (11).

We observed that LPS induces the rapid release of IL-10 in vivo in mice (17,34). Serum IL-10 was already detected 90 min after LPS injection and was still present at 6 h. These data show that IL-10 is released at the same time as TNF and IFN-γ during murine endotoxemia, suggesting that the production of these two pro-inflammatory cytokines could be regulated by IL-10. We tested this hypothesis by injecting mice with rat anti-mouse IL-10 mAb (JES5-2A5) 2 h before LPS. An irrelevant mAb was used as negative control (LO-DNP). We found that neutralization of endogenously produced IL-10 resulted in an increased production of both TNF and IFN-γ after LPS injection. Moreover, we observed that anti-IL-10 mAb administration was associated with a higher mortality (17). As shown in Fig. 2, neutralization of TNF activity prevented the increased mortality found in anti-IL-10-treated mice, indicating that endogenous IL-10 controls LPS toxicity at least in part through the inhibition of TNF release. The injection of the control mAb did not influence either cytokine production or lethality induced by LPS. These data indicate that IL-10 production during endotoxemia is an important protective mechanism against LPS toxicity and are in keeping with results obtained by Ishida et al. in mice chronically injected from birth with anti-IL-10 mAb (35). Interestingly, similar results were obtained by van der Poll et al. in another mouse model of septic shock, where administration of anti-IL-10 mAb before caecal ligation and puncture increased TNF levels and lethality associated with septic peritonitis (36). The role of TNF in these type of experimental sepsis models is still controversial, as passive immunization against TNF does not have the same protective effect as in endotoxemia (37).

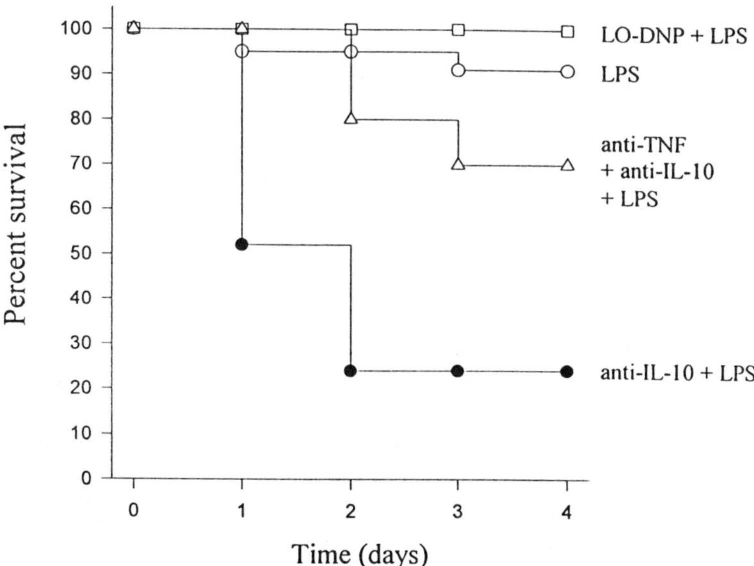

Figure 2 Role of TNF in lethality associated with IL-10 neutralization during murine endotoxemia. Mice were injected with 500 μg of LPS without ($n = 22$) or with pretreatment with neutralizing anti-IL-10 mAb (JES5-2A5, 2 mg per mouse, $n = 21$), isotype-matched control mAb (LO-DNP, $n = 10$), or a combination of anti-IL-10 and neutralizing anti-TNF mAb (TN3, 500 μg per mouse, $n = 10$) 2 h before LPS challenge. Anti-IL-10 + LPS versus LPS alone or LO-DNP + LPS: $p < 0.01$. Anti-IL-10 + anti-TNF + LPS versus anti-IL-10 + LPS: $p < 0.05$.

C. TNF and Interleukin-10 Are Differentially Regulated During Murine Endotoxemia

The central role played by TNF in mediating LPS toxicity has led to the evaluation of various inhibitors of LPS-induced TNF production for their ability to mitigate LPS toxicity in vivo. Glucocorticoids (GC), chlorpromazine (CPZ), and pentoxifylline (PTX) are potent inhibitors of TNF production by LPS-activated monocytes and macrophages and were shown to improve survival of endotoxemic mice (7,38,39). As endogenous IL-10 protects mice from endotoxin shock, Mengozzi et al. and our group investigated the effects of GC, CPZ, and PTX on LPS-induced IL-10 release in vivo. Pretreatment with GC or CPZ almost completely abrogated TNF production, whereas PTX was a less potent inhibitor (40,41). Interestingly, it was found that CPZ and GC administration up-regulated LPS-induced IL-10 production, while PTX pretreatment did not influence IL-10 release (40,41). Cyclosporin A was shown to inhibit TNF production during murine endotoxemia (42). Interestingly, Durez et al. observed that cyclosporin A also increased LPS-induced IL-10 release in vivo in mice (34). Taken together, these data show that TNF and IL-10 can be differentially regulated during murine endotoxemia. The lack of inhibition of IL-10 production could play a role in the protective effect of these drugs against LPS toxicity.

IV. INTERLEUKIN-10 PRODUCTION DURING HUMAN SEPTICEMIA AND SEPTIC SHOCK

The protective role of endogenously produced IL-10 during endotoxin shock and septic peritonitis led us to evaluate the production of IL-10 in patients with severe bacterial infection. IL-10 plasma levels were measured in 69 patients (9 surgical and 60 medical) with culture-proven gram-negative ($n = 25$) or gram-positive ($n = 44$) septicemia. (43). Seventeen patients had septic shock at the time of sampling. As shown in Fig. 3, we found high IL-10 levels in 57% of septicemic patients. Patients with septic shock had higher IL-10 levels than patients without shock (median: 58 versus 11 pg/mL, $p < 0.001$). Similar IL-10 plasma levels were found in gram-positive or gram-negative septicemia (43). Plasma IL-10 was detected in few patients with similar underlying disease but without any sign of infection and not in healthy volunteers (Fig. 3), demonstrating that IL-10 production was related to bacterial infection. Recently, Derkx et al. measured IL-10 plasma levels in children with fulminant meningococcal septic shock. They found that IL-10 is massively produced during the initial phase of meningococcal septic shock, median IL-10 levels being 10-fold higher than in adults with septic shock (44). Our experimental data suggest that IL-10 production during septicemia and septic shock could control the release of inflammatory cytokines in these settings. The higher IL-10 release observed in severely affected patients as well as in meningococcal sepsis suggest that the intensity of the antiinflammatory response is related to the importance of the inflammatory phenomenon. Interestingly, van Deuren et al. recently showed that monocytes from patients with meningococcal infection have a defect in LPS-induced TNF production, whereas the release of IL-lra is increased as compared to healthy volunteers (45). As IL-10 differentially regulates TNF and IL-lra production by LPS-stimulated monocytes, its massive release could play a role in monocyte abnormalities found during meningococcal infections.

Similar impairment of monocyte responses to in-vitro stimulation by LPS have also been described in other types of septic shock (46). Interestingly, Simpson et al. showed that alveolar macrophages from adult septic shock patients display a similar decrease in LPS-induced TNF production, indicating that LPS-unresponsiveness affecting circulating monocytes is not related to their recent migration from bone marrow, as it also affects differentiated cells (47).

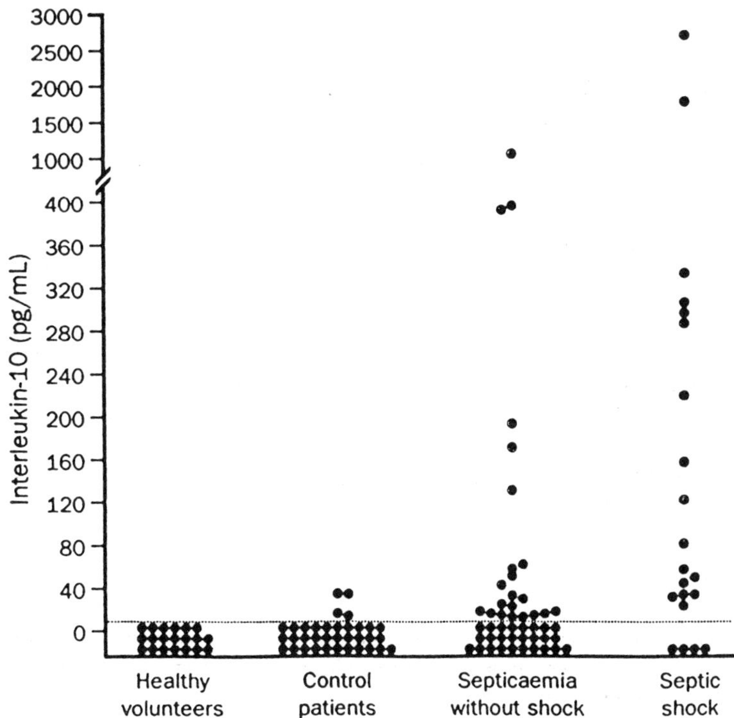

Figure 3 Plasma immunoreactive IL-10 in healthy volunteers, control patients without infection, and septicemic patients with and without shock. IL-10 plasma levels were determined by immunoenzymatic methods (Medgenix, Fleurus, Belgium). (From Ref. 43.)

V. CONCLUSIONS

IL-10 is a potent macrophage-deactivating factor. In vivo, IL-10 decreases LPS-induced TNF and IFN-γ production and protects mice from lethality associated with endotoxin shock. These data indicate that rIL-10 could be useful for the treatment of inflammatory disorders associated with macrophage activation, including sepsis, if administered early during the course of the disease. Endogenously produced IL-10 controls the secretion of pro-inflammatory cytokines and prevents LPS-induced lethality. The presence of circulating IL-10 in patients with septicemia and septic shock suggests that it might also control the production of inflammatory cytokines in these settings. Along this line, the impairment of TNF production by monocytes from septic shock patients suggests that mechanisms controlling monocyte activation are effective during sepsis, but the role of IL-10 in this decreased monocyte responsiveness to LPS requires further investigations.

Understanding the pathophysiology of sepsis needs the study of the mechanisms developed by the immune system to control the inflammatory response. The progression of critically ill patients from sepsis to multiple organ failure and death despite monocyte and macrophage deactivation may suggest that cell types other than monocytes, such as vascular endothelial cells, could play an important role in the pathophysiology of the disease and represent relevant targets for new therapeutic approaches to sepsis.

ACKNOWLEDGMENTS

Anti-IL-10, LO-DNP, and anti-TNF mAbs were kindly provided by T. Mosmann (Edmonton, Canada), H. Bazin (Louvain, Belgium), and Cell Tech (Berkshire, United Kingdom), respectively. This work was supported by the Fonds National de la Recherche Scientifique/Télévie, the Association Contre le Cancer, Brussels, Belgium, and by a the Immunotoxicology Biotech Project of the EEC Commission. Arnaud Marchant is a research assistant of the Fonds National de la Recherche Scientifique, Belgium.

REFERENCES

1. Glauser MP, Heumann D, Baumgartner JD, Cohen J. Pathogenesis and potential strategies for prevention and treatment of septic shock: an update. Clin Infect Dis 1994; 18 (suppl 2):S205–S216.
2. Beutler B, Milsark IW, Cerami AC. Passive immunisation against cachectin/tumor necrosis factor protects mice from lethal effect of endotoxin. Science 1985; 229:869–871.
3. Tracey KJ, Fong Y, Hesse DG, et al. Anti-cachectin/TNF monoclonal antibodies prevent septic shock during lethal bacteriaemia. Nature 1987; 330:662–664.

4. Mathison JC, Wolfson E, Ulevitch RJ. Participation of tumor necrosis factor in the mediation of gram-negative bacterial lipopolysaccharide-induced injury in rabbits. J Clin Invest 1988; 81:1925–1937.

5. Silva AT, Bayston KF, Cohen J. Prophylactic and therapeutic effects of a monoclonal antibody to tumor necrosis factor-alpha in experimental gram-negative shock. J Infect Dis 1990; 162:421–427.

6. Dinarello CA, Thompson RC. Blocking IL-1: interleukin 1 receptor antagonist in vivo and in vitro. Immunol Today 1991; 12:404–410.

7. Gonzalez JC, Johnson DC, Morrison DC, Freudenberg MA, Galanos C, Silverstein R. Endogenous and exogenous glucocorticoids have different roles in modulating endotoxin lethality in D-galactosamine-sensitized mice. Infect Immun 1993; 61:970–974.

8. te Velde AA, Huijbens RJ, Heije K, de Vries JE, Figdor CG. Interleukin-4 (IL-4) inhibits secretion of IL-1 beta, tumor necrosis factor alpha, and IL-6 by human monocytes. Blood 1990; 1392–1397.

9. Fiorentino DF, Zlotnik A, Mosmann TR, Howard M, O'Garra A. IL-10 inhibits cytokine production by activated macrophages. J Immunol 1991; 147:3815–3822.

10. Bogdan C, Vodovotz Y, Nathan C. Macrophage deactivation by interleukin 10. J Exp Med 1991; 174:1549–1555.

11. de Waal Malefyt R, Abrams J, Bennett B, Figdor CG, de Vries JE. Interleukin-10 (IL-10) inhibits cytokine synthesis by human monocytes: an autoregulatory role of IL-10 produced by monocytes. J Exp Med 1991; 174:1209–1220.

12. Fiorentino DF, Bond MW, Mosmann TR. Two types of mouse helper T cell. IV. Th2 clones secrete a factor that inhibits cytokine production by Th1 clones. J Exp Med 1989; 170: 2081–2095.

13. Fiorentino DF, Zlotnik A, Vieira P, et al. Il-10 acts on the antigen presenting cell to inhibit cytokine production by Th1 cells. J Immunol 1991; 146:3444–3451.

14. de Waal Malefyt R, Figdor C, Huijbens R, et al. Effects of IL-13 on phenotype, cytokine production, and cytotoxic function of human monocytes. J Immunol 1993; 151:6370–6381.

15. Pradier O, Gérard C, Delvaux A, et al. Interleukin-10 inhibits the induction of monocyte procoagulant activity by bacterial lipopolysaccharide. Eur J Immunol 1993; 23:2700–2703.

16. Gazzinelli RT, Oswald IP, James SL, Sher A. IL-10 inhibits parasite killing and nitrogen oxide production by IFN-γ activated macrophages. J Immunol 1992; 148:1792–1796.

17. Marchant A, Bruyns C, Vandenabeele P, et al. Interleukin-10 controls interferon-γ and tumor necrosis factor production during experimental endotoxemia. Eur J Immunol 1994; 24:1167–1171.

18. Jephthah-Ochola J, Urmson J, Farkas S, Halloran PF. Regulation of MHC expression in vivo: bacterial lipopolysaccharide induces class I and II MHC products in mouse tissues by a T cell-independent, cyclosporine-sensitive mechanism. J Immunol 1988; 141:792–800.

19. D'Andrea A, Aste-Amezaga M, Valiante NM, Ma X, Kubin M, Trinchieri G. Interleukin 10 (IL-10) inhibits human lymphocyte interferon gamma-production by

suppressing natural killer cell stimulatory factor/IL-12 synthesis in accessory cells. J Exp Med 1993; 178:1041–1048.

20. Tripp CS, Wolf SF, Unanue ER. Interleukin-12 and tumor necrosis factor α are costimulators of interferon γ production by natural killer cells in severe combined immunodeficiency mice with listeriosis, and interleukin-10 is a physiologic antagonist. Proc Natl Acad Sci USA 1993; 90:3725–3729.

21. Gérard C, Bruyns C, Marchant A, et al. Interleukin-10 reduces the release of tumor necrosis factor and prevents lethality in experimental endotoxemia. J Exp Med 1993; 177:547–550.

22. Heinzel FP. The role of IFN-gamma in the pathology of experimental endotoxemia. J Immunol 1990; 145:2920–2924.

23. Silva AT, Cohen J. Role of interferon-γ in experimental gram-negative sepsis. J Infect Dis 1992; 166:331–335.

24. Doherty GM, Lange JR, Langstein HN, Alexander HR, Buresh CM, Norton JA. Evidence of IFN-γ as a mediator of the lethality of endotoxin and tumor necrosis factor-α. J Immunol 1992; 149:1666–1670.

25. Howard M, Muchamuel T, Andrade S, Menon S. Interleukin 10 protects mice from lethal endotoxemia. J Exp Med 1993; 177:1205–1208.

26. van der Poll T, Levi M, Hack CE, et al. Elimination of interleukin 6 attenuates coagulation activation in experimental endotoxemia in chimpanzees. J Exp Med 1994; 179:1253–1259.

27. Schindler R, Mancilla J, Endres S, Ghorbani R, Clark SC, Dinarello CA. Correlations and interactions in the production of interleukin-6 (IL-6), IL-1, and tumor necrosis factor (TNF) in human blood mononuclear cells: IL-6 suppresses IL-1 and TNF. Blood 1990; 75:40–47.

28. Aderka D, Le J, Vilcek J. IL-6 inhibits lipopolysaccharide-induced tumor necrosis factor production in cultured human monocytes, U937 cells, and in mice. J Immunol 1989; 143:3517–3523.

29. Sironi M, Munoz C, Pollicino T, et al. Divergent effects of interleukin-10 on cytokine production by mononuclear phagocytes and endothelial cells. Eur J Immunol 1993; 23:2692–2695.

30. Bean AGD, Freiberg RA, Andrade S, Menon S, Zlotnik A. Interleukin-10 protects mice against staphylococcal enterotoxin B-induced lethal shock. Infect Immun 1993; 61:4937–4939.

31. Bermudez LE, Champsi J. Infection with mycobacterium avium induces production of interleukin-10 (IL-10), and administration of anti-IL-10 antibody is associated with enhanced resistance to infection in mice. Infect Immun 1993; 61:3093–3097.

32. Denis M, Ghadirian E. IL-10 neutralization augments mouse resistance to systemic mycobacterium avium infections. J Immunol 1993; 151:5425–5430.

33. Frei K, Nadal D, Pfister HW, Fontana A. Listeria meningitis: identification of a cerebrospinal fluid inhibitor of macrophage listericidal function as interleukin-10. J Exp Med 1993; 178: 1255–1261.

34. Durez P, Abramowicz D, Gérard C, et al. In vivo induction of Interleukin-10 by anti-CD3 monoclonal antibody or bacterial lipopolysaccharide: differential modulation by cyclosporin A. J Exp Med 1993; 177:551–555.

35. Ishida H, Hastings R, Thompson-Snipes L, Howard M. Modified immunological status of anti-IL-10 treated mice. Cell Immunol 1993; 148:371–384.

36. van der Poll T, Marchant A, Berman L, et al. Endogenous interleukin-10 protects against death in septic peritonitis in mice. Surg Forum (in press).

37. Zanetti G, Heumann D, Gérain J, et al. Cytokine production after intravenous or peritoneal gram-negative bacterial challenge in mice. J Immunol 1992; 148:1890–1897.

38. Gadina M, Bertini R, Mengozzi M, Zandalasini M, Mantovani A, Ghezzi P. Protective effect of chlorpromazine on endotoxin toxicity and TNF production in glucocorticoid-sensitive and glucocorticoid-resistant models of endotoxic shock. J Exp Med 1991; 173:1305–1310.

39. Schade UF. Pentoxifylline increases survival in murine endotoxin shock and decreases formation of tumor necrosis factor. Circ Shock 1990; 31:171–181.

40. Mengozzi M, Fantuzzi G, Faggioni R, et al. Chlorpromazine specifically inhibits peripheral and brain TNF production, and up-regulates IL-10 production, in mice. Immunology 1994; 82:207–210.

41. Marchant A, Bruyns C, Vandenabeele P, et al. The protective role of interleukin-10 in endotoxin shock. In: Levin J, van Deventer S, van der Poll T, Sturk A, eds. Bacterial Endotoxins: Basic Science to Anti-Sepsis Strategies. New York: Wiley-Liss, 1994:417–423.

42. Nguyen DT, Eskandai MK, DeForge LE, et al. Cyclosporin A modulation of tumor necrosis factor gene expression and effects in vitro and in vivo. J Immunol 1990; 144:3822–3828.

43. Marchant A, Devière J, Byl B, De Groote D, Vincent JL, Goldman M. Interleukin-10 production during septicaemia. Lancet 1994; 343:707–708.

44. Derkx B, Marchant A, Goldman M, Bijlmer R, van Deventer S. High levels of interleukin-10 during the initial phase of fulminant meningococcal septic shock. J Infect Dis 1995; 171:229–232.

45. van Deuren M, van der Ven-Jongekrijg J, Demacker PNM, et al. Differential expression of proinflammatory cytokines and their inhibitors during the course of meningococcal infections. J Infect Dis 1994; 169:157–161.

46. Munoz C, Carlet J, Fitting C, Misset B, Bleriot JP, Cavaillon JM. Dysregulation of in vitro cytokine production by monocytes during sepsis. J Clin Invest 1991; 88:1747–1754.

47. Simpson SQ, Modi HN, Balk RA, Bone RC, Casey LC. Reduced alveolar macrophage production of tumor necrosis factor during sepsis in mice and men. Crit Care Med 1991; 19:1060–1066.

18

Hydrazine Sulfate: A Deceptively Simple Molecule Combining Endocrine and Immunological Protective Mechanisms Against Endotoxin Lethality

Richard Silverstein
University of Kansas Medical Center
Kansas City, Kansas

I. INTRODUCTION

Hydrazine, H_2NNH_2, is the smallest molecule currently known to protect against the lethal effects of endotoxin. That finding was first reported by our laboratory in 1989 (1). Those studies were predicated upon a series of reports from several laboratories dating back to the early part of the century, which, on the surface, appear to have little to do with therapeutic sepsis intervention. Underhill (2–4) and others (5) demonstrated that a single high-level dose of hydrazine sulfate administered to dogs, rabbits, or rats resulted in death within a matter of hours. This was preceded by an acute drop in blood sugar. These animals evidently proceeded through a crisis inasmuch as the survivors soon exhibited normal blood sugar levels and otherwise manifested no apparent aftereffects.

In 1970, evidence for a possible biochemical explanation for these observations was published. Lardy had been studying the gluconeogenic regulatory enzyme phosphoenolpyruvate carboxykinase (PEPCK), including its modulation by a number of low-molecular-weight nitrogen compounds. In an elegant set of in vitro and in vivo studies with fasted rats, he and his co-workers were able to confirm rapid and reversible changes in blood glucose in response to hydrazine. They also demonstrated that, prior to the drop in blood glucose, hydrazine precipitated a metabolic crossover in the gluconeogenic pathway at the PEPCK locus (6). When PEPCK was isolated from the livers of these animals, its concentration in that tissue was shown to be increased as a function of time following hydrazine sulfate administration, at least through the first few hours. The authors suggested that this might have resulted from an adrenal response to the drop in blood glucose. By 5 h after admininstration of hydrazine, glucose levels had returned to normal values. Finally, it was demonstrated that hydrazine inhibited PEPCK in vitro in a reversible and noncompetitive manner and at concentrations of hydrazine consistent with the in vivo crossover. Hydrazine-mediated hypoglycemia, therefore, became associated with gluconeogenesis, its enzyme machinery, and, specifically, the enzyme PEPCK.

The first indication that hydrazine sulfate might, under some circumstances, elicit a beneficial effect toward disease did not come from sepsis research, but rather from studies of cancer cachexia, another serious medical problem with broad pathological manifestations. As early as 1968, Gold had argued that pharmacological agents that inhibit gluconeogenesis might be useful in the treatment of cancer (7). In subsequent studies, his efforts focused on one particular agent, hydrazine sulfate, and on the cachexia associated with cancer. While it is not the focus of this review to critically assess these studies here, it should be noted that several laboratories have subsequently reported positive manifestations of hydrazine sulfate as an anticancer cachexia agent (8–12). In contrast, other investigators have not found a significant therapeutic value in its application (13–15).

Gold's rationale for hydrazine sulfate as an anticachexia agent centers on its antigluconeogenic action against PEPCK, and in that respect, hydrazine sulfate has been shown to have potential metabolic benefits in cancer patients related to glucose tolerance and to metabolic turnover (10,16).

Our understanding of the underlying causes of cancer cachexia, though still not entirely clear, has evolved to include not only metabolic and endocrine considerations, but also immunological modulation. As reviewed recently by Beutler (17), there is increasing evidence for a cytokine role in mediating cancer cachexia and, in particular, involvement of TNF. Though it should be emphasized that these viewpoints of cachexia need not be mutually exclusive, it was amid that background that the first studies from this laboratory were carried out to test whether hydrazine sulfate would protect mice against the lethal effects of LPS, a prime source of host TNF.

II. HYDRAZINE SULFATE PROTECTS MICE AGAINST LPS AND TNF LETHALITY

A. The Strategy for Hydrazine Sulfate Administration: A Concern with Hydrazine Toxicity

In the normal mouse endotoxin lethality model, endotoxin is injected into mice intraperitoneally in a single bolus dose. Mice that are given an LPS dose approximating the LD_{50} (100–500 µg) proceed to a lethal crisis between 24 and 36 h. By 48–72 h, the surviving mice appear normal and the final numbers of survivors can be estimated with reasonable confidence that no additional deaths will occur. The possibility that hydrazine sulfate treatment might compound LPS toxicity was of potential concern inasmuch as LPS is, itself, hypoglycemic, down-regulating PEPCK at the level of its transcription (18). In an effort to circumvent possible hydrazine sulfate toxicity, it was administered 5 h prior to LPS challenge. This allowed sufficient time for glucose levels to return to normal before the animals would be required to respond to the LPS challenge.

It was found that the 5-h pretreatment time with hydrazine sulfate was an optimum period for the protection, as were doses of hydrazine sulfate of 30–80 mg/kg. Pretreatment with higher doses increased the number of deaths even though as much as 120 mg/kg hydrazine sulfate did not, of itself, lead to an irreversible decrease in blood glucose. When we eliminated the pretreatment period, hydrazine sulfate significantly increased endotoxin lethality, even within the 30–80 mg/kg hydrazine sulfate dose range (1).

B. Protection Against TNF

The initial focus for the studies to investigate hydrazine protective efficacy against LPS was the possibility that hydrazine might act against TNF, a cachexia-eliciting agent (19). Galanos and Freudenberg's laboratory had developed a murine model, the D-galactosamine model, that exquisitely sensitizes against TNF and, in the process, also sensitizes against LPS (20,21). Using this endotoxin-hypersensitive mouse model, we were able to show that hydrazine sulfate protected mice against both TNF- and LPS-mediated lethality (22). The timing and dosage of hydrazine sulfate administration that we had earlier shown would determine whether hydrazine sulfate would either protect against or intensify the harmful effects of LPS in normal mice were similar in this model as well. Also, the protection against LPS lethality was even more pronounced than in normal mice. In the latter, hydrazine sulfate protected at or near the LD_{50}. For example, in one of the published studies, none of 16 hydrazine sulfate–treated mice died in response to LPS at the control LD_{50} (12/24 deaths) (1). Among D-galactosamine–sensitized mice, protection held not only at the LD_{50}, but even when the dose of LPS was raised by more than four orders of magnitude relative to the LD_{50} (22).

III. MECHANISM

A. Introduction

Three different approaches were explored to define the potential mechanism for the observed protective efficacy of hydrazine sulfate. The first focused on hydrazine involvement in metabolic regulation (glucose, PEPCK, glucocorticoid). A second focused on the role of hydrazine sulfate in modulating the expression of LPS-derived inflammatory mediators. A third dealt directly with hydrazine chemistry. It was established that, in healthy animals, hydrazine will modulate PEPCK with some measure of enzyme and metabolic specificity, even though the relationship of that effect to hydrazine chemistry as yet remains unresolved. It was also reasonably clear from the research of Berry (23) and McCallum (24), that PEPCK is an important parameter in the endotoxin cascade. We therefore chose to focus first on the relationship between hydrazine and PEPCK, including the possibility of glucocorticoid mediation.

B. Glucocorticoid Participates in Hydrazine Sulfate Protection Against LPS

Hydrazine sulfate is known to up-regulate hepatic PEPCK, as documented by substantial and significant increases in PEPCK specific activity (units/mg total protein) in isolated liver homogenates and cytosol. This had earlier been reported in both normal (6,25) and cancerous (25) rodents. PEPCK is known to be modulated by several hormones, including significant up-regulation by glucocorticoid. Interestingly, glucocorticoids have long been associated with protection against LPS lethality, with pretreatment being critical to that protection (26). Thus, one possibility for hydrazine sulfate protection against LPS might be via glucocorticoids. It will be established in this and succeeding sections of this report that glucocorticoid is, in fact, a necessary component of hydrazine sulfate protection against LPS. It will also be shown, however, that there is a significant glucocorticoid-*independent* component to the protection.

Several pieces of both negative and positive experimentation suggest glucocorticoid involvement in hydrazine sulfate protection against LPS. For example, removal of the pituitary abrogates hydrazine sulfate protection (22), as does removal of the adrenals (27). In normal mice, an elevated serum glucocorticoid can be demonstrated within 1 h after injection of a protective dose of hydrazine sulfate (22). Perhaps the most definitive evidence derives from corticosterone replacement studies (27). As is well known, adrenalectomized mice manifest a markedly increased sensitivity to the lethal effects of LPS. Corticosterone and/ or mineralocorticoid supplementation, by injection and/or drinking water, will increase the LD_{50}. However, LD_{50} levels are still substantially less than those seen in normal mice, and even that measure of increased defense requires substantial supplementation (28). Lower doses of *natural* glucocorticosteroid, which by itself provides no apparent benefit against LPS lethality, were nevertheless able to restore hydrazine sulfate protection.

It can therefore be concluded that (1) hydrazine sulfate treatment results in an up-regulation of circulating glucocorticoid levels, (2) hydrazine sulfate protection against LPS requires glucocorticoid, and (3) hydrazine sulfate up-regulates PEPCK in normal and cancerous rodents. Thus, a testable endocrine-metabolic hypothesis for hydrazine sulfate protection can be stated as follows:

> During the pretreatment period, hydrazine provokes a decrease in blood sugar that triggers a glucocorticoid response. The elevated glucocorticoid, in turn, leads to an increase in PEPCK. By the time of LPS challenge, glucose levels return to normal and the increased glucocorticoid and PEPCK bolster host defense.

To further explore such a possibility, it is necessary to consider the impact of hydrazine sulfate on hepatic PEPCK, not just in normal mice, but also during and immediately preceding endotoxic shock.

C. Hydrazine Sulfate and PEPCK in Endotoxin Shock

When mice are challenged with an LPS LD_{50} (200 μg) in the absence of hydrazine sulfate pretreatment, hepatic PEPCK levels are significantly reduced at 6 h and remain so through 12 h, consistent with earlier reports from the literature (24). Administration of 50 mg/kg hydrazine sulfate 5 h prior to LPS challenge results in an up-regulation of PEPCK at 6 h and 12 h post-LPS but not above that of normal untreated mice (1).

More recently, we have determined PEPCK and glucose levels not only at 6 h post-LPS, but also at the close of the 5-h pretreatment period, i.e., at 0 h in terms of LPS, as well as at 4 h post-LPS. These determinations were carried out in both the normal and D-galactosamine murine LPS lethality models. Once again, a significant decrease in PEPCK is attributable to LPS at 6 h, and a significant improvement among the hydrazine sulfate–pretreated groups has been observed. The levels of PEPCK do not, however, increase before that time, either at the end of the pretreatment phase or even 4 h into the challenge (R. Silverstein, W. Ewing, unpublished results) (Fig. 1). Such a result remains consistent with the previous study from Lardy's laboratory, where a sustained and continued increase in PEPCK was brought about by hydrazine as early as 2 h following hydrazine sulfate injection. In that study, the hydrazine sulfate dose used was 260 mg (2 mmol)/kg. In our experiments, the hydrazine sulfate dose was 80 mg/kg. We also established that, with the 80 mg/kg hydrazine sulfate, glucose levels were unaffected even during the pretreatment period (data not shown).

We therefore conclude that hydrazine sulfate modulation of PEPCK during protection against endotoxic shock is not a result of its ability to inhibit PEPCK directly and thereby bring about a hypoglycemic response. That would require significantly higher hydrazine sulfate dosage. More likely, it includes effects against one or more mediators of the endotoxin cascade, as discussed below. It is further concluded that the fundamental cause of hydrazine toxicity (without

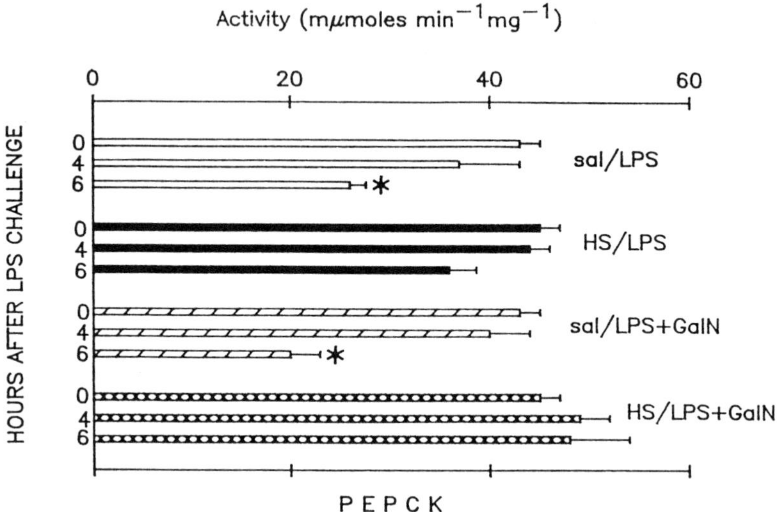

Figure 1   Effect of a 5-h 80 mg/kg hydrazine sulfate (HS) versus saline vehicle (sal) pretreatment on hepatic PEPCK activity before (0 h) and 4 h and 6 h after challenge of CF1 mice with 200 μg LPS, *S. enteritidis* (sal/LPS versus HS/LPS) or LPS plus 20 mg D-galactosamine (sal/LPS + GalN versus HS/LPS + GalN). Four mice per group. Data are ± SEM. Significance, $p < .05$, determined by Student's *t*-test.

pretreatment) is not limited to hypoglycemia, and indeed, under some circumstances, blood glucose modulation may not be involved at all.

D. Hydrazine Sulfate Acts Against the Release and Action of TNF

As discussed above, the hypothesis that both glucocorticoid and PEPCK are involved in hydrazine sulfate protection against LPS has proven correct, but not as originally conceived, that is, *not* through hydrazine's capacity to directly modulate gluconeogenesis. A second focus of our studies has been the relationship between hydrazine sulfate protection and cytokine mediators of endotoxin shock. We shall show from our own studies, as well as those from another laboratory (29), that modulation of TNF is in fact implicated. It will also become evident that the glucocorticoid requirement for protection may take place apart from hydrazine sulfate modulation of TNF activity.

1. Hydrazine Sulfate Selectively Attenuates the Release of TNF from Macrophages

Circulating levels of TNF and of IL-6 have been assessed in mice challenged with LPS, and then with or without pretreatment with a protective dose of hydrazine sulfate. These experiments were conducted with different strains of mice, different sources of LPS, and different modes of TNF assay (bioassay, immunoassay). In each instance, LPS-induced serum TNF was significantly reduced in hydrazine sulfate–pretreated mice relative to controls, whereas that of IL-6 was not (27).

To determine whether this attenuation was a consequence of hydrazine sulfate action at the level of the macrophage, complementary experiments were conducted in vitro with cultured macrophages (J774 cells). A selective decrease in LPS-dependent TNF secretion was again observed, and a hydrazine sulfate pretreatment period of several hours was required for the effect (30).

The attenuation of the TNF response to LPS occurs independently of glucocorticoid. It is seen not only in vitro and without glucocorticoid supplementation, but also in vivo in hypophysectomized or adrenalectomized mice (27).

2. Hydrazine Sulfate Acts Against TNF

The evidence that hydrazine acts not only against the release of TNF from its site of origin, but also against its subsequent pathophysiological effects is drawn from various observations and sources. First, as summarized above, hydrazine sulfate protects against the lethal effects of exogenous TNF as tested in the D-galactosamine model (22). Second, we have shown using C3H/HeJ mice, which are resistant to LPS at the level of the macrophage, that hydrazine sulfate pretreatment, followed by adoptive transfer of endotoxin-responsive macrophages, also results in protection. These LPS-responsive macrophages were either stimualted with LPS immediately before transfer or given to the C3H/HeJ mice simultaneously with LPS. The fact that hydrazine sulfate pretreatment remained protective even under these circumstances (27) allows the conclusion that hydrazine sulfate protection occurs, in part, subsequent to initial stimulation of the macrophage by LPS and, most likely, at one or more TNF targets.

A third piece of evidence derives from published studies of another laboratory (and which we have since fully confirmed) that demonstrate hydrazine sulfate protection of actinomycin D–sensitized L929 fibroblasts against TNF cytotoxicity (29).

Finally, there is increasing evidence that down-regulation of PEPCK by LPS not only requires one or more factors originating from the macrophage (26) but, in fact, is cytokine-mediated (18). Hydrazine sulfate counteraction of the PEPCK response to endotoxin is consistent with its being protective at the level of cytokine production and/or activity.

E. Modulation of Gene Expression

The ability of D-galactosamine to sensitize animals to LPS and TNF derives from its capacity to deplete hepatocyte UTP levels and thereby block RNA and protein synthesis in that cell (20). In the model developed by Galanos, and which was one of those employed in our lethality studies, D-galactosamine is administered simultaneously with LPS or TNF. Hydrazine sulfate pretreatment protects dramatically against LPS in this model, increasing the LD_{50} by several orders of magnitude. Hydrazine sulfate is administered 5 h prior to LPS, and therefore 5 h prior to D-galactosamine. Accordingly, a test was made of the hypothesis that hydrazine sulfate might be responsible for inducing the expression of one or more genes during the pretreatment period, which might somehow prime the animal for the inhibitory effects of D-galactosamine upon subsequent challenge (31).

It was first shown that hydrazine sulfate pretreatment did not affect the level of TNF and IL-1 mRNA produced by liver Kupffer cells in response to LPS challenge 5 h later. It was also shown that expression of metallothionein mRNA produced by the hepatocyte in response to LPS was unaffected. Such findings, nevertheless, do not preclude the possibility of one or more as-yet-unidentified genes in the hepatocyte being directly, or indirectly, triggered by hydrazine sulfate during the pretreatment period. That possibility receives a measure of support from the fact that when D-galactosamine is also present during the pretreatment period, protection is not only reduced, it is eliminated (22).

IV. WHY IS HYDRAZINE SULFATE DIFFERENT FROM ALL OTHER PROTECTING AGENTS? OR IS IT?

One of the most important and consistent findings of these studies is the fact that a pretreatment period is a necessity for protection. At least part of the explanation for this fact seems straightforward, namely a hydrazine-mediated hypoglycemia. Yet a pretreatment period is *always* required for hydrazine sulfate beneficial action, even in the in vitro macrophage and fibroblast experiments. Moreover, within the dose range shown to be effective against LPS lethality, hydrazine sulfate is *not* detectably hypoglycemic. Collectively, these observations lead to the interesting speculation that the underlying basis for hydrazine toxicity overlaps that for LPS toxicity. Such a concept would have three immediate implications:

1. Administration of hydrazine sulfate at the same time as LPS would serve to enhance toxicity in vivo and in vitro. To achieve protection, a pretreatment period would be practically and theoretically unavoidable.
2. LPS at sublethal doses would protect against LPS. A pretreatment period would be required.
3. Hydrazine sulfate pretreatment protection and LPS pretreatment protection would overlap in mechanism.

The first prediction is supported by all findings with hydrazine sulfate to date. The second prediction is supported by the concept, by now well established, of early endotoxin tolerance (21). The third point is not inconsistent with our studies of hydrazine sulfate (27) and those of others of early endotoxin tolerance (32), showing a glucocorticoid-dependent and glucocorticoid-independent character to both protective effects.

V. FUTURE DIRECTIONS

In the event that hydrazine sulfate protection and early endotoxin tolerance might be interrelated mechanistically, certain directions for future studies are suggested. It should first be noted that there is evidence for cross-tolerance in vivo between LPS and TNF (21). As pointed out above, hydrazine is a much simpler molecule than LPS, so it would seem reasonable to sharpen the focus on its structure and chemical properties. Hydrazine, as a weak base, could be expected to act as a lysosomotropic amine, and such low-molecular-weight amines have already been reported to be protective against TNF cytotoxicity (33). Another possibility is suggested by a recent report from Baeuerle's laboratory pointing to a possible role for hydrogen peroxide in LPS-mediated signal transduction (34). Hydrazine has long been known to possess a chemistry in certain respects similar to that of hydrogen peroxide (35,36). Also, hydrazine derivatives have earlier been shown to be irreversible inhibitors of the decomposition of hydrogen peroxide by catalase (37). Recently, we have shown that hydrazine itself is a potent, kinetically reversible catalase inhibitor (R. Silverstein, M. P. Sherman, D. C. Johnson, D. C. Morrison, unpublished results). The relationship between H_2NNH_2 and LPS, and perhaps also between H_2NNH_2 and HOOH, may continue to develop, possibly as one additional and novel route toward increased understanding and control of LPS pathophysiology.

ACKNOWLEDGMENT

This research was supported by NIH Grant AI30500. The author also wishes to acknowledge the support, encouragement, and collaboration of a number of colleagues, in particular Drs. David C. Morrison, Donald C. Johnson, Michael P. Sherman, Glen K. Andrews, Chris Galanos, and Marina A. Freudenberg. The author also acknowledges Dr. Fenglan Jia for the in-vitro studies with J774 macrophages.

REFERENCES

1. Silverstein R, Christofferson CA, Morrison DC. Modulation of endotoxin lethality in mice by hydrazine sulfate. Infect Immun 1989; 57:2072–2078.
2. Underhill FP. Studies in carbohydrate metabolism. I. The influence of hydrazine upon the organism, with special reference to the blood sugar content. J Biol Chem 1911; 10:159–168.

3. Underhill FP, Fine MS. Studies in carbohydrate metabolism. II. The prevention and inhibition of diabetes. J Biol Chem 1911; 10:271–285.

4. Underhill FP. The influence of hydrazine upon blood concentration and blood sugar content. J Biol Chem 1923; 58:147–151.

5. Fortney SR, Clark DA, Stein E. Inhibition of gluconeogenesis by hydrazine adminnistration in rats. J Pharmacol Exp Ther 1967; 156:277–284.

6. Ray PD, Hanson RL, Lardy HA. Inhibition by hydrazine of gluconeogenesis in the rat. J Biol Chem 1970; 245:690–696.

7. Gold J. Proposed treatment of cancer by inhibition of gluconeogenesis. Oncology 1968; 22:185–207.

8. Gold J. Use of hydrazine sulfate in terminal and preterminal cancer patients: results of investigational new drug (IND) study in 84 evaluable patients. Oncology 1975; 32:1–10.

9. Gershanovich ML, Danova LA, Ivin BA, Filov VA. Results of clinical study of antitumor action of hydrazine sulfate. Nutr Cancer 1981; 3:7–12.

10. Chlebowski RT, Heber D, Richardson B, Block JB. Influence of hydrazine sulfate on abnormal carbohydrate metabolism in cancer patients with weight loss. Cancer Res 1984; 44:857–861.

11. Chlebowski RT, Bulcavage L, Grosvenor M, et al. Hydrazine sulfate in cancer patients with weight loss. Cancer 1987; 59:406–410.

12. Chlebowski RT, Bulcavage L, Grosvenor M, et al. Hydrazine sulfate influence on nutritional status and survival in non-small cell lung cancer. J Clin Oncol 1990; 8:9–15.

13. Lerner HJ, Regelson W. Clinical trial of hydrazine sulfate in solid tumors. Cancer Treat Rep 1976; 60:959–960.

14. Loprinzi CL, Kuross SA, O'Fallon JR, et al. Randomized, placebo-controlled evaluation of hydrazine sulfate in patients with advanced colorectal cancer. J Clin Oncol 1994; 12:1121–1129.

15. Loprinzi CL, Goldberg RM, Su JQ, et al. Placebo-controlled trial of hydrazine sulfate in patients with newly diagnosed non-small-cell lung cancer. J Clin Oncol 1994; 12:1126–1129.

16. Tayer JA, Heber D, Chlebowski RT. Effect of hydrazine sulphate on whole-body protein breakdown measured by ^{14}C-lysine metabolism in lung cancer patients. Lancet 1987; 2:241–243.

17. Beutler B. Cytokines and cancer cachexia. Hosp Pract April 15, 1993, pp. 45–52.

18. Hill MR, McCallum RE. Identification of tumor necrosis factor as a transcriptional regulator of the phosphoenolpyruvate carboxykinase gene following endotoxin treatment of mice. Infect Immun 1992; 60:4040–4050.

19. Tracey KJ, Wei H, Manogue KR, et al. Cachectin/tumor necrosis factor induces cachexia, anemia, and inflammation. J Exp Med 1988; 167:1211–1227.

20. Galanos C, Freudenberg MA, Reutter W. Galactosamine-induced sensitization to the lethal effects of endotoxin. Proc Natl Acad Sci USA 1979; 11:5939–5943.

21. Galanos CA, Freudenberg MA, Katschinski T, Salomao R, Mossmann H, Kumazawa Y. Tumor necrosis factor and host response to endotoxin. In: Ryan JL, Morrison DC, eds. Bacterial endotoxic lipopolysaccharides. Vol. 2. Boca Raton, FL: CRC Press, 1992:75–104.

22. Silverstein R, Turley BR, Christoffersen CA, Johnson DC, Morrison DC. Hydrazine sulfate protects D-galactosamine–sensitized mice against endotoxin and tumor necrosis factor/cachectin lethality: evidence of a role for the pituitary. J Exp Med 1991; 173:357–365.

23. Rippe DF, Berry LJ. Study of the inhibition of induction of phosphoenolpyruvate carboxykinase by endotoxin with radial immunodiffusion. Immunity 1972; 6:766–772.

24. McCallum RE, Seale TW, Stith RD. Influence of endotoxin treatment on dexamethasone induction of hepatic phosphoenolpyruvate carboxykinase. Infect Immun 1983; 39:213–219.

25. Silverstein R, Bhatia P, Svoboda DJ. Effect of hydrazine sulfate on glucose-regulating enzymes in the normal and cancerous rat. Immunopharmacology 1989; 17:37–43.

26. Silverstein, R. The endocrine response to endotoxin. In: Ryan JL, Morrison DC, eds. Bacterial endotoxic lipopolysaccharides. Vol. 2. Boca Raton, FL: CRC Press, 1992:295–309.

27. Johnson DC, Freudenberg MA, Jia F, et al. Contribution of tumor necrosis factor-α and glucocorticoid in hydrazine sulfate–mediated protection against endotoxin lethality. Circ Shock 1994; 43:1–8.

28. Silverstein R, Hannah PD, Johnson DC. Natural adrenocorticoids do not restore resistance to endotoxin in the adrenalectomized mouse. Circ Shock 1993; 41:162–165.

29. Hughes TK, Cadet P, Larned CS. Modulation of tumor necrosis factor activities by a potential anticachexia compound, hydrazine sulfate. Int J Immunopharm 1989; 5:501–507.

30. Jia F, Morrison DC, Silverstein R. Hydrazine sulfate selectively modulates the TNF response to endotoxin in mouse macrophages. Circ Shock 1994; 42:111–114.

31. De SK, Silverstein R, Andrews GK. Hydrazine sulfate protection against endotoxin lethality: analysis of effects on expression of hepatic cytokine genes and an acute-phase gene. Microb Pathogen 1992; 13:37–47.

32. Evans GF, Zuckerman SH. Glucocorticoid-dependent and -independent mechanisms involved in lipopolysaccharide tolerance. Eur J Immunol 1991; 21:1973–1979.

33. Watanabe N, Niitsu Y, Neda H, et al. Cytocidal mechanism of TNF: effects of lysosomal enzyme and hydroxyl radical inhibitors on cytotoxicity. Immunopharmacol Immunotoxicol 1988; 10:109–116.

34. Schreck R, Rieber P, Baueurle PA. Reactive oxygen intermediates as apparently widely used messengers in the activation of the NF-kappa B transcription factor and HIV-1. EMBO J 1991; 10:2247–2258.

35. Walling C. Free radicals in solution. New York: Wiley, 1957:524.

36. Pauling L. The Nature of the Chemical Bond, 3rd ed. Ithaca, NY: Cornell University Press, 1960:85.

37. Margoliash E, Novogrodsky A, Ashejter A. Irreversible reaction of 3-amino-1:2:4-triazole and related inhibitors with the protein of catalase. J Biol Chem 1960; 74:339–348.

19

Variations in β-Lactam Antibiotic-Induced Release of Endotoxin: In Vivo Relevance

J. J. Jackson and H. Kropp
Merck Research Laboratories
Rahway, New Jersey

I. ENDOTOXIN IS IMPLICATED IN SEPTIC SHOCK

Despite discoveries of numerous specific and broad-spectrum antibiotics, in addition to improved adjunctive supportive therapy, mortality and morbidity associated with gram-negative-related septic shock remain unacceptably high. A similar statement may apply to infections due to gram-positive bacteria. While "appropriate antibiotic therapy" significantly reduces mortality, excess endotoxin (lipopolysaccharide, LPS) spontaneously released from gram-negative bacteria (during the normal bacterial growth cycle or as a consequence of interactions of normal serum with gram-negative bacteria), or following antibiotic treatment, has been implicated in septic shock (1–5). Endotoxin(s), which may vary considerably in bioreactivity and concentration, circulate in the milieu and trigger a cascade of events in septic shock through binding of its lipid A moiety to receptors on the surfaces of a variety of host cells (primarily macrophages/monocytes), thereby stimulating the production and release of excess immunomodulatory proteins (cytokines). It is the serial production of excess cytokines and mediators (TNF-α. IL-1β, PAF, IFN-γ, IL-8, IL-6, etc.) that primarily propagates secondary inflammatory mediators as a consequence of extended exposure to relatively high LPS concentrations, which result in host immunosuppression and tissue destruction that contribute to pathogenesis associated with septic shock (6–8).

Aside from cellular targets, excess LPS also impacts the host negatively through excess activation of humoral targets such as the complement and coagulation systems (cascades), which contribute to vasodilation, disseminated intravascular coagulation (DIC), capillary leakage, and neutrophil chemotaxis. This, combined with cellular-mediated effects, can lead to the septic syndrome, hypotension, adult respiratory distress syndrome (ARDS), multiple organ failure (MOF), and possibly death. Other non-LPS bacterial products (peptidoglycan, teichoic acids, non-LPS toxins, etc.) have variable effects but are less significant (individually) in pathogenesis associated with septic shock than endotoxin.

Difficulty of Establishing in-Vitro/in-Vivo Correlation of Antibiotic-Induced LPS Release

Clinical attempts to establish an in-vitro/in-vivo correlation between gram-negative bacteremia, antibiotic-induced endotoxin liberation, or cytokine levels and poor patient outcome are complicated by (a) the lack of homogeneity in the lethalities or cytokine-stimulatory properties of endotoxins from bacterial isolates of the same and different species; (b) differences in modes of action of antibiotics being compared—differences which affect the quantity and time of endotoxin release and the magnitude of cytokines produced; (c) local versus systemic sampling techniques; and (d) underlying infections due to fungi, viruses, protozoa, or gram-positive bacteria (and their non-LPS subcellular components), each of which is also capable of stimulating cytokine production (although to a somewhat lesser extent than endotoxin released from gram-negative bacteria) (9). The manner of reporting endotoxin levels may add further to this controversy. For example, when antibiotic-induced LPS release is reported as percentage of total LPS instead of absolute amount of free endotoxin, the cell (bio) mass (i.e., number of bacteria in the infection), which is responsible for LPS production, becomes irrelevant. This is misleading, especially when antibiotics with different modes of action and fast killing rates are compared to those with delayed killing actions [which allow continued increased bacterial cell mass with concomitant continued endotoxin synthesis) (10)]. Retrospective studies are complicated by the lack of standardization of antibiotic regimens, intentional or inadvertent delays of such treatments, in addition to the vast numbers of antibiotic regimens to which an individual patient may have been exposed.

II. DO β-LACTAM ANTIBIOTICS LIBERATE MORE LPS THAN OTHER ANTIBIOTIC CLASSES?

Despite the above complexities, it is generally accepted that all antibiotics studied thus far can induce the release of variable amounts of endotoxin under appropriate circumstances and that excess antibiotic-liberated (free) endotoxin is deleterious to the welfare of the patient. More than any other, β-lactam (cell-wall-active) antibiotics as a class are widely considered the antibiotics most responsible for excessive endotoxin liberation (6,11–21) in response to their cell-wall-destructive modes of activities. The antimicrobial actions of all β-lactams on gram-negative bacteria are the result of their differential binding to important enzymes in cell-wall synthesis referred to as penicillin-binding proteins (PBPs), found in the periplasmic space of the outer membranes of gram-negative bacteria. Although the PBPs may number as many as nine, depending on the bacterial species and individual isolates, only three or four are considered important targets of β-lactams (PBPs 1, 2, 3, and perhaps 7).

A. β-Lactam Antibiotics Act Through PBP Binding

Most β-lactam antibiotics have multiple and variable binding affinities for PBPs, and thus enzymatic inhibition occurs through the saturation of one or more PBPs to differentially induce morphological changes in bacteria which are important for growth, shape, and bacterial lysis (22,23). Saturation of PBP 1 induces cell lysis compared to spheroplast (round or oval shape) formation stimulated by inhibition of PBP 2 and filament (cell elongation without septation) induction upon saturation of PBP 3 (24). (See Fig. 1 for a diagram of representative morphologies.) PBP 7 is thought to be important in antibiotic penetration of slow- or nongrowing bacteria—a property associated with imipenem (IPM), nocardicin, GCP14233, etc. (25). The ultimate morphology obtained, however, is the sum of the inhibitory actions on these PBPs (24).

For example, in the absence of host factors, in-vitro filaments induced by saturation of PBP 3 exist until lysed by antibiotic saturation of PBP 1. Filaments have been shown to last ≥24 h following treatment of certain gram-negative bacteria (i.e., *Pseudomonas aeruginosa*) with subMIC levels of antibiotics that have high primary but not exclusive PBP 3 affinity (i.e., ceftazidime, CTZ and aztreonam, AZT). Thus, the initial inhibition of PBP 1 or 2 may preclude the potential development of filaments induced by delayed saturation of PBP 3. Antibiotics with relatively high binding affinities for more than one primary PBP (i.e., PBPs 2 and 3) may demonstrate both morphologies (i.e., filaments and spheroplasts), depending on antibiotic concentration and provided the affinity for PBP 1 is significantly below that of both PBP 2 and PBP 3 (26). The numerous β-lactam antibiotics are further divided into subclasses (i.e., carbapenems, cephalosporins, monobactams, and penicillins), depending on side-group modifications of their β-lactam core structure. As a result, they show wide variability in binding affinities for a number of high- and low-molecular-weight PBPs. It should be noted that none of the β-lactam antibiotics being discussed in this report has affinity for only one PBP. Thus, reference to the PBP specificity of a particular antibiotic (e.g., PBP 3-specific) simply identifies the PBP for which the relevant antibiotic has the highest affinity.

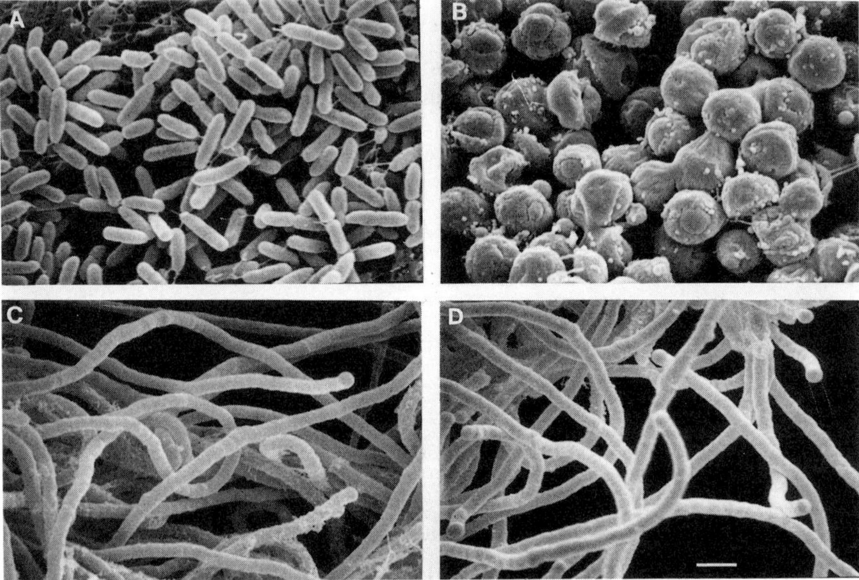

Figure 1 Scanning electronmicrographs of *P. aeruginosa* MB3286 exposed to: A, no antibiotic; B, imipenem 2 μg/mL (2 × MIC) for 3 h; C, ceftazidime 4 μg/mL (2 × MIC) for 7 h; D, aztreonam 16 μg/mL (2 × MIC) for 7 h. Magnification 10,000. Bar = 1 μm.

B. Relationship of PBP Specificity to Endotoxin Liberation

Recent in-vitro data using a variety of gram-negative bacteria show that some, but not all, β-lactam antibiotics induce the release of LPS above that released by antibiotics of other classes (i.e., aminoglycosides, quinolones, and bacteriostatic agents) (11–21). In fact, differences in the relative propensities of β-lactam antibiotics to release LPS also exist among and within the subclasses of β-lactam antibiotics and have been demonstrated in studies using *Pseudomonas aeruginosa*, *Escherichia coli*, *Enterobacter cloacae*, *Haemophilus influenza*, and *Klebsiella pneumoniae* (6,7,11,15,21,23,27,28).

1. SubMIC Antibiotic Levels Effectively Demonstrate Relationship Between PBP 3-Specific Antibiotic-Induced Filamentation and LPS Release

Studies with subminimal inhibitory antibiotic concentrations (subMIC) show that antibiotic-induced endotoxin release is not solely dependent on the cell-wall-destructive actions of β-lactams and that the induction of filament formation may be partially responsible (11,15,27–29). In these studies it has been determined that low antibiotic levels (11) or subMIC [15] amounts of β-lactam antibiotics that primarily exhibit high affinity for PBP 3, including cephalosporins [e.g., ceftazidime (CTZ) and cefuroxime (CFX)] and monobactams [e.g., aztreonam (AZT)], induce liberation of endotoxin in amounts at least equivalent to, but more frequently in excess of, that released via correspondingly higher inhibitory quantities ($2\times$ to $800\times$ MIC) of the same antibiotics. Additionally, it is shown that fast-killing spheroplast-inducing β-lactam antibiotics (e.g., imipenem) do indeed release near-maximum amounts of LPS at earlier times than slower-killing filament-inducing β-lactams (i.e., certain cephalosporins, monobactams, and penicillins), which will ultimately liberate even greater total quantities of free LPS at later time points than IPM (11,15). In this respect LPS release is associated with bacterial biomass.

Thus, exclusive reliance on colony counts as an indication of cell number (biomass) gives the illusion that filament-inducing β-lactam antibiotics rapidly inhibit bacterial growth, whereas in fact, individual rod growth (increased cell mass) and concomitant increased endotoxin synthesis is continued for extended periods of time—a phenomenon that is not unique to β-lactam antibiotics. For example, Van den Berg et al. recently showed filamentation of *E. coli* following a 6-h treatment with a fluoroquinolone, ciprofloxacin (CIP). Quinolones, unlike β-lactam antibiotics, do not bind to PBPs but inhibit DNA-gyrase activity which causes induction of the SOS response that leads to filamentation. Consequently, under these circumstances *E. coli* exposed to CIP lose their capacity to reproduce but grow individually as filaments to reach a total cell mass that approaches that of non-antibiotic-treated cultures (27). It is hypothesized that free LPS activity is proportional to bacterial biomass. This, however, may not be entirely true, since bacteria allowed to form filaments at subMIC levels of β-lactam antibiotics with high PBP 3 affinity (at concentrations in which no cell lysis occurs) can release even more free LPS (in a yet-unexplained manner) than that liberated spontaneously by exponentially growing non-antibiotic-treated bacteria. Thus, the release of excess LPS through treatment with subMIC antibiotic levels may be the result of nonlytic bacterial wall damage in addition to filament induction.

The relationship between bacterial cell mass and antibiotic-induced LPS release may be determined via combination studies using optical density measurements of antibiotic-treated cultures, microscopic observations, and by determining free endotoxin levels of bacterial filtrates and of EDTA-treated filter residues of bacteria previously exposed to antibiotics over time. Up to 50% of endotoxin is releasable from gram-negative bacteria by treatment with a Ca^{2+} and Mg^{2+} chelating agent (0.01% EDTA) at room temperature for as little as 10 min. EDTA treatment of 0.45-μm filter residues of gram-negative bacteria exposed to inhibitory amounts of CTZ or IPM show that reduced amounts of free LPS are liberated by IPM lysis of spheroplasts compared to high LPS amounts released from filaments induced by CTZ treatment. This effect is not the result of an unusual or unexplainable action by these antibiotics. Rather, LPS-release analysis of EDTA filter residues simply show that fewer bacteria (smaller cell mass) remain in the bacterial filter retentate. Therefore, less LPS is available to be released following IPM exposure than is obtained from similar CTZ treatment of the same organism (15). The bacterial cell masses of *Pseudomonas* cultures treated with IPM and CTZ differ so vastly that any detectable differences in the percentage of free LPS release from total endotoxin by these antibiotics becomes irrelevant (10).

2.   In-Vitro Liberated Endotoxin Determined via Chromogenic Limulus Amebocyte Lysate (C-LAL) Assay Correlates with LPS Lethality In Vivo

The above in-vitro studies include monitoring changes in bacterial-associated LPS (free and bound) and colony-forming units, morphological variations, and cytokine production. For the most part, endotoxin quantifications are made using an LPS-enzyme-stimulated C-LAL assay that cleaves a chromogenic substrate. Importantly, membrane 0.45-μm filtrates of antibiotic-treated bacterial isolates grown in standard culture media are used as the endotoxin source. At high bacterial concentrations (i.e., 10^8-10^9 CFU), use of 0.2-μm filters causes bacterial shearing with subsequent release of large amounts of endotoxins that are not related to antibiotic treatment. Membrane shearing of LPS usually occurs during attempts to filter non-antibiotic-treated control cultures near their late log or stationary phase and may yield erroneously high amounts of free LPS. To confirm that differential C-LAL-positive 0.45-μm filtrates of antibiotic-treated cultures correlate with endotoxin lethality, 0.2-mL samples of 10-fold serial dilutions of filtrates obtained from cultures treated with spheroplast-forming IPM or filament-inducing CTZ discussed above are administered into the tail veins of CD1 mice. Before administration of the bacterial filtrates, mice are made hypersensitive to LPS by administering 20 μg of actinomycin D. The in-vivo toxicity of filtrates determined over 24–48 h confirm that IPM (a carbapenem which has the following PBP affinities, $2 > 1 > 3$) liberates 40- to 80-fold less lethal endotoxin than ceftazidime (a cephalosporin which has high primary affinity for PBP 3 which is $> 1 > 2$) despite comparable MICs. Along with this, the lethality in hypersensitive mice is consistent with differential endotoxin levels obtained in the C-LAL assay (15).

C.   How Does LPS Manifest Its Toxic Effect?

Endotoxin is innately nontoxic but manifests its lethality primarily through excessive cytokine production by a variety of host cells, including endothelial but principally LPS-stimulated macrophages/monocytes. Using a macrophagelike cell line (THP-1), Simon et al. (7), demonstrated that filtrates of imipenem-treated *E. coli* liberate less endotoxin than is obtained by similar treatments with cefotaxime (CFTX), CTZ, AZT, and CIP as measured by TNF-α production. At the same time, TNF-α levels induced by filtrates of IPM-exposed cultures were equivalent to low amounts released by amikacin (aminoglycoside) treatment. These data show that TNF-α levels correlate well with the amounts of LPS being liberated by the corresponding antibiotics and that minimum TNF-α/ LPS levels released in these studies also correlate with rapid bacterial death (reduced cell mass) following treatment with amikacin and imipenem. Similar observations were made by Dofferhoff et al. in LPS (11) and TNF-α release (30) studies with IPM-, CTZ-, CFX-, tobramycin (TOB)-, and chloramphenicol-treated *E. coli*. In the latter studies, even bacteriostatic chloramphenicol liberated more LPS than low levels released by fast-killing TOB or IPM. Although, the neuro- and nephrotoxic potentials of aminoglycosides are enhanced by the presence of free endotoxin (31,32), it is important to note that aminoglycosides (i.e., tobramycin, amikacin) used in combination with cephalosporins (i.e., cefuroxime, ceftazidime, cefotaxime), penicillins (i.e., ampicillin) (11,14,33), and perhaps monobactams (i.e., aztreonam), but not with carbapenems (i.e., imipenem), prevent the release of excessive free LPS liberated by the above antibiotics when used alone. Reduced endotoxin release by combinations with aminoglycosides may have been accomplished in part by rapid inhibition of cell growth in addition to possible direct LPS neutralization by aminoglycosides. Although impractical, we suspect that combination of fast-killing imipenem with slower cell mass-reducing cephalosporins, etc., may also yield low levels of LPS (similar in quantity to that liberated by IPM alone) as well, even though, unlike aminoglycosides, imipenem does not bind and neutralize endotoxin.

Arditi et al. extended the studies of Simon et al. (7) by comparing the amounts of TNF-α produced by normal physiologically relevant whole blood levels of macrophages/monocytes stimulated by exposure to LPS which passes through Transwell filters from ceftriaxone- or imipenem-treated *H. influenza* (6). The authors confirm the propensities of cephalosporins to liberate LPS levels in excess of those released by carbapenems and non-antibiotic-treated controls and in addition show that the amounts of TNF-α correspond to the killing capacity of the antibiotics, which may vary with the bacterial inoculum size.

Assuming that antibiotic-induced release of LPS is the major subcellular gram-negative bacterial inducer of cytokine production, the next logical step is to measure TNF-α levels stimulated by endotoxin liberated differentially from antibiotic-treated bacteria in whole blood or plasma containing normal levels of macrophages/monocytes rather than under optimal laboratory conditions using culture media. This would seem plausible because both differential antibiotic-induced bacterial clearance and endotoxin liberation have been reported in systemic (i.p. but not i.v.) or local infections of healthy animals using a variety of gram-negative bacteria (see Ref. 28).

The feasibility of using ''normal, healthy'' whole blood/plasma in such studies would, however, be questionable, since both serum-sensitive and -resistant bacteria are either lysed and/or rapidly cleared by normal, healthy (immunoglobulin- and complement-replete) whole blood/serum/plasma in the absence of antibiotic treatment. Removal of bacteria in this manner also releases excessive amounts of endotoxin, which makes it difficult to observe differential antibiotic-induced bacterial killing or endotoxin release. Perhaps the use of blood/plasma of infected patients or "somewhat compromised blood/plasma" rather than that of normal/ healthy individuals would be more appropriate (e.g., pretreatment of blood/ plasma with gram-positive bacteria or non-LPS subcellular bacterial fragments, etc., to "condition blood" prior to exposure to gram-negative bacteria and antibiotics). Further studies are required in this area.

D. Filamentation Occurs in Vivo

In-vitro and ex-vivo studies reported above suggest that circumstances in which antibiotic-induced filamentation is likely to occur are also conditions that yield release of excessive amounts of endotoxin. However, little in-vivo (17,28,34–38) or clinical evidence (1–3,11,39) has accumulated to suggest that antibiotic-induced LPS release is not simply an in-vitro phenomenon but has relevance in endotoxin-induced septic shock. Until recently, little published data even supported the occurrence of antibiotic-induced filamentation in the infected host. A current photograph submitted by Whelan et al. demonstrated *E. coli* filamentation in a poorly responding premature infant treated with vancomycin and CTZ. Filaments were not, however, observed when the infant later responded to combination antibiotic treatments with CTZ and amikacin (33). The Whelan observations agree with animal results obtained in the aminoglycoside-cephalosporin combination studies of Dofferhoff et al. (11) and in aminoglycoside-penicillin studies reported by Bingen et al. (14). Walterspiel et al. also report the presence of filaments in *H. influenza*-infected meningitis patients (personal communication), while Dofferhoff et al. recently showed filamentation of *E. coli* in the peritoneum of rats treated with CTZ (40). Finally, Bucklin and Morrison most recently demonstrated that *E. coli*-infected mice treated with CTZ and IPM (with similar MICs) differentially release LPS and, compared to low-LPS-inducing IPM, CTZ releases larger quantities of LPS, which results in an adverse effect on antibiotic efficacy as demonstrated by its comparatively poor response to more severe infections (13).

III. ANTIBIOTICS WITH EQUIVALENT MICs DIFFER DRAMATICALLY IN IN-VIVO EFFICACY REQUIREMENTS

Consistent with the results of Bucklin and Morrison (13), routine in-vivo efficacy comparison studies in our laboratories with normal CD1 mice severely infected by the i.p. route with a serum-sensitive laboratory isolate of s-LPS (smooth, complete or wild-type endotoxin) *P. aeruginosa* MB3286 showed that (despite comparable MICs) the amounts of CTZ required to protect mice (50% effective dose, ED_{50}) was unexpectedly 865-to 1057-fold greater than that of IPM following a single antibiotic treatment (Table 1, Exp. 1). Similar observations (451-fold above IPM-treated groups) were made in mice infected with a clinical s-LPS isolate (CL2343) in Exp. 2 and in mice immunocompromised (380- to 851-fold higher than that of IPM, Exp 3) with cyclophosphamide (CY) which was supplemented with ferric iron (Fe^{3+}) to enhance bacterial virulence of MB3286. Surprisingly, the increased amounts of CTZ necessary for protection against infection with CTZ-sensitive *Pseudomonas* MB3286 was of the same order of magnitude as that needed to protect normal mice against infection with CTZ-resistant (CTZ-R) *Pseudomonas* MB3286 (1571- to 1700-fold above that afforded by similar IPM treatment, Exp 4). Similar antibiotic treatment of normal mice infected with IPM-resistant (IPM-R) *Pseudomonas* CL2341 (Exp 5) showed, conversely, that the ED_{50} for CTZ more closely approaches that of IPM-treated mice (the CTZ need was only 36-fold greater than that of IPM), due primarily to a 90-fold increased need in the IPM protective dose compared to a 5-fold increased need in the amount of CTZ necessary for equivalent protection (compare Exp. 2 and Exp 5, Table 1). The above unexpected findings could be due to a variety of reasons, among which excess endotoxin released following antibiotic therapy could be at least partially responsible.

Table 1 Antibiotic Efficacy in Mice

CD1 mice versus *P. aeruginosa*	Challenges No. of LD_{50}s	ED_{50}, mg/kg (MIC)		ED_{50} ratio
		Imipenem	Ceftazidime	
1. MB3286—smooth	1000	0.2 (1–2)	173 (2)	865
	286	~0.1	148	1057
2. CL2343—smooth	1341	~0.1 (0.5)	65 (4)	451
3. MB3286 + CY/Fe^{3+}	700	~0.9	357	380
	70	~0.7	613	851
4. MB3286—Smooth, CTZ-R	1000	~0.4 (1)	613 (32)	1571
	574	~0.1	119	1700
5. CL2341—Smooth, IPM-R	32	9.1 (8)	334 (4)	36

Comparative in-vivo antibiotic efficacy (ED_{50}, single s.c. dose) of IPM plus cilastatin or CTZ in CD1 mice severely infected with a variety of laboratory and clinical isolates of s-LPS-liberating antibiotic-sensitive and -resistant *P. aeruginosa*. Mice in Exp 3 were immunosuppressed with cytoxan (CY) at 250 mg/kg 4 days prior to infection. Fe^{3+} (as ferric ammonium citrate) at 10 mg/kg was given as an admix of bacteria on the day of infection. All other experiments were conducted with normal mice. CTZ-R = ceftazidime-resistant and IPM-R = imipenem-resistant *P. aeruginosa*. Numbers in parenthesis = minimal inhibitory antibiotic concentrations (MICs).

A. Differential Antibiotic-Induced LPS Liberation via Imipenem (IPM), Ceftazidime (CTZ), and Meropenem (MERO) Treatments Is Concentration- and PBP-Specific

Using a variety of laboratory and clinical s-LPS (MB3286, CL2343, and MB5120) and one r-LPS mutant (MB5121) isolate of *P. aeruginosa*, it was established that (a) PBP 3-specific ceftazidime liberates up to 20- to 40-fold more free LPS than PBP 2-specific IPM or non-antibiotic-treated controls from both s-LPS and r-LPS mutants; (b) differential in-vitro LPS liberation correlates with lethality in mice; and (c) excess LPS release can occur in the relative absence of bacterial lysis (15,21). We conclude (as stated above) that the amount of antibiotic-released LPS correlates with the primary PBP-specificity/affinity (filamentation) and antibiotic concentration. We also suggest that a β-lactam antibiotic with primary affinity for a single PBP (i.e., represented by PBP 2-specific imipenem, a carbapenem) may liberate minimal endotoxin compared to excessive amounts released by other β-lactam antibiotics that have primary affinity for PBP 3. These data, while confirmed by others (6,7,11–15,20), may have inadvertently suggested that all carbapenems liberate minimal endotoxin even though most LPS-release studies only report results of noncarbapenem β-lactam antibiotics. To date, meropenem (or MERO, which has high affinities for both PBPs 2 and 3) is the only other carbapenem reported in LPS-release studies (41). The latter report, however, makes no comparison between carbapenems.

SubMIC data with β-lactams suggest that antibiotic concentration may be important in endotoxin liberation, as is the case with inductioin of foilamentation which has been associated with antibiotic-induced LPS release (15). It was established by Sumita et al. (26), in comparison studies with IPM, that MERO induces filamentation with *P. aeruginosa* at subMIC (½×) and (1× and 2×) MIC antibiotic levels and spheroplast formation at higher MICs (≥4× MIC), unlike IPM which induces only spheroplasts at both subMIC (½×) and MIC (1×, 2×, and ≥4× MIC) levels. The dual morphologies shown with MERO at different antibiotic concentrations are attributable to its high dual affinities for PBPs 2 and 3. Therefore, to confirm the importance of the PBP 2 specificity of IPM and determine if other carbapenems also release minimum free LPS, the relative propensities of PBP 2-specific IPM, PBP 3-specific CTZ, and PBPs 2- and 3-specific MERO to induce morphological changes and differentially release endotoxin from antibiotic-sensitive and -resistant *P. aeruginosa* at antibiotic concentrations of 100×, 2×, 1×, ½×, and ¼× MIC were compared. These MIC values are representative of those shown in the pharmacokinetic antibiotic spectrum (Fig. 2). The in-vitro morphological observations of Sumita were confirmed with IPM and MERO in studies with laboratory and clinical, antibiotic-sensitive and (surprisingly) -resistant *P. aeruginosa* isolates as well. These studies also reaffirm that CTZ induces filaments at subMIC (¼×, ½×) and inhibitory (1×, 2×, and 100× MIC) concentrations (which allows continuous individual rod growth and endotoxin synthesis).

Thus, there appears to be a direct correlation between PBP 3-specific antibiotic concentration and induction of filament formation. It should be noted that the potential development of this morphological variation (i.e., filamentation) may also vary for each individual antibiotic as well as for the bacterial species being evaluated as a result of differential PBP affinities of each antibiotic in addition to the quantity of PBP to be saturated for a particular isolate. For example, aztreonam (AZT), which has relatively low affinities for PBP 1 and 2 but high affinity for PBP 3, forms filaments readily with most gram-negative bacteria regardless of antibiotic concentration, while CTZ is more selective and induces filaments with *P. aeruginosa*, *E. cloacae*, etc., more readily than with *E. coli* at high MICs. However, at low to subMIC antibiotic levels CTZ and AZT induce filament formation equally well with most gram-negative organisms. SubMIC β-lactam antibiotic levels generally appear to consistently induce filaments and readily release excessive amounts of LPS from most gram-negative bacteria. A considerable number of β-lactam antibiotics, however, more often than not, induce filaments well above their MICs (42). Yet induction of specific morphologies may vary considerably among PBP 3-specific β-lactam antibiotics for a

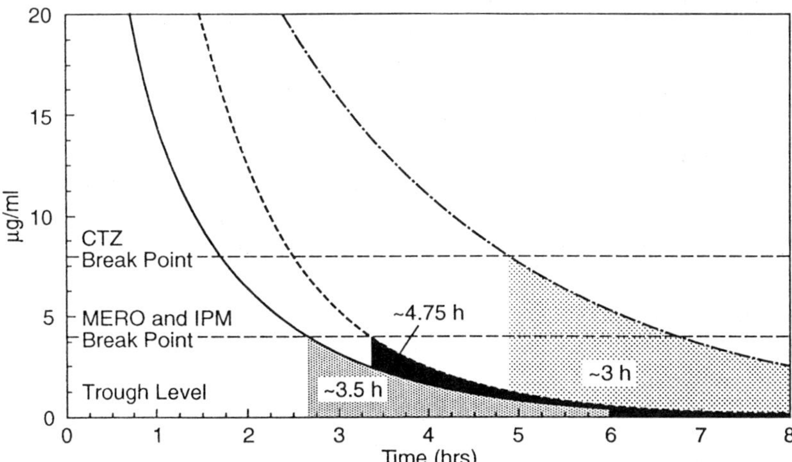

Figure 2 Human pharmacokinetic plasma antibiotic concentrations of imipenem (IPM, ——) administered in 0.5-g doses (4 × day or every 6 h) while meropenem (MERO, – – – –) and ceftazidime (CTZ, –•–•–) are given as 1-g doses (3 × day or every 8 h). Shaded areas represent time in hours in which antibiotics are below their respective inhibitory concentrations (subMIC) following antibiotic administration.

specific bacterial isolate. In contrast, PBP 2-specific imipenem induces only spheroplast formation in a wide variety of gram-negative bacteria at subMIC and high-MIC antibiotic levels.

B.   Subinhibitory Antibiotic Concentrations Exist in Vivo

Subinhibitory antibiotic concentrations occur in vivo. The manufacturers of the IPM, MERO, and CTZ antibiotics recommend a dosing regimen of 3–4 times/day or every 6–8 h. In humans, imipenem is usually administered in 0.5-g doses 4 times daily (every 6 h), while both MERO and CTZ are administered primarily in 1- to 2-g doses 3 times daily or at 8-h intervals. Following a single antibiotic treatment, the antibiotic level rapidly increases to a maximum concentration (C_{max}) or "peak" level, which then rapidly and progressively declines over the next 6–8 h to fall below a mean therapeutic level ("break point") and ultimately reach a subinhibitory or "trough" level prior to the next dosage. Human pharmacokinetic data (Fig. 2) therefore suggest that subinhibitory concentrations may occur in vivo for periods of one-third to one-half of the recommended dosing schedule (~3.5 of 6 h, 4.75 of 8 h, and 3 of 8 h, respectively, for IPM, MERO, and CTZ) (43–45).

C.   Comparative LPS Release from *Pseudomonas* Induced by IPM, MERO, and CTZ

The relative propensities of IPM, MERO, and CTZ to liberate endotoxin at doses representative of "peak," "break point," and "trough" antibiotic concentrations ($100\times$, $2\times$, $\frac{1}{2}\times$, and $\frac{1}{4}\times$ MICs) were compared in IMP-, MERO- and CTZ-sensitive and -resistant *Pseudomonas* cultures. The relative MICs of IPM, MERO, and CTZ for antibiotic-sensitive MB3286 and the IPM-, CTZ-, and MERO-resistant clinical isolate (CL2533) were very similar in concentration, although ~8- to 16-fold higher for the resistant *Pseudomonas* isolate.

In-vitro LPS-release studies with the above sensitive and resistant *Pseudomonas* organisms show that β-lactam antibiotic PBP specificity correlates well with the propensities of these antibiotics to liberate endotoxin, as shown by representative data in Figs. 3–5. Not only morphology but also the ability of MERO to release LPS are also antibiotic concentration-dependent. For example (against antibiotic-sensitive *P. aeruginosa*, MB3286), at a high antibiotic concentration, MERO not only shows similar morphology to IPM, it also liberates minimal amounts of endotoxin. Lower MIC and subMIC amounts of MERO, like CTZ, induce filaments (26) and liberate excessive amounts of free LPS. Unlike IPM, MERO displays a greater antibiotic dependence on concentration at both the 4-h and 8-h time points, while CTZ liberates excessive amounts of LPS at both subMIC ($\frac{1}{2}\times$) and at multiples of the MIC (up to $100\times$) concentrations. Furthermore, in all instances, the amount of free LPS was more pronounced upon continued antibiotic exposure for up to 8 h, the recommended dosing interval (t.i.d.) for CTZ and MERO. This evidence, along with the above human pharmacokinetic data, suggest that more frequent or higher doses of CTZ and/ or MERO would perhaps yield higher prolonged antibiotic blood levels that could potentially reduce the release of endotoxin, whereas, conversely, the current recommended dosage prolongs the time the antibiotic levels remain below their inhibitory concentrations (MIC) and thereby potentially maintain sustained liberation of excessive free endotoxin.

The morphologies and the abilities to liberate LPS were similar for laboratory antibiotic-sensitive (MB3286) and clinically antibiotic-resistant (CL2533) *P. aeruginosa* isolates exposed to IPM, MERO, and CTZ. LPS-release data with antibiotic-resistant *Pseudomonas* emphasizes that inappropriate treatment of infections due to antibiotic-resistant bacteria may carry additional burdens (release toxins) aside from the possible lack of therapeutic efficacy as an antibiotic. Inappropriate antibiotic therapy is akin to delayed treatment and may result in enhancing the deleterious effects of the infecting pathogen via prolonged release of excess freed toxins. These data thus reemphasize *"frappez fort et vite"*

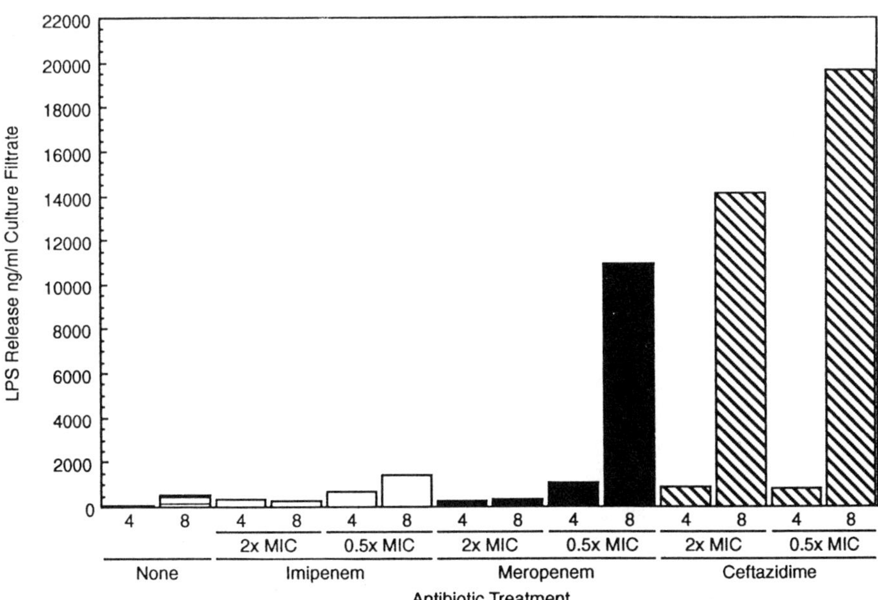

Figure 3   Relative antibiotic-induced release of free LPS from antibiotic-sensitive *P. aeruginosa* MB3286 cultured in trypticase soy broth (TSB). Each antibiotic was given at both ½ and 2 × MIC. Samples were taken at 4- and 8-h intervals during incubation at 35°C. MICs are 1–2 μg/mL, 1 μg/mL, and 2 μg/mL, respectively for IPM □, MERO ■, CTZ ▨, and non-antibiotic-treated controls ▤.

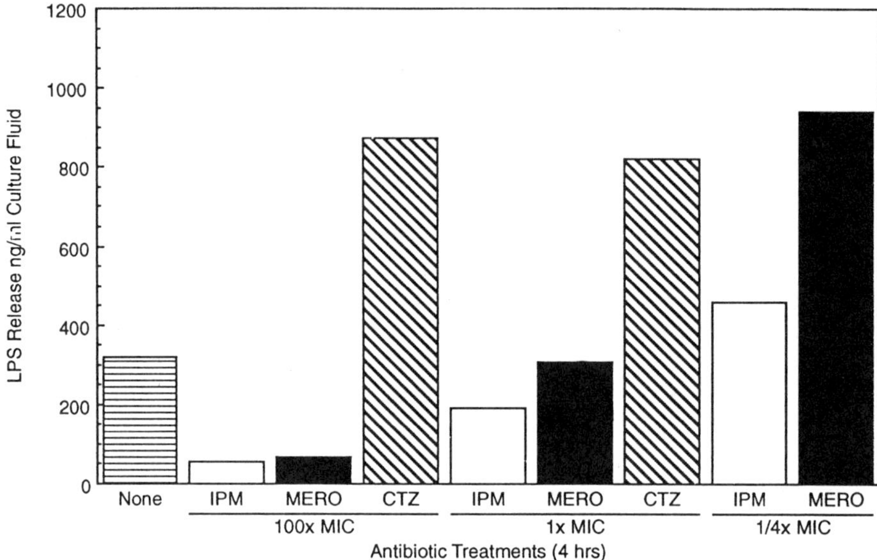

Figure 4 Relative antibiotic-induced LPS release from antibiotic-sensitive *P. aeruginosa* MB3286 following antibiotic exposure for 4 h at 35°C. Bacteria were exposed to 100 ×, 1 ×, and ¼ × MIC of IPM □, MERO ■, CTZ ◪, and untreated ▤. MICs are shown in Fig. 3.

("hit vigorously") instead of *"frappez doucement"* ("hit gently"), as reported recently by Prins et al. (28).

Despite accumulating in-vitro evidence, there are little data to support the clinical relevance of antibiotic-induced endotoxin release to patient outcome. Additionally, it seemed unlikely that nanogram amounts of LPS liberated by CTZ mentioned above could account for the unexpected increased CTZ requirements shown in Table 1—especially since mice are innately more resistant to the lethal effects of endotoxin and require hundreds of micrograms to reach lethality in normal noninfected mice. Once infected, however, mice are as sensitive to smooth LPS as are other mammals—including humans (48)—requiring only nanogram quantities of free endotoxin to reach a toxic state.

IV. ESTABLISHING AN IN-VIVO ROLE FOR ANTIBIOTIC-RELEASED ENDOTOXIN

It is generally known that LPS-liberating gram-negative bacteria are more virulent than their nonliberating variants, that bacteria that liberate smooth LPS (s-LPS)

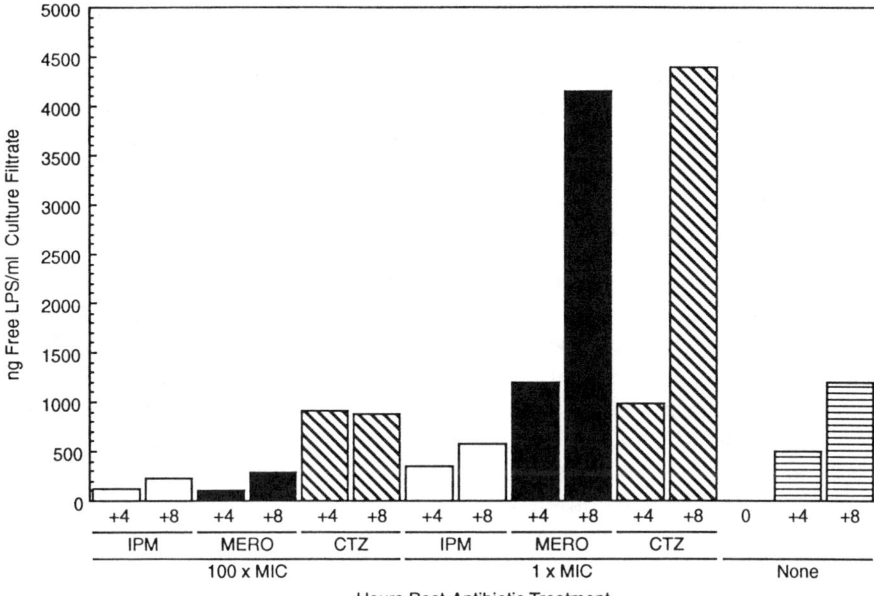

Figure 5 Relative antibiotic-induced LPS release from a clinical antibiotic-resistant *P. aeruginosa* CL2533 isolate following antibiotic exposure for 4 and 8h at 100 × and 1 × MIC of IPM □, MERO ■, CTZ ◨, and untreated ▤. MICs were 8 μg/mL, 16 μg/mL, and 8 μg/mL, respectively, for IPM, MERO, and CTZ.

are more virulent that those that release rough-LPS (r-LPS), and that purified smooth LPS is more lethal than (poorly bioreactive) rough endotoxin (15). In order to determine the importance of antibiotic-induced endotoxin release to the unexpected 100- to 1000-fold decrease in in-vivo CTZ efficacy reported in Table 1, in-vivo efficacy studies with CTZ and IPM were repeated in mice infected with either an s-LPS parent *P. aeruginosa* isolate (MB5120) or its r-LPS mutant (MB5121), which differed from its parent only in the absence of the O-side chain of its LPS.

A. CTZ and IPM Differentially Induce Release of LPS from Both the Smooth Parent and Its Rough-LPS Variant Strain

In LPS-release studies it was established that the rough-LPS mutant spontaneously releases 30-fold more LPS than the smooth parent (495 ng/mL versus 16 ng/mL, respectively, for the r-LPS mutant and its s-LPS parent). In addition, CTZ induces liberation of 20- and 30-fold more LPS from the rough and smooth isolates, respectively, Table 2. With the increased liberation of excessive amounts of poorly bioreactive r-LPS from the rough mutant compared to that released from its smooth parent, it was of interest to determine the relative in-vivo effects of differential antibiotic-induced release of these physiochemically distinct endotoxins on antibiotic efficacy in the mouse assay described in Table 1.

B. Evidence for in-Vivo Relevance of Antibiotic-Induced LPS Release

In follow-up studies of single antibiotic treatment with either IPM or CTZ, it was determined that the amount of CTZ required to protect mice infected with the s-LPS parent (MB5120) was 290-fold greater than that for IPM. Mice challenged with the r-LPS mutant (MB5121), on the other hand, required only 5-fold more CTZ than IPM for equivalent protection, despite the release of excessive amounts of rough LPS (Table 2). The ED_{50}s for CTZ were 142 versus 2.3 mg/kg against infections due to s-LPS *Pseudomonas* parent and its rough mutant, respectively. The smaller differences between the ED_{50}s of IPM and CTZ (0.44 versus 2.3 mg/kg, respectively) in mice infected with the rough mutant were due to a 62-fold decrease in the ED_{50} for high-LPS-releasing CTZ (compared to that of its smooth parent). At the same time, there was little to no change in the efficacy of IPM with either s-LPS or r-LPS *P. aeruginosa*—the ED_{50}s for IPM were 0.49 versus 0.44 mg/kg for smooth and rough *Pseudomonas*, respectively.

Although rough-LPS-liberating bacteria are generally clinically irrelevant, these data demonstrate that, in addition to quantity, the physiochemical composition of the endotoxin being liberated may influence the host's ability to defend against the infecting organism. Also, unlike large amounts of bioreactive s-LPS released from the parent isolate, the release of even greater amounts of poorly

Table 2 Antibiotic Efficacy of CTZ and IPM and LPS Release Versus Bacterial Challenge Against Smooth- and Rough-LPS *Pseudomonas aeruginosa* Isolates

	Smooth-LPS parent (MB5120)			Rough-LPS mutant (MB5121)			
Treatment	LPS (ng/mL)	ED_{50} (mg/kg)	MIC (μmg/mL)	LPS (ng/mL)	ED_{50} (mg/kg)	MIC (μmg/mL)	
None[a]	16	—	—	495	—	—	
IPM	63	0.49	0.5	140	0.44	1.0	
CTZ	1900	142	2.0	2800	2.3	2.0	
CTZ/IPM ratio	—	—	—	290-fold	—	—	—	5-fold

Relative antibiotic efficacy (ED_{50}) of a single treatment of CTZ or IPM plus cilastatin in normal CD1 mice infected with either *P. aeruginosa* MB5120 (smooth-LPS-liberating) or MB5121, its rough-LPS-liberating mutant.
[a]LPS release data were obtained in vitro.

bioreactive r-LPS into the host as a result of exposure to CTZ has little impact on the virulence of the infecting bacteria or on the amount of CTZ necessary to inhibit its growth (Table 2). These data also suggest a possible endotoxin threshold below which the host maintains its normal defenses against bacterial invasion and above which the host is somehow defective in bacterial clearance. Therefore, in-vivo differential antibiotic-induced release of free bioreactive LPS manifests itself in the form of variations in in-vivo antibiotic efficacy. For example, to achieve protection against gram-negative invasion, greater amounts of those antibiotics which release excessive amounts of highly bioreactive endotoxin are required compared to a smaller need in those antibiotics which liberate only minimal amounts of LPS with the same bioreactivity. These data (although in a somewhat indirect manner) therefore suggest a role for differential antibiotic-released endotoxin in the unexpectedly high CTZ requirement found in the mouse experiments in Table 1.

C. Further Proof of Endotoxin Relevance in Vivo

To further establish an in-vivo role for endotoxin, we considered that endotoxin in itself is nontoxic but mediates its lethality through the production of a cascade of cytokines (primarily from macrophages) following lipid A binding to cell surface receptors (46). This toxic process makes it difficult to predict the in-vivo time of maximum LPS release and cytokine production following antibiotic exposure. In-vivo LPS release induced by β-lactam antibiotics which differ in their modes of actions among and within the subclasses further complicates this process. Thus, in the absence of reagents with very long half-lives that could either readily neutralize endotoxin in mice during its release over an extended period of time or inhibit LPS binding to lipid A receptors on surfaces of cells that mediate the lethal effects of LPS, mice were pretreated with a low dose of a macrophage-specific toxin (carrageenan, CGN). Treatments with CGN 1–4 days prior to infection with s-LPS-liberating serum-sensitive *P. aeruginosa* destroys a "biologically significant number of macrophages." Infection was subsequently followed by comparison studies in groups of mice individually treated with a single dose of β-lactam antibiotics that differed widely in their potential to release free LPS (i.e., CTZ and IPM).

The reduction of an "appropriate number of macrophages" was previously determined in infectivity studies in mice systemically (i.p.) challenged with either *P. aeruginosa* (cleared primarily by neutrophils) or *Listeria monocytogenes* (cleared primarily by macrophages) following pretreatment with various doses of CGN. It was determined that 5–20 mg/kg of CGN given 1–2 days before infection would increase the infectivity of *Listeria* in mice by 5–6 logs without any increased susceptibility to infection due to challenge with either s-LPS *P. aeruginosa* or *E. coli* (also neutrophil cleared). Similar pretreatment with CGN at higher doses of 50 mg/kg administered 4 days before bacterial challenge yielded equivalent results. In addition, the above CGN pretreatments also significantly decreased the lethality of smooth pure LPS in normal mice and in mice chemically rendered hypersensitive to the lethal effects of endotoxin (CGN data not reported). Bacterial infection susceptibility studies with CGN-pretreated mice clearly show a biologically significant reduction in macrophage/monocyte numbers as shown by reduced natural host bacterial clearance.

Antibiotic efficacy studies with CTZ and IPM described in Table 1 for normal mice were repeated in the macrophage-depleted CGN mouse model. Results show that normal (non-CGN-treated) mice infected with smooth *P. aeruginosa* require 157- to 227-fold higher amounts of CTZ for protection equivalent to that obtained with IPM, while CGN-pretreated mice (15 mg/kg i.p. on day 1) need only ~8-fold more CTZ than IPM for equivalent protection—a 19- to 27-fold decrease in the CTZ dose requirement (Table 3). Thus, removal of "significant" numbers of cells that mediate endotoxin lethality reduces the lethal effects of excess s-LPS liberated by filament-inducing CTZ and thereby requires lesser amounts of CTZ to afford protection in CGN-pretreated mice. Since the macrophage/monocyte population is perhaps only partially destroyed, these data coupled with those from the smooth/rough studies above suggest that an endotoxin threshold may indeed exist and that excessive amounts of antibiotic-induced bioreactive LPS liberated in vivo may have biological relevance, at least as demonstrated in our antibiotic efficacy animal studies.

Changes in antibiotic efficacy probably reflect the effects of endotoxin or the corresponding inducible cytokines on host susceptibility to infection (host defenses) or their effects on increased virulence of the infecting pathogens. This may be possibly through direct binding of cytokines to the bacteria which is reported to increase bacterial growth (49) or as a result of cytokine-enhanced bacterial invasiveness (48,49). Such an effect would require an increased protec-

Table 3 Antibiotic Efficacy in Mice

CD1 mice versus *P. aeruginosa*	Challenges No. of $LD_{50}s$	ED_{50}, mg/kg (MIC)		ED_{50} ratio CTZ/IMP
		Imipenem	Ceftazidime	
1. MB3286—smooth	55	~1.0 (1–2)	151.0 (2)	157.0
MB3286 + CGN	74	~0.7	~5.8	8.4
2. MB3286—smooth	111	5.7	1291.0	227.0
MB3286 + CGN	13	4.6	38.8	8.4

Comparative antibiotic efficacy in non- and carrageenan-treated CD1 mice. Carrageenan administered at 15 mg/kg 1 day (i.p.) prior to infection (i.p.) with *P. aeruginosa* MB3286. CTZ or IPM plus cilastatin was administered s.c. once at 1 h postinfection. Two experiments are shown. Numbers in parenthesis = minimal inhibitory concentrations (MICs).

tive amount of CTZ. In our judgment, these data at least partially explain our original observation of the need of higher (100- to 1000-fold) CTZ levels to overcome the deleterious effects of antibiotic-induced release of excessive amounts of bioreactive endotoxin by this antibiotic.

V. CONCLUSIONS

While many studies suggest rather strongly that antibiotic-induced free endotoxin release does indeed play a significant role in the effectiveness of antibiotic therapy in mice, only careful clinical evaluations will determine its true relevance in patients with possible underlying secondary infections and other complications. The use of fast-acting, low-LPS-releasing antibiotics may indeed facilitate a reduction in the added burden placed on the infected host due to excess endotoxin liberation. However, (existing) severe infections may also require the use of adjunctive therapy in the form of anticytokines, antireceptors, anti-lipid A, antagonist, or combinations of the above to radically decrease the mortality and morbidity associated with gram-negative-and/or perhaps even gram-positive-related septic shock. The potential role of antibiotic-induced liberation of free endotoxin in shock associated with gram-negative sepsis may explain the lack of improved survival in some patients despite decreased infection rates observed following antibiotic therapy.

Finally, it is becoming increasingly accepted that TNF-α enhances viral replication. Therefore, should a role for differential antibiotic-induced LPS release prove to be important in septic shock, it may be of interest to consider more carefully the possible role of antibiotics in exacerbating conditions in bacterial-infected AIDS patients due to LPS stimulation of TNF-α production.

ACKNOWLEDGMENTS

We thank Charlie Gill, Nova Walker, and Jon Sundelof for support in in-vitro and in-vivo evaluations, Solomon Scott for electron micrographs, Michele McColgan for graphics, and John L. Ryan for critical comments and advice.

REFERENCES

1. Dofferhoff, ASM, Bom VJJ, van Ingen J, et al. Patterns of cytokines, plasma endotoxin and acute phase proteins during the treatment of severe sepsis in humans. Prog Clin Biol Res 1991; 367:43–54.
2. Shenep JL, Flynn PM, Barrett FF, Stidham GL, Westenkirchner DF. Serial quantitation of endotoxemia and bacteremia during therapy for gram-negative bacterial sepsis. J Infect Dis 1988; 157:565–568.
3. Arditi M, Ables L, and Yogev R. Cerebrospinal fluid endotoxin levels in children

with *H. influenza* meningitis before and after administration of intravenous ceftriaxone. J Infect Dis 1989; 160: 1005–1011.

4. Brandtzaeg P, Kierulf P, Gaustad P, et al. Plasma endotoxin as a predictor of multiple organ failure and death in systemic meningococcal disease. J Infect Dis 1989; 159:195–204.

5. Fry DE, Pearlstein L, Fulton RL, Polk HC. Multiple system organ failure. Arch Surg 1971; 115: 136–140.

6. Arditi M, Kabat W, Vogev R. Antibiotic-induced bacterial killing stimulates tumor necrosis factor-α release in whole blood. J Infect Dis 1993; 167: 240–244.

7. Simon DM, Koenig G, Trenholme GM. Differences in release of tumor necrosis factor from THP-1 cells stimulated by filtrates of antibiotic killed *Escherichia coli*. J Infect Dis 1991; 164:800–802.

8. Burroughs M, Cabellos C, Prasad S, Toumanen E. Bacterial components and the pathophysiology of injury to the blood brain barriers: does cell wall add to the effects of endotoxin in gram-negative meningitis? J Infect Dis 1992; 165(suppl 1):S82–S85.

9. Ferrante A, Staugas REM, Rowan-Kelly B, et al. Production of tumor necrosis factor alpha and beta by human mononuclear leukocytes stimulated with mitogen, bacteria and malarial parasites. Infect Immun 1990; 58:3996–4003.

10. Jackson JJ, Kropp H. Influence of antibiotic class and concentration on the percentage of release of lipopolysaccharide from *Escherichia coli*. J Infect Dis 1994; 169:471–472.

11. Dofferhoff ASM, Nijland JH, de Vries-Hospers HG, Mulder POM, Weits J, Bom VJJ. Effects of different types and combinations of antimicrobial agents on endotoxin release from gram-negative bacteria: an in-vitro and in-vivo study. Scand J Infect Dis 1991; 23:745–754.

12. Eng RH, Smith SM, Fan-Harvard P, Ogbara T. Effects of antibiotics on endotoxin release from gram-negative bacteria. Diagn Microbiol Infect Dis 1993; 16:185–189.

13. Bucklin SE, Morrison D. Contributions of antibiotic-derived endotoxin to lethality in experimental bacteremia and sepsis (abstr 1419). 33rd Interscience Conference on Antimicrobial Agents and Chemotherapy (ICAAC), New Orleans, LA, Oct 17–20, 1993.

14. Bingen E, Goury V, Bennani H, Lambert-Zechovsky N, Aujard Y, Darbord JC. Bactericidal activity of β-lactam antibiotics and amikacin against *Haemophilus influenza:* effect on endotoxin release. J Antimicrob Chemother 1993; 30:165–172.

15. Jackson JJ, Kropp. β-Lactam antibiotic-induced release of free endotoxin: in-vitro comparison of penicillin-binding protein (PBP) 2-specific imipenem and PBP 3-specific ceftazidime. J Infect Dis 1992; 165:1033–1041.

16. Flynn PM, Shenep JL, Gigliotti F, Davis DS, Hildner WK. Immunolabelling of LPS liberated from antibiotic-treated *Escherichia coli*. Infect Immun 1988; 56:2760–2762.

17. Shenep JL, Barton RP, Morgan KA. Role of antibiotic class in the rate of liberation of endotoxin during therapy for experimental gram-negative bacterial sepsis. J Infect Dis 1985; 151:1012–1018.

18. Andersen BM, Solberg O. Release of endotoxin from *Neisseria meningitidis*. A

short survey with a preliminary report on virulence in mice. NIPH Ann 1980; 3:49–55.

19. Andersen BM, Solberg O. The endotoxin liberating effect of antibiotics on meningococcus in-vitro. Acta Path Microbiol Scand 1980; 88:231–236.

20. Walterspiel JW, Kaplan SL, Mason EO. Protective effect of subinhibitory polymyxin B alone and in combination with ampicillin for overwhelming *Haemophilus influenza* type B infection in the infant rat: evidence for in-vivo and in-vitro release of free endotoxin after ampicillin treatment. Pediatr Res 1986; 20:237–241.

21. Jackson JJ, Kropp H. Decrease of endotoxin release in *Pseudomonas aeruginosa* after imipenem treatment and its influence on efficacy in mice (abstr 755). 30th Interscience Conference on Antimicrobial Agents and Chemotherapy (ICAAC), Atlanta, GA, Oct 21–24, 1990.

22. Neu, HC. Carbapenems: special properties contributing to their activity. Am J Med 1985; 78:33–40.

23. Jackson JJ, Kropp H. Reply: β-lactam antibiotic-induced release of lipopolysaccharide. J Infect Dis 1993; 167:775–777.

24. Wientjes FB, Nanninga N. On the role of high molecular weight penicillin-binding proteins in the cell cycle of *Escherichia coli*. Res Micribiol 1991; 142:333–344.

25. Tuomanen E, Tomasz A. Induction of autolysis in nongrowing *Escherichia coli*. J Bacteriol 1986; 167:1077–1080.

26. Sumita Y, Fukasawa M, Okuda T. Comparison of two carbapenems, SM-7338 and imipenem; affinities for penicillin-binding proteins and morphological changes. J antibiotics 1990; 43:314–320.

27. Van den Berg C, De Neeling WNM, Schot CS, Hustinx WNM, Wemer J, De Wildt DJ. Delayed antibiotic-induced lysis of *E. coli* in-vitro is correlated with enhancement of LPS release. Scand J Infect Dis 1992; 24:619–627.

28. Prins JM, vanDeventer SJH, Kuijper EJ, Speelman P. Minireview. Clinical relevance of antibiotic induced endotoxin release. Antimicrob Agents Chemother 1994; 38:1211–1218.

29. Hurley JC. Antibiotic-induced release of endotoxin: a reappraisal. Clin Infect Dis 1992; 15:840–854.

30. Dofferhoff ASM, Esselink MT, de Vries-Hospers HG, et al. The release of endotoxin from antibiotic-treated *Escherichia coli* and the production of tumor necrosis factor by human monocytes. J Antimicrob Chemother 1993; 31:373–384.

31. Tune Bruce M, Hsu C-Y. Augmentation of antibiotic nephrotoxicity by endotoxin in the rabbit. J Pharmacol Exp Therapeut 1984; 234:425–430.

32. Joly V, Bergeron Y, Bergeron MG, Carbon C. Endotoxin-tobramycin additive toxicity on renal proximal tubular cells in culture. Antimicrob Agents Chemother 1991; 35:351–357.

33. Whelan, AC. *E. coli* damaged by antibiotics. ASM News 1993; 59:225.

34. Shenep JL, Morgan KA. Kinetics of endotoxin release during antibiotic therapy for experimental gram-negative bacterial sepsis. J Infect Dis 1991; 150:380–388.

35. Tauber MG, Shibl AM, Hackbarth JW, Larrick JW, Sande MA. Antibiotic therapy, endotoxin concentration in cerebrospinal fluid, and brain edema in experimental *Escherichia coli* meningitis in rabbits. J Infect Dis 1987; 15:456–462.

36. Røkke O, Revhaug A, Osterud B, Giercksky. Increased plasma levels of endotoxin and corresponding changes in circulatory performance in a porcine sepsis model: the effect of antibiotic administration. Prog Clin Biol Res 1988; 272:247–262.
37. Mustafa MM, Ramilo O, Mertsola J, et al. Modulation of inflammation and cachectin activity in relation to treatment of experimental *Haemophilus influenza* type b meningitis. J Infect Dis 1989; 160:818–825.
38. Mertsola J, Ramilo O, Mustafa MM, Saez-Llorens X, Hansen EJ, McCracken GH Jr. Release of endotoxin after antibiotic treatment of gram-negative meningitis. Pediatr Infect Dis J 1989; 8:904–906.
39. Hurley JC, Louis WJ, Tosolini FA, Carlin JB. Antibiotic-induced release of endotoxin in chronically bacteriuric patients. Antimicrob Agents Chemother 1991; 35:2388–2394.
40. Dofferhoff, ASM. Abstract 1420. 33rd Interscience Conference on Antimicrobial Agents and Chemotherapy (ICAAC), New Orleans, LA, Oct 17–20, 1993.
41. Friedland IR, Jafari H, Ehrett S, et al. Comparison of endotoxin release by different antimicrobial agents and the effect on inflammation in experimental *Escherichia coli* meningitis. J Infect Dis 1993; 168:657–662.
42. Hanberger H, Nilsson LE, Nilsson M, et al. Post antibiotic effect of beta-lactam antibiotics on gram-negative bacteria in relationship to morphology, initial killing and MIC. Eur J Microbiol Infect Dis 1991; 10:927–934.
43. Drusano GL, Standiford HC, Bustamante C, et al. Multiple-dose pharmacokinetics of imipenem-cilastatin. Antimicrob Agents Chemother 1984; 26:715–721.
44. Bax RP, Bastain W, Featherstone A, Wilkinson DM, Hutchinson M, Haworth SJ. The pharmacokinetics of meropenem in volunteers. J Antimicrob Chemother 1989; 24 (suppl A):311–320.
45. Harding SM, Monro AJ, Thornton JE, Ayrton J, Hogg MIJ. The comparative pharmacokinetics of ceftazidime and cefotaxime in healthy volunteers. J Antimicrob Chemother 1981; 8(suppl B):263–272.
46. Matsuura M, Galanos C. Induction of hypersensitivity to endotoxin and tumor necrosis factor by sublethal infection with *Salmonella typhimurium*. Infect Immun 1990; 58:935–937.
47. Porat, R, Clark BD, Wolff SM, Dinarello CA. Enhancement of growth of virulent strains of *Escherichia coli* interleukin-1. Science 1991; 254:430–432.
48. Luo G, Niesel DW Shaban RA, Grimm EA, Klimpel GR. Tumor necrosis factor alpha binding to bacteria: evidence for high-affinity receptors and alteration of bacterial virulence properties. Infect Immun 1993; 61:830–835.
49. Koch T, Duncker HP, Axt R, Schieffer HG, van Ackerman K, Neuhof H. Alterations of bacterial clearance induced by endotoxin. Infect Immun 1993; 61:3143–314.

Index

About the Editors

DAVID C. MORRISON is the Kansas Masons Distinguished Professor of Cancer Research in the Department of Microbiology, Molecular Genetics, and Immunology at the University of Kansas Medical Center, Kansas City. The author or coauthor of over 180 book chapters, professional papers, and reviews, he is Cofounder and President Elect of the International Endotoxin Society, a Fellow of the Infectious Diseases Society of America and the American Academy of Microbiology, and a member of the American Society for Biochemistry and Molecular Biology, the Society of Leukocyte Biology, and the Shock Society, among other organizations. The holder of a prestigious MERIT Award from the National Institutes of Health, Dr. Morrison received the B.S. degree (1963) in physics from the University of Massachusetts, Amherst, and the Ph.D. degree (1969) in molecular biology and biophysics from Yale University, New Haven, Connecticut.

JOHN L. RYAN is Vice President of Clinical Development at the Genetics Institute, Inc., Cambridge, Massachusetts. A member of the American Association of Immunologists, the American Association of Pathologists, the American Society for Microbiology, the Infectious Diseases Society of America, and the International Endotoxin Society, among other organizations, he is the author or coauthor of over 130 professional papers, book chapters, reviews, and abstracts.

Dr. Ryan received the B.S. degree (1964) in biophysics and the Ph.D. degree (1969) in molecular biology and biophysics from Yale University, New Haven, Connecticut, and the M.D. degree (1972) from the University of California, San Diego. He is a diplomate of the American Board of Internal Medicine and the American Board of Infectious Diseases.